MAXLOVE PROJECT · LOVE · HOPE · THRIVE ®

# The Fierce Foods Kitchen

## Healing Through Culinary Medicine

*The Fierce Foods Kitchen: Healing Through Culinary Medicine*




First Printing Edition, 2024
ISBN: 979-8-218-37338-2

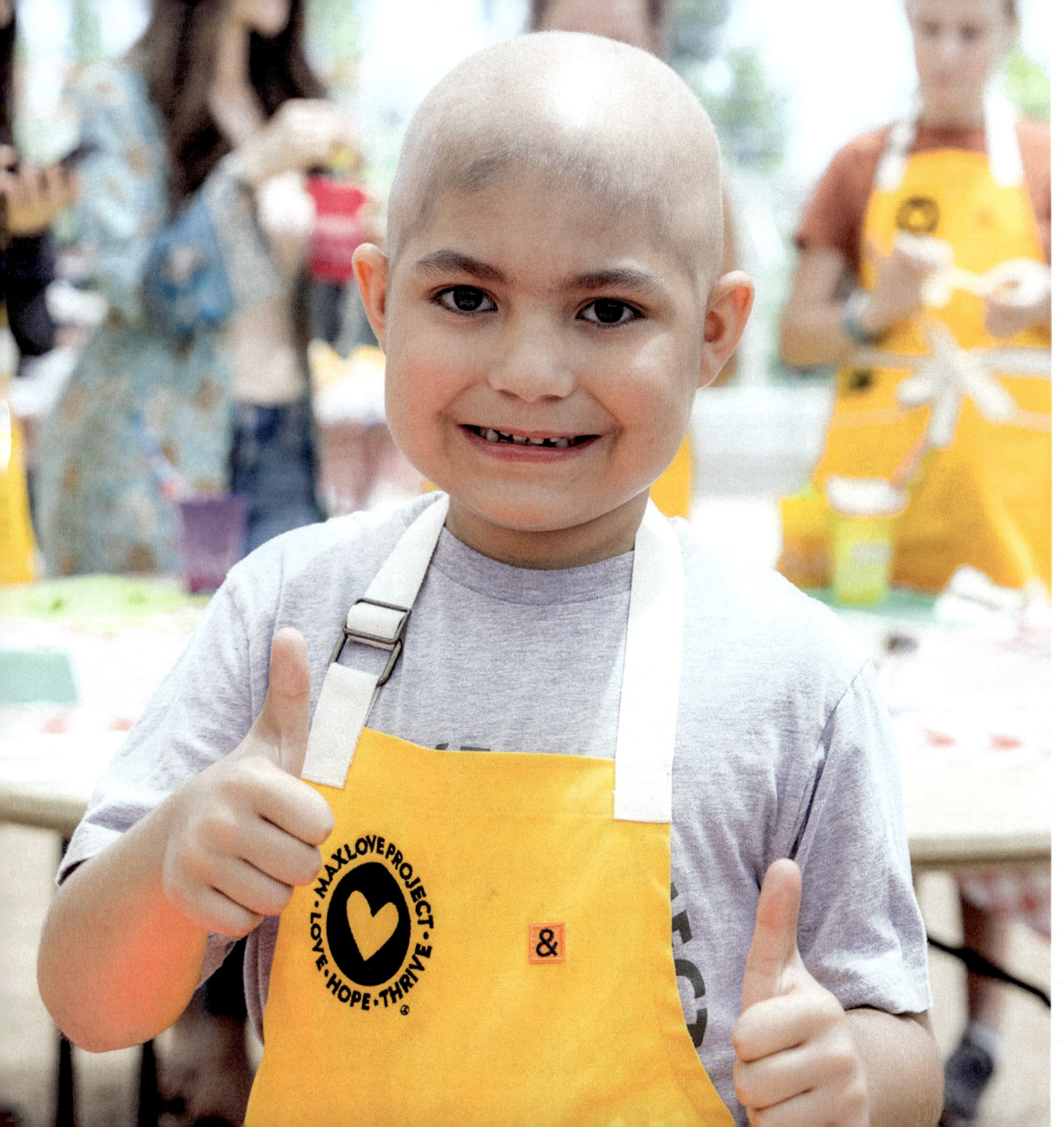
MAXLOVE PROJECT
LOVE · HOPE · THRIVE
&

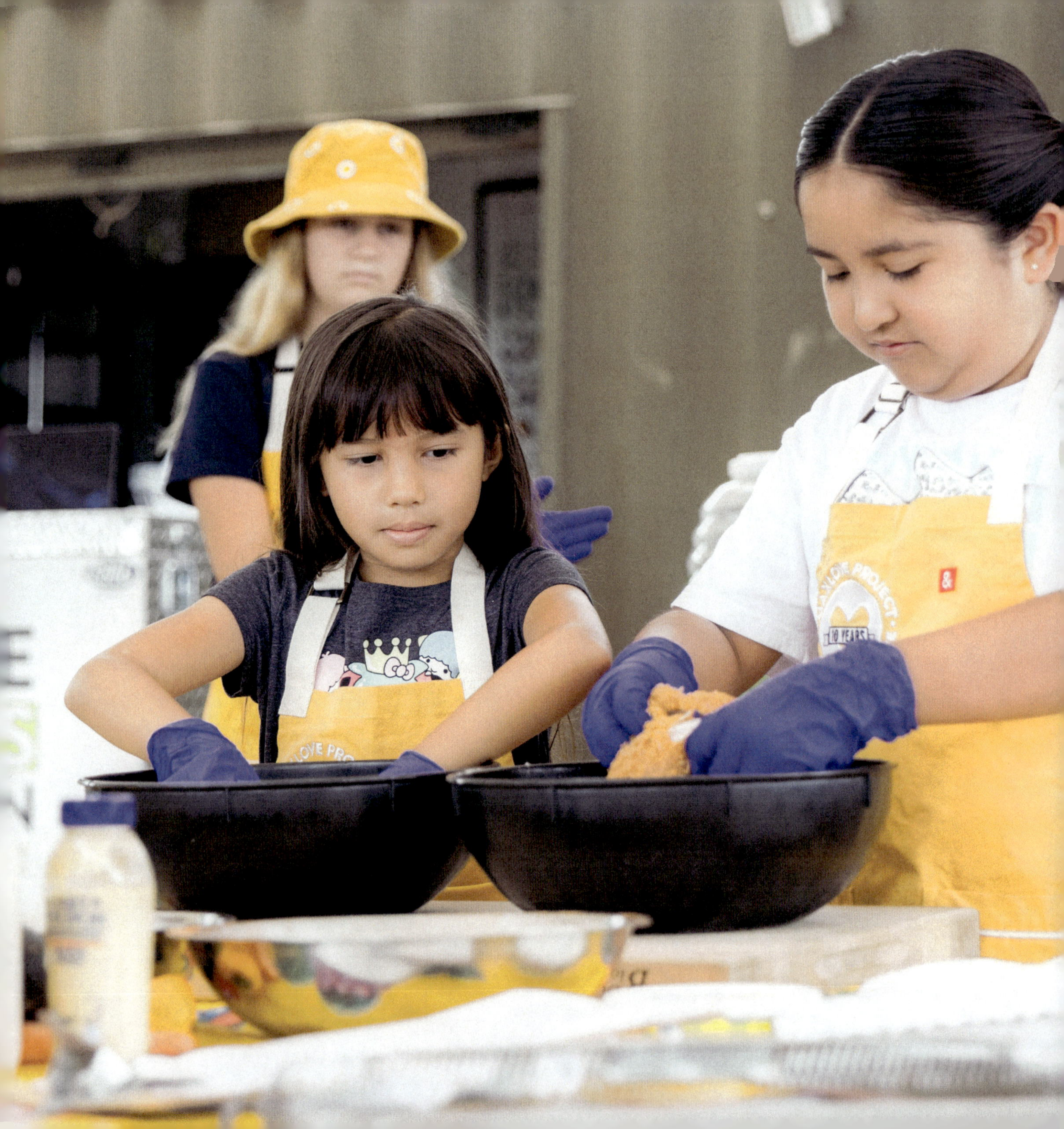
10 YEARS

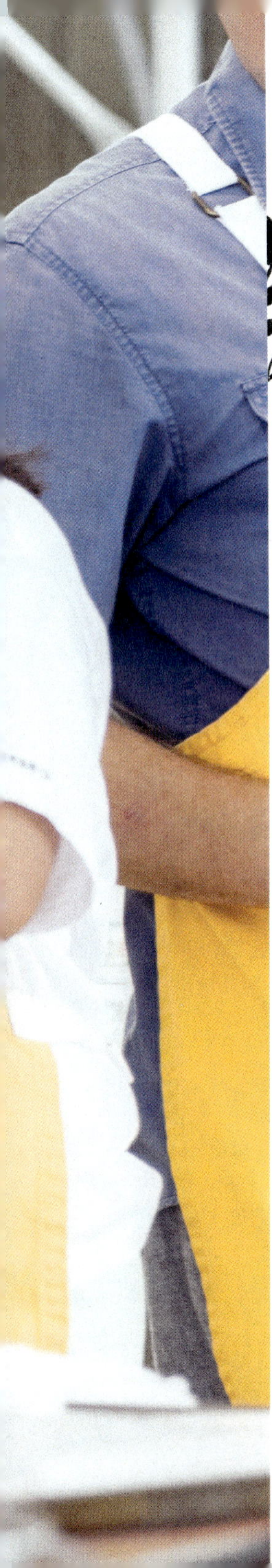

# Table of Contents

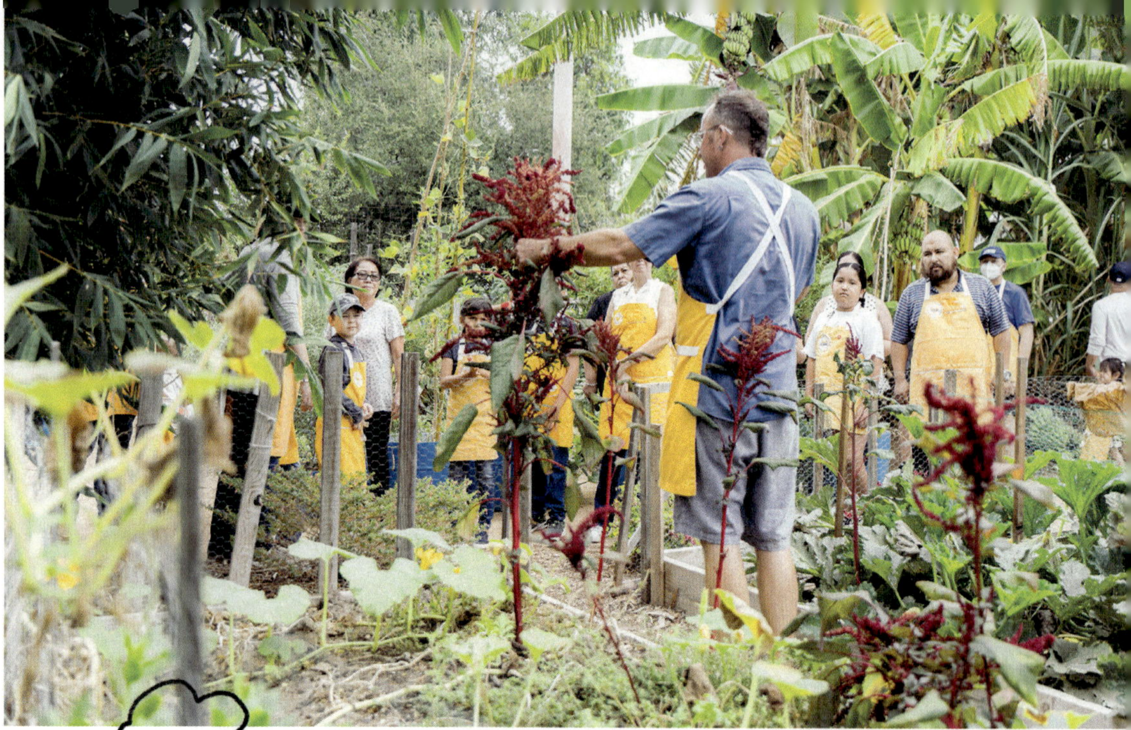

# The MaxLove Project

**MaxLove Project is a 501c3 nonprofit organization** based in Orange, California, that has been serving families facing pediatric cancer and rare diseases across the nation for over 10 years. It's our mission to increase the quality of life and reduce health risks for all children surviving cancer, in treatment and beyond.

We empower families fighting childhood cancers and related life-threatening conditions with quality-of-life care, culinary medicine, mental wellness, integrative health resources, education, and research. We believe that true health starts when families are empowered to be active partners in their child's healing.

The standard of care treatment protocols for childhood cancer and most related rare pediatric diseases focus on quantity over quality of life. This results in both immediate and late-onset treatment effects, psychological difficulties, and illness that can be supported with palliative, integrative, and quality-of-life-focused care. Furthermore, most kids diagnosed with cancer go on to survive through adulthood but experience significantly reduced quality of life and enormous health risks for everything from heart disease and obesity to secondary cancers and early death.

MaxLove Project is the only childhood cancer non-profit that focuses exclusively on improving quality of life and reducing long-term health risks for all families affected by childhood cancer and related pediatric rare diseases. Our goal is to ensure that every **family** facing a childhood cancer or pediatric **rare disease** diagnosis is equipped with **the tools to thrive**, in treatment and beyond.

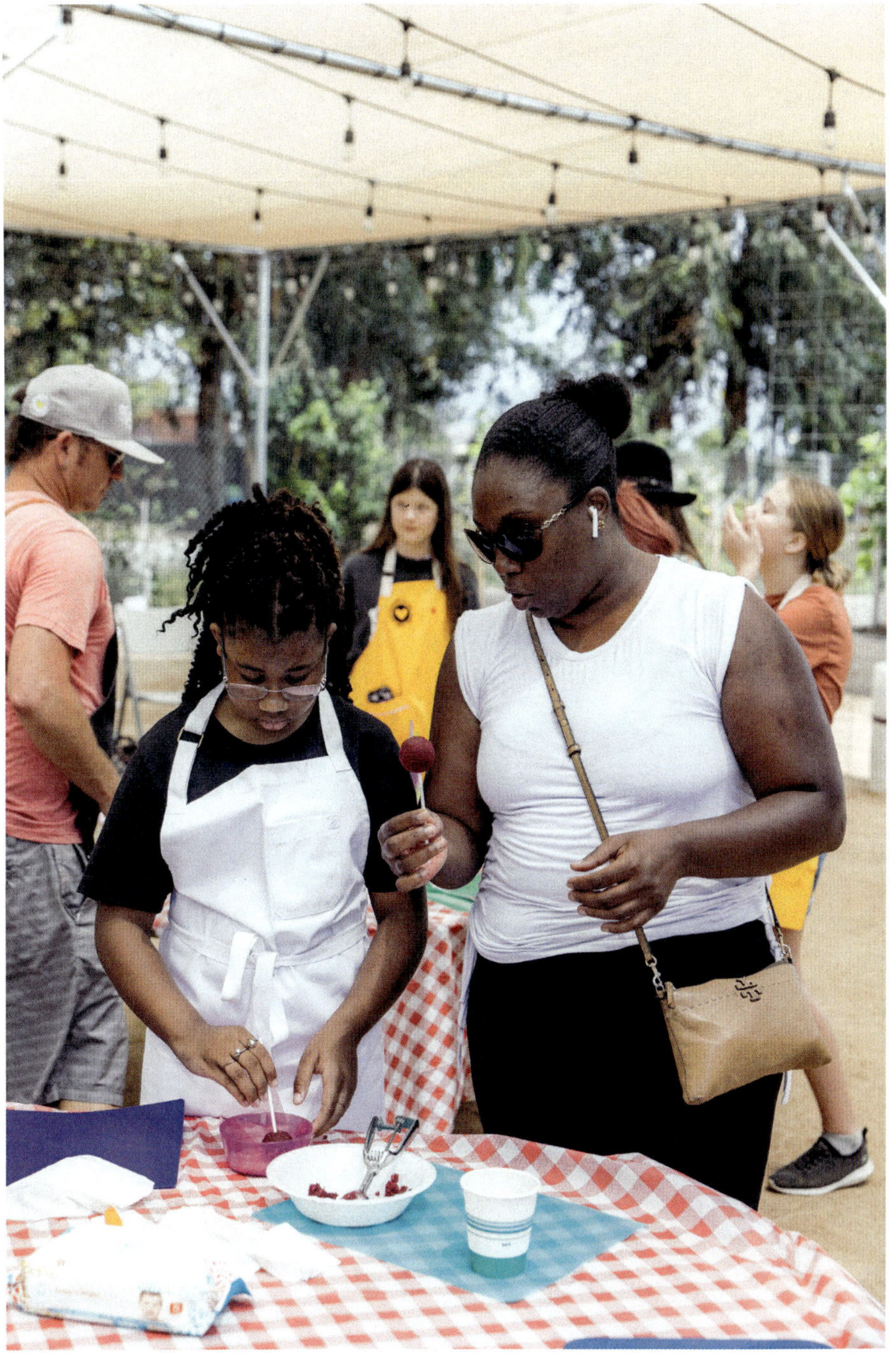

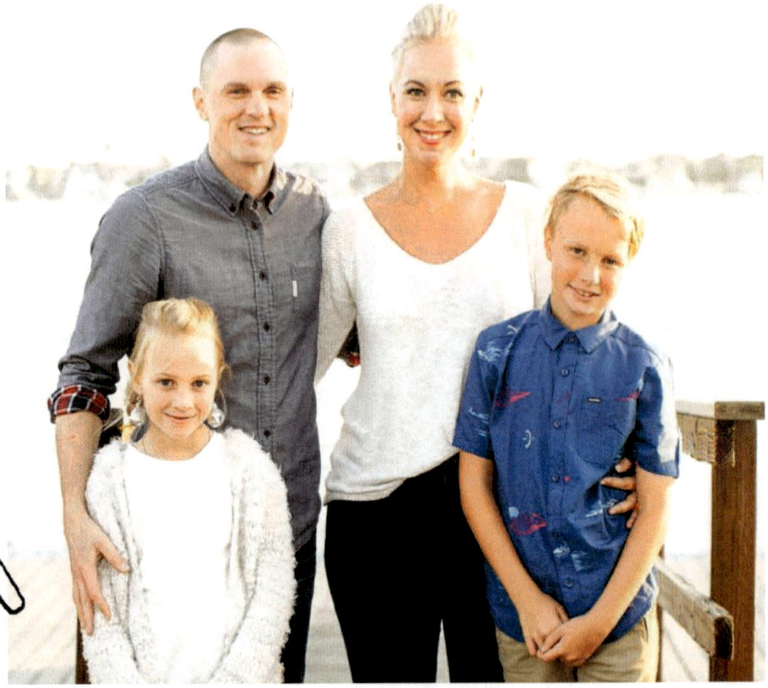

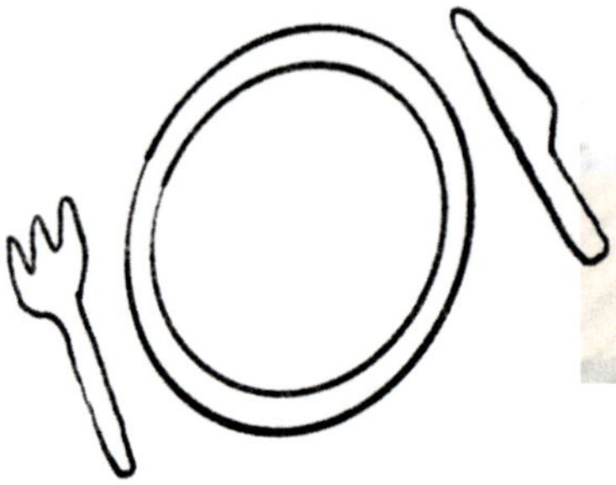

# Our Story

**After his fourth birthday, our son Max** started to show balance problems. They were barely detectable at first, but they got worse and worse over time. He became afraid to go downstairs, could no longer climb on the playground, wouldn't ride his scooter, and would suddenly lose his balance and fall.

He never complained and would often laugh about it. So even though we took him to the pediatrician several times for symptoms like early morning debilitating headaches and vomiting (and he checked out fine each time), we weren't panicked. But when he fell off his bunk bed ladder one morning and couldn't get back up, our pediatrician ordered an MRI for the following day.

I took the day off work and planned to take Max to see a movie right after the MRI. We were expecting they'd show a sinus infection or ear problem. Instead, as I was in the waiting room, the anesthesiologist came out to tell me that my son needed to be immediately rushed by ambulance to our local children's hospital.

The rest was a blur. We were surrounded by nurses and the chaplain was called in. Our pediatrician called and told me that Max had a brain tumor and needed immediate surgery to save his life from emergent hydrocephalus. Max was taken into surgery early the next morning.

Two days later, my husband Justin and I were standing next to Max's hospital bed as he lay unconscious and intubated. He had much of the accessible part of the tumor removed, but a substantial amount remained inside of his brainstem, and we were just wrapping our heads around the fact that we had a long, terrible road ahead of us.

Our neurosurgeon came in to discuss Max's case and the results of the surgery. He told us to focus on Max's quality of life. Treatment, he told us, would only do so much in Max's case. He asked us to agree that at the point when treatment starts to compromise Max's quality of life, we need to stop. This conversation planted a powerful seed. It was the first time that quality of life was mentioned to us and, in that, we found hope.

For the next several days, Justin and I took turns sobbing and putting our bravest faces on. Finally, about five days after that MRI, we were all cried out and exhausted with the fake, cheery smiles. We looked at each other and we promised that together, we were going to do whatever it takes to make sure Max has the best quality of life no matter what.

Of course, we had no idea what this would entail. We just knew we weren't going to simply rely on the standard of care. Of course, we weren't rejecting the standard of care, but rather it was the foundation on which we'd do everything else.

At this point, the surgery had left Max unable to move the left side of his body or talk, and he couldn't walk at all. We were stuck in the hospital for the foreseeable future until Max could move well enough to go home. So, we looked around for anything we could do right then to start shifting the odds in his favor, to give him the best quality of life possible.

As if on cue, we noticed the hot dogs and mac and cheese on order from room service. We looked at each other and we decided our fight for Max would start with food—Fierce Foods.

We didn't know where to start, so we immediately requested the support of a hospital dietitian. We wanted help finding the best nutrition to support a brain tumor patient who needs to get his mobility and strength back. The nurse and doctor looked at us like we were crazy: Why would we need a dietitian when Max could physically eat? Dietitians are for clinical eating problems, not whatever it is we were asking for.

Coming into our childhood cancer journey, we didn't know much about nutrition. I trained as a cook in my undergraduate college days but had zero training in nutrition. What Justin and I knew about nutrition at the time was that one day fat was bad for you, then sugar, then eggs. And then we'd see a news segment that fat is good for you, sugar maybe not so bad, and eggs were the best!

They humored us and sent us the special hospital smoothie menu, explaining that these are great ways to get a lot of calories into kids at once. The next thing we know, they bring in a cup of hot water and a packet of powdered broth, with corn syrup as the first ingredient. We sent it back and decided we'd have to figure nutrition out on our own. Things have changed at this and other children's hospitals since then, but at that moment we knew we'd have to let the surgeons and oncologists do their thing, and we would have to take figure out how to use food as medicine on our own.

We knew that food wasn't the reason for Max's diagnosis, and it wasn't going to cure him, but it had to be a part of the answer for helping him thrive through treatment and, hopefully, beyond.

Fortunately, Justin had just earned his PhD in the social sciences and was teaching at UCLA. He had access to any scientific research articles we needed. And we started reaching out to researchers and dietitians to get a clearer picture of what a pediatric cancer patient should eat. We slowly cut through conflicting dietary opinions by digging into the research literature and listening to as many of the experts as we could, and we started to see a few really important nutrition principles emerge. When we collected them together into a comprehensive nutritional approach, we called them Fierce Foods.

## Fierce Foods Principles

**Prioritize** whole foods over processed foods

**Reduce** sugar and other refined carbohydrates (e.g. crackers, chips, and bread)

**Emphasize** protein in each meal

**Focus** on your cultural heritage recipes that are nutrient-dense

I vividly remember learning these principles and making snacks for Max to have at chemo. Sliced veggies, sugar-free protein snacks, and seaweed chips. His nurse told us that, although she was impressed by Max's eating, if he lost any weight she'd have to tell us to stop and he'd need to eat "regular" food.

Not only did he keep his weight on, but he looked healthier the longer his chemo protocol continued. As we worked these principles into our family's meals, we saw Max thrive through treatment, and Justin and I got healthier as well. We lost weight, we had more energy, and we felt physically better than we had in years.

When we started MaxLove Project just a few months after Max's diagnosis, we were focused on helping childhood cancer families thrive through sleep and integrative therapies like acupuncture. But as we developed a Fierce Foods approach for Max, we started working with dietitians on MaxLove cooking classes. We called each class a Fierce Foods Academy, and it was a mix of nutrition education and using new culinary skills to make the fiercest and most delicious recipes we could find.

Parents loved the social connection and learning new ways to make healthy foods at home, and kids loved getting their hands dirty with each other as they got to feel and see how Fierce Foods are made. We saw first-hand how a whole-food, nutrient-dense approach not only made families healthier during cancer treatment, but could also bring families together for powerful emotional support.

This cookbook is the result of over a decade of collaborating with forward-thinking doctors, dietitians, amazing researchers, and open-hearted chefs. But most of all, it's a *big thank* you to all the childhood cancer families who joined us in teaching kitchens, farms, and hospital community areas to learn about the healing power of fierce foods and fierce friendship.

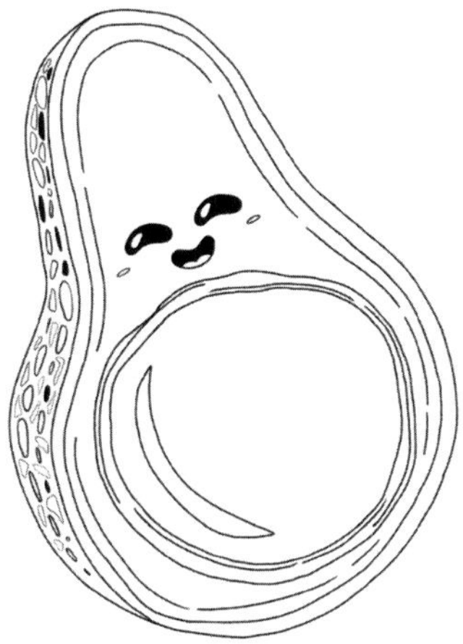

# Fierce Foods Approach

## Our Fierce Foods Philosophy

Up until 50 to 100 years ago, most people ate local, whole foods. They didn't do it because they were health-conscious foodies. They did it because it was all they had. Today, however, we're constantly surrounded by ultra-processed foods that are designed to hook us and make us overeat. This combination of industrial production with sophisticated food laboratory design has made people around the world addicted, sick, and confused.

The situation is even worse for childhood cancer survivors who, because of different cancer treatments, face long- term health risks like diabetes, heart disease, stroke, a weakened immune system, and early aging.

A poor diet on top of these cancer-related risks only increases the chance that survivors will have to deal with lifelong chronic diseases as they age. Fortunately, the nutritional answer to this problem is pretty straightforward: prioritize whole foods and increase our meals' nutrient density as much as possible. We call this approach Fierce Foods.

Although the details can get complex, the solution to our sick food environment is really this simple: eating whole, real food plays a significant role in improving quality of life, reducing long-term health risks, and in some cases, boosting the effect of cancer treatments.

### Increase in Health Risks for Childhood Cancer Survivors

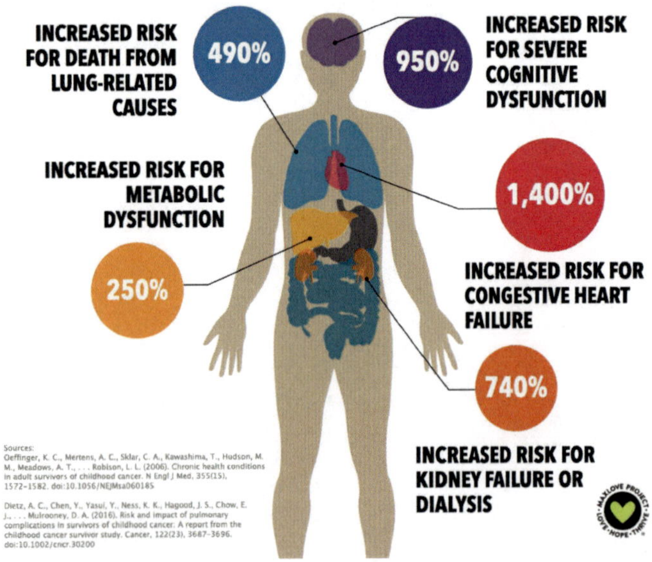


## Fierce Foods: The Foundation

Eating Fierce Foods is all about sticking to science-backed nutrition principles to achieve the health goals we have for our kids and ourselves. These goals can include fighting current diseases, improving energy, and reducing future health risks. And we can achieve these goals by eating foods that help:

- Reduce inflammation in the body
- Eliminate spikes in blood sugar and insulin
- Increase different types and amounts of nutrients in our bodies
- Boost the immune system
- Heal and protect the gut

The Fierce Foods approach has four principles that ultimately revolve around whole vegetables and fruit, lots of high-quality protein, herbs, spices, and healthy fats like olive oil. At the same time, it steers us away from unhealthy processed foods like added sugars and highly refined grains.

These are just the broad outlines, and we're not dogmatic about anything. Our Fierce Foods philosophy is meant to be a guide for daily food choices, not a strict set of rules. We believe that Fierce Foods is a journey, not a destination. And we're just getting started...

## Fierce Foods Principle #1: Prioritize whole foods over processed foods

Nutrition science can get pretty confusing and contentious: vegan vs. keto vs. plant-based vs. paleo vs. low-carb vs. you-name-it. It can easily get overwhelming. The good news is that the one thing that all the major nutrition scientists agree on is the best diets are those that are full of whole foods.

Whole foods are plants (like vegetables, fruits, and grains), animal products (like meat, fish, eggs, and dairy), or minimally processed fats from plants or animals (like olive oil, avocado oil, and butter).

Not all whole foods work for every-body: some have a dairy intolerance or food allergies. But regardless of the restrictions some of us have, what ends up on our plate should be minimally processed.

The most widely praised whole foods are vegetables and low-sugar fruit. Vegetables, like broccoli and cauliflower, and low-sugar fruit, like avocado and olives, pack a huge amount of nutrients into small bites. They have a great amount of fiber, they don't raise blood sugar, and they contain special micronutrients that have been shown to improve immunity, cognition, mood, weight, and heart health.

An equally important whole food, however, is animal protein. Unprocessed and well-raised beef, chicken, pork, fish, lamb, and eggs are important sources of healthy protein, fat, and micronutrients. Studies have shown that diets containing animal protein, including red meat, support a range of health outcomes from weight to cholesterol to inflammation. Animal protein may also be important for mental health concerns, such as depression and cognition. It also appears to be crucial for children's development.

## The Meat Mix-up:
### How nutrition science got the health effects of animal protein wrong

The confusion around the health benefits of animal protein comes from observational studies that show that the average person who eats more meat has worse health outcomes. Observational studies just ask people what they eat and what sort of health problems they have, then researchers crunch the numbers and look for statistical associations.

The associations these studies found between meat and different diseases were correlational, not causal. That is, just because two things can be found together (like ice cream consumption and heat stroke) doesn't mean one causes the other (it's warm weather that is causing both).

Observational nutrition studies consistently show that people who eat a lot of meat also do many things that are known to harm health, like eating a lot of processed foods, smoking cigarettes, and drinking a lot of alcohol.

Public health officials and doctors have urged Americans to reduce meat consumption over the past 60 years. So people who listened to medical advice and wanted to improve their health also reduced meat consumption.

But they were not just reducing meat consumption; they were also doing many other things to improve their health, like going to the doctor more, eating more unprocessed foods, exercising, quitting smoking, drinking less, and so on.

This is what scientists call the healthy adherer bias. The healthy adherer bias is when: 1) You measure some action that people who care about their health do or don't do; and 2) You find a statistical association between that action (like eating more veggies than meat) and health outcomes like heart disease and cancer. But that association is not causation.

For example, people who care about their health also use seat belts more often, but seat belt use does not cause better heart health. To determine causation, we need to look at randomized controlled trials where participants were randomly assigned to different groups who either do or don't eat meat. When studies like this have been done, unprocessed meat has been shown to be a healthy whole food.

## Fierce Foods Principle #2: Reduce sugar and other refined carbohydrates

When we consume foods high in sugar and refined carbohydrates, the levels of sugar (also known as glucose) in the blood rapidly rises. This "spike" forces our body to respond by producing a hormone called insulin. Insulin helps lower the sugar levels in the blood by helping it get into cells.

We're okay if this happens once in a while, but over the long term, these repeated spikes are harmful to the body and increase the risk for diabetes, obesity, and heart disease, for which childhood cancer survivors are at even greater risk. There is also evidence that diets high in sugar and refined carbohydrates contribute to

# The Fierce Foods Wheel

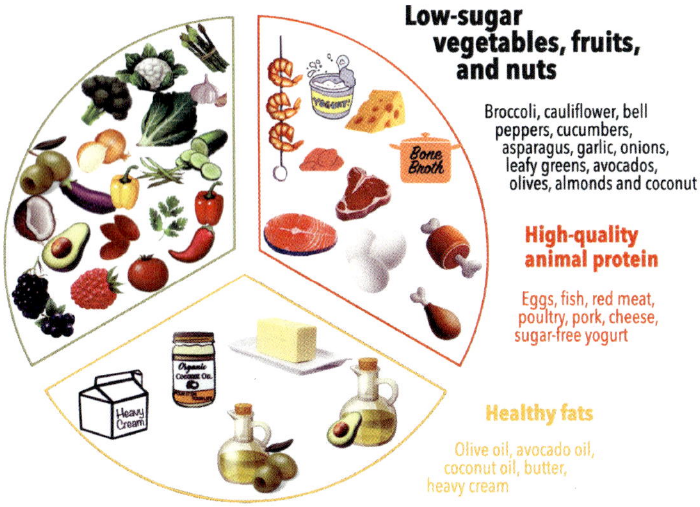


problems in school, depression, and other mental health challenges.

Refined carbohydrates (also known as simple carbohydrates) are carbohydrates that are low in nutritional value, digest quickly, and lead to spikes in blood glucose. They include foods high in simple sugars, like candy, cookies, fruit juice, and soda, as well as foods that contain a lot of starch, like bread, pasta, crackers, and potatoes. Vegetables and fruit are also carbohydrates, but they also contain fiber. Fiber slows the body's digestion of sugars and helps prevent spikes in blood glucose when we eat these whole and nutritious foods.

Sugar comes in many different forms and names. Regardless of its source, too much can wreak havoc on our metabolism. Consistently elevated blood sugar and insulin may also be linked to health problems like premature aging.

Pediatrician and researcher Robert Lustig argues that: "Sugar turns on the aging programs in your body. The more sugar you eat, the faster you age."

Sugar has also been linked to fatty liver disease in children, a condition that in the past was only seen in adult alcoholics. Because childhood cancer survivors may be at greater risk for premature aging and liver diseases, it's even more important for families to adopt a Fierce Foods approach that eliminates sugar from the diet.

# Nutrients: Macro and Micro

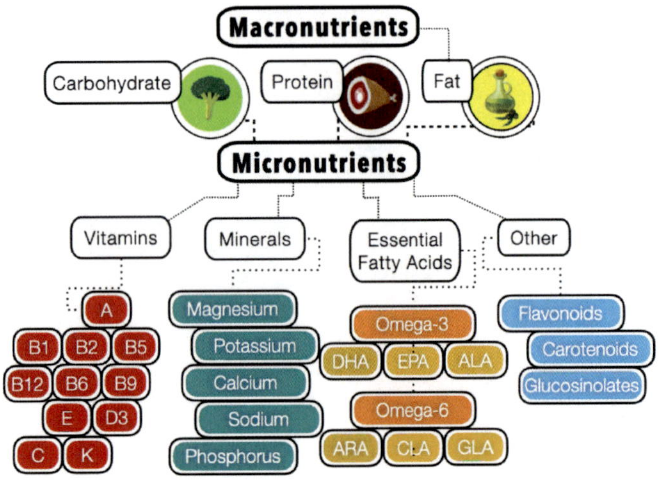


**Fierce Foods Principle #3: Focus on your cultural heritage recipes that are nutrient-dense**

Every culture around the world has a deep history of Fierce Foods. We only have to go back a few generations in our own culinary traditions—whether they're Chinese, Mexican, Afro-Caribbean, Indian, mid-Western Anglo-American or any other tradition—to find recipes and meals complete with Fierce Foods.

*Examples include:*

- Cruciferous vegetables (e.g. cauliflower, cabbage, bok choy, and collard greens)
- Allium vegetables (e.g. onions, garlic, leeks, and shallots)
- Spices (e.g. cinnamon, turmeric, paprika, black pepper, cumin, and coriander)
- Herbs (e.g. basil, cilantro, oregano, dill, and parsley)
- Unprocessed animal protein (e.g. eggs, lamb, chicken, beef, and seafood)

What all of these culinary heritage foods have in common is that they have a ton of nutrients packed into each calorie. When a food has a lot of nutrients per calorie, we call it "nutrient-dense," which is a way of saying that our culinary traditions pack the most nutritional punch in the smallest bite.

Nutrients are the natural chemical compounds that make up all food. They provide humans with energy, are building blocks for muscle, skin, and bones, and are chemical messengers that help cells function and stay healthy. Scientists break nutrients down into two types: macronutrients and micronutrients. The three main macronutrients are carbohydrates, fat, and protein. Of the three, protein is the most important. We could also include fiber and water because they are necessary for human health and longevity.

Fierce Foods focuses on culinary heritage because traditional recipes center on whole foods that include a lot of essential nutrients in a relatively small serving size.

First, let's think about macronutrients, of which protein is the most important. Sure, it's possible to get protein from ultra-processed foods like potato chips, but we only get 1.3 grams of protein for every 100 calories of chips we eat, while 100 calories of chicken give us 11.3 grams of protein. Of course, we don't only need protein.

What about fiber? Collard greens have 12 times, cabbage 10 times, and bok choy 8 times more fiber per calorie than potato chips.

Micronutrients are just as important! From essential vitamins (like A, C, D, and the B vitamins)

## Whole Plants + Animal Protein

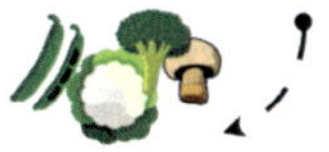

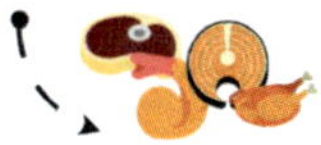

**Fiber and Micronutrients** | **Essential proteins and fatty acids**

When we eat whole plants and animal protein, our bodies get all the nutrients it needs. This not only makes us healthier but it makes us feel full for longer.

## Nutrient Sparsity = Simple Carbs + Dietary Fat

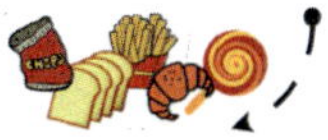

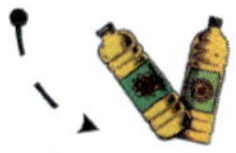

**Flour, sugar, processed corn and potatoes** | **Soybean oil, corn oil, canola oil**

Eating simple (starchy and refined) carbs *with* dietary fat tells the body that it should store body fat. It also makes us hungrier later because our bodies are still searching for nutrients.

to essential minerals (like magnesium, sodium, and potassium) to essential fatty acids (omega-3s and 6s), heritage Fierce Foods provide all of the necessary chemical messengers to help our cells work in tip-top shape.

Deficiencies in these micronutrients can cause some serious health consequences. Beyond the essentials, there are special micronutrients found in herbs and spices that can boost immunity and brain health and potentially improve cancer outcomes. These provide so many delicious ways to super-boost a meal.

We can ensure we're getting all the micronutrients we need by focusing on Fierce Food heritage staples like eggs (yolks are a great source of vitamins), salmon (super for omega-3 fatty acids), and low-starch vegetables like broccoli and cauliflower (great for vitamins and minerals). And nearly every heritage recipe boosts these essential nutrients with even more micronutrients from herbs and spices.

The best thing about the nutrient density of heritage foods is that they're naturally bundled with macro- and micro-nutrients that have evolved to work together. While we can get as biochemically complex about these foods as we want, their real genius lies in the fact that all we need to do to benefit from them is just sit down and eat.

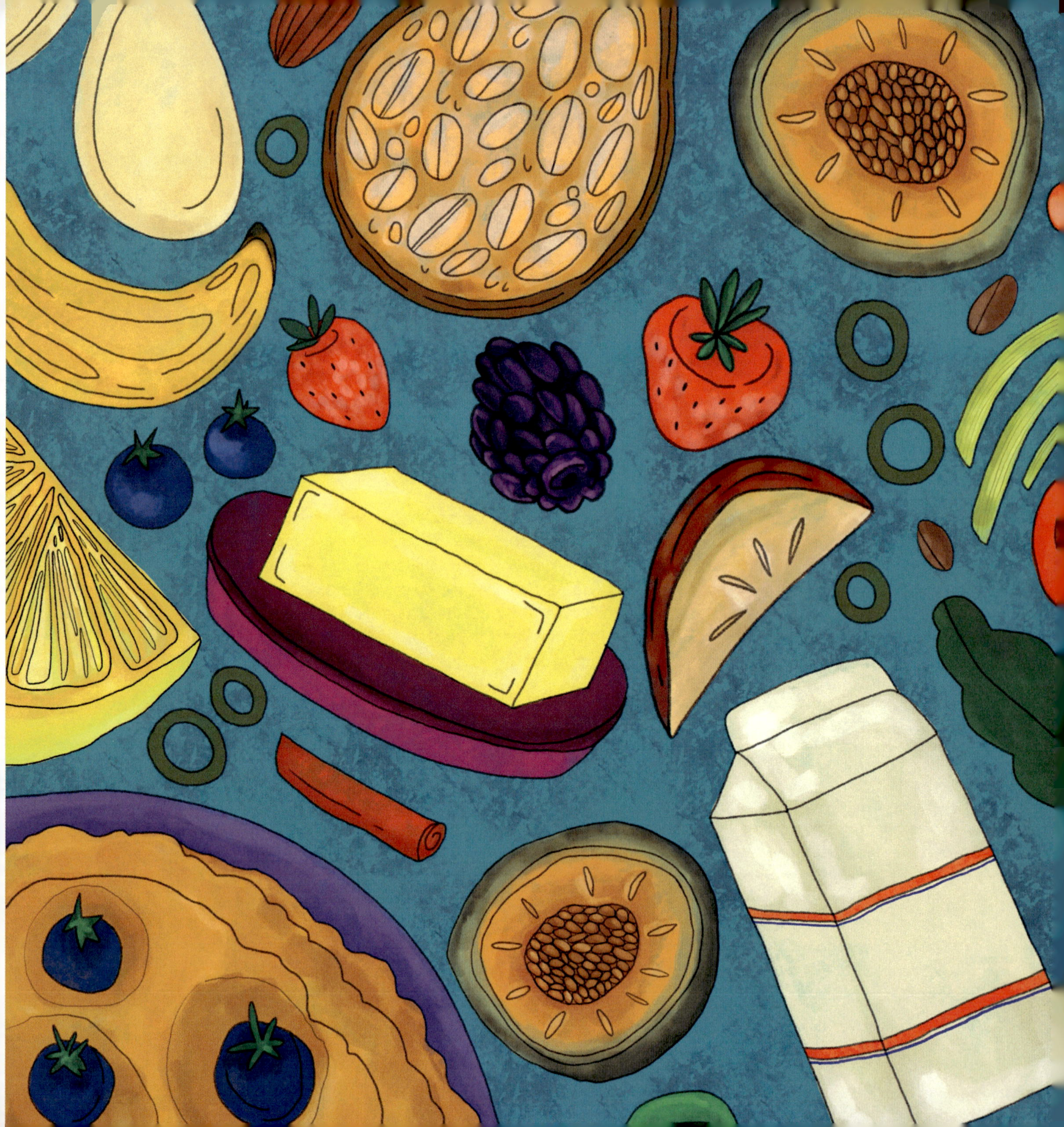

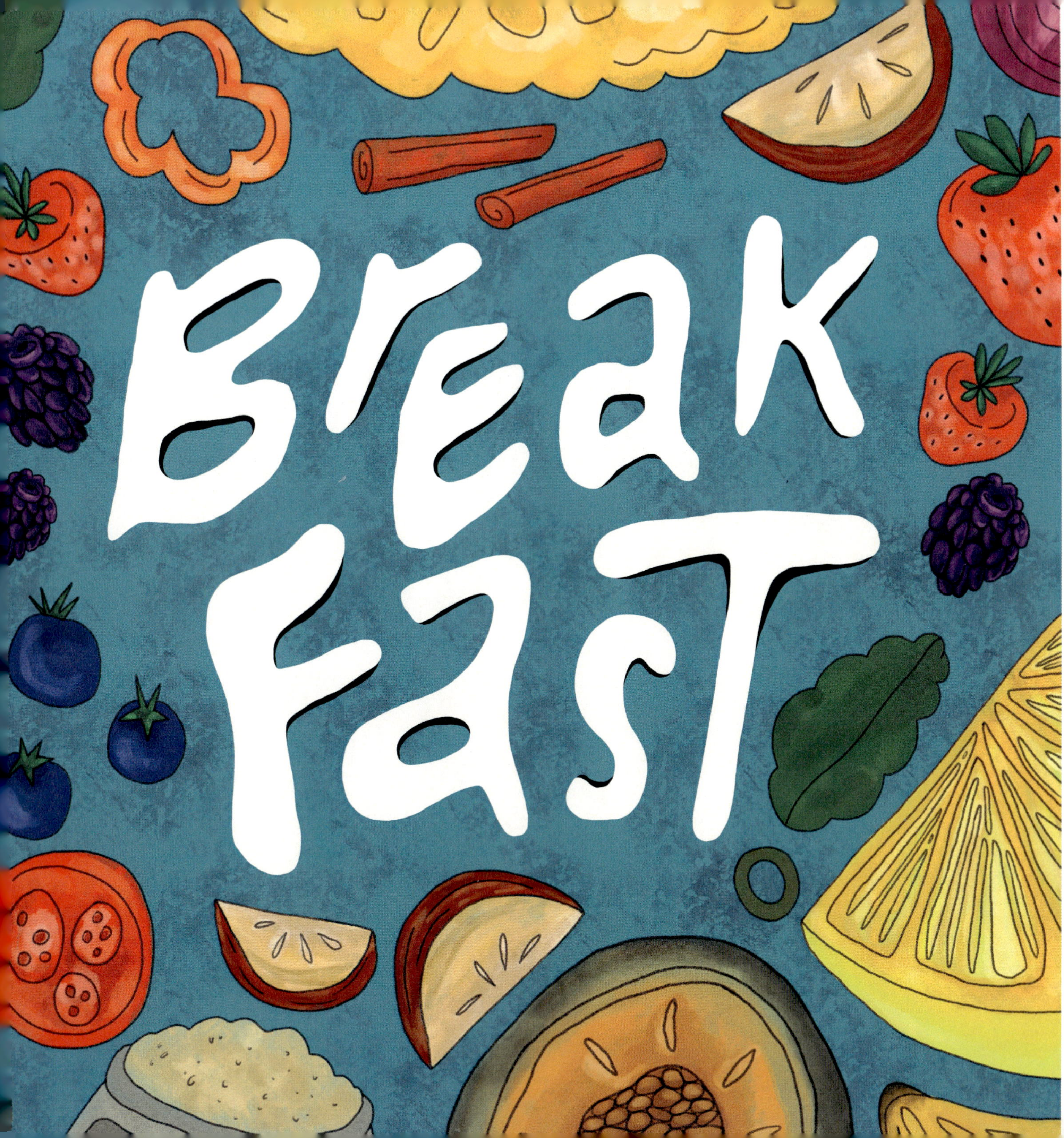
Break
Fast

# Breakfast



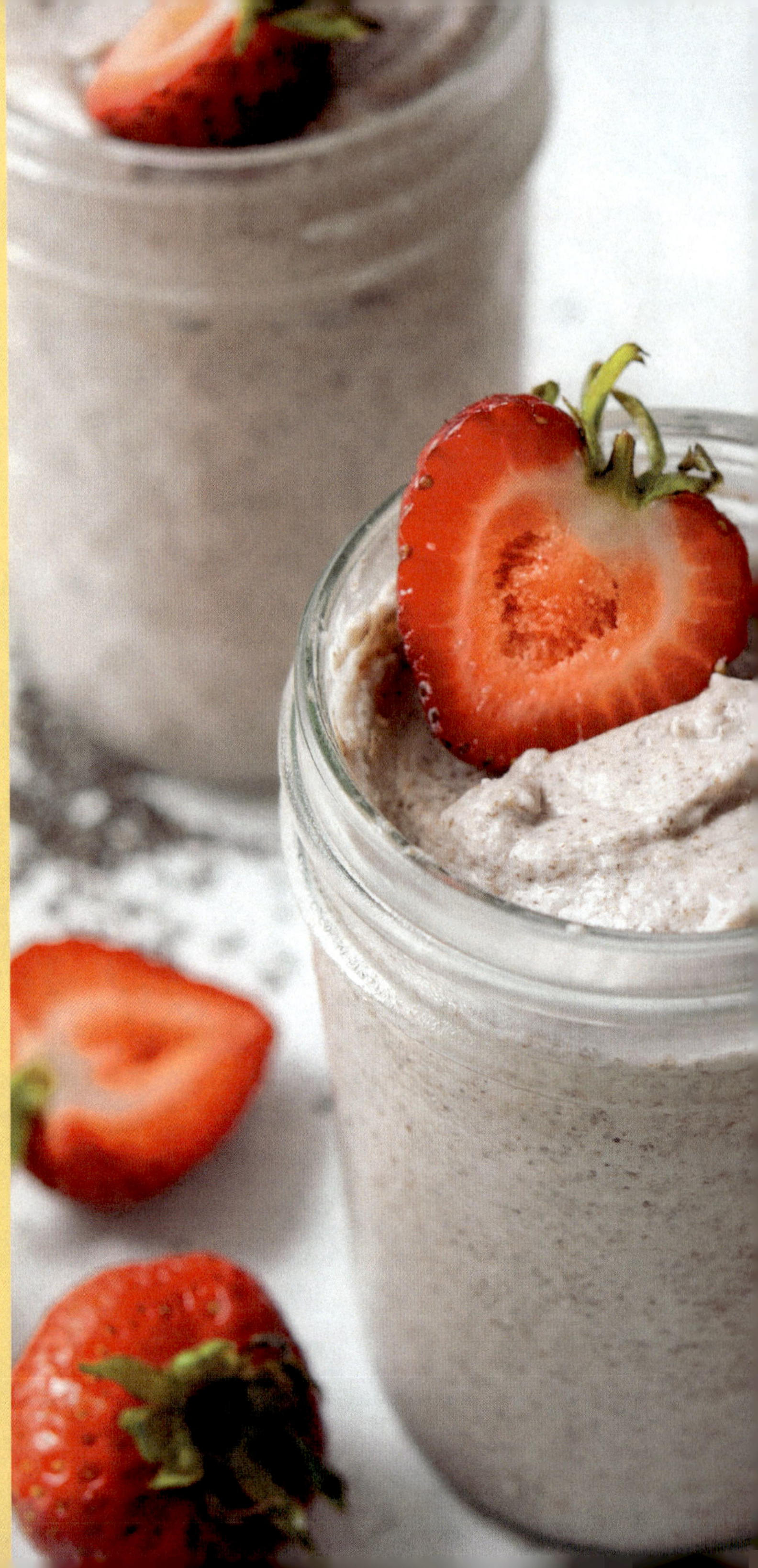

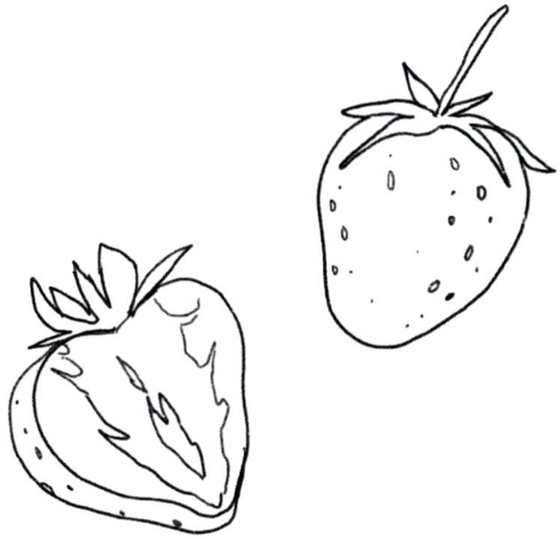

There is a right way to "break a fast," whether it happens immediately upon waking or when you're ready to start eating after a long period without food. Regardless, the best way to approach breaking a fast is by stabilizing blood sugar.

We do this by making sure we have macronutrient balance. Providing balance in that first meal is key. Quality carbohydrates like fruits and vegetables provide much-needed energy, plenty of protein provides building blocks for every cell in the body, and a healthy dose of anti-inflammatory and satiating fat insulates the brain and provides a calm focus for the rest of the day.

The point of breakfast is to provide long-lasting fuel to keep the body prepared and energized and the mind optimistic and centered, without creating an unnecessary spike in blood sugar followed by an unnecessary energy crash.

Whole, natural, and unprocessed foods can do all of these things for us by providing a nutrient density that ultra-processed foods just can't. Real food will provide all of the necessary tools such as vitamins, minerals, anti-oxidants, and phytonutrients to help our bodies rebuild, repair, and recover from the damage caused by necessary medical treatments and will also prepare the body with a resilience to successfully manage the stressors of everyday life.

Each of the recipes in this chapter provides a wide variety of fruits and vegetables, nutrient-dense proteins, and anti-inflammatory fats. They are also designed to be accessible—empowering impacted families with batch cook ideas to stock the freezer and prepare in advance for times when cooking is just plain hard to do.

Chef Alexia Hall, RDN

# Easy Banana Pancakes

**Makes 1 serving:** 5 pancakes each, 203 grams

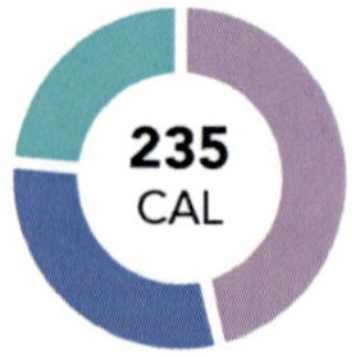


10g **Fat**
20g **Net Carb**
13g **Protein**

## Ingredients

1 small banana

2 large eggs

¼ tsp vanilla extract

¼ tsp ground cinnamon

## Directions

**1.** In a mixing bowl, use a fork to mash the bananas. With a whisk, whip the eggs in a small bowl, then add to the mashed banana. Mix until well blended, and add the vanilla extract and ground cinnamon.

**2.** Heat griddle to 350°F. Pour 2½ tablespoons of batter on the hot griddle and cook until golden brown on both sides. Serve hot, and top with nuts, seeds, or berries.

**3.** Double or triple the recipe for additional servings.

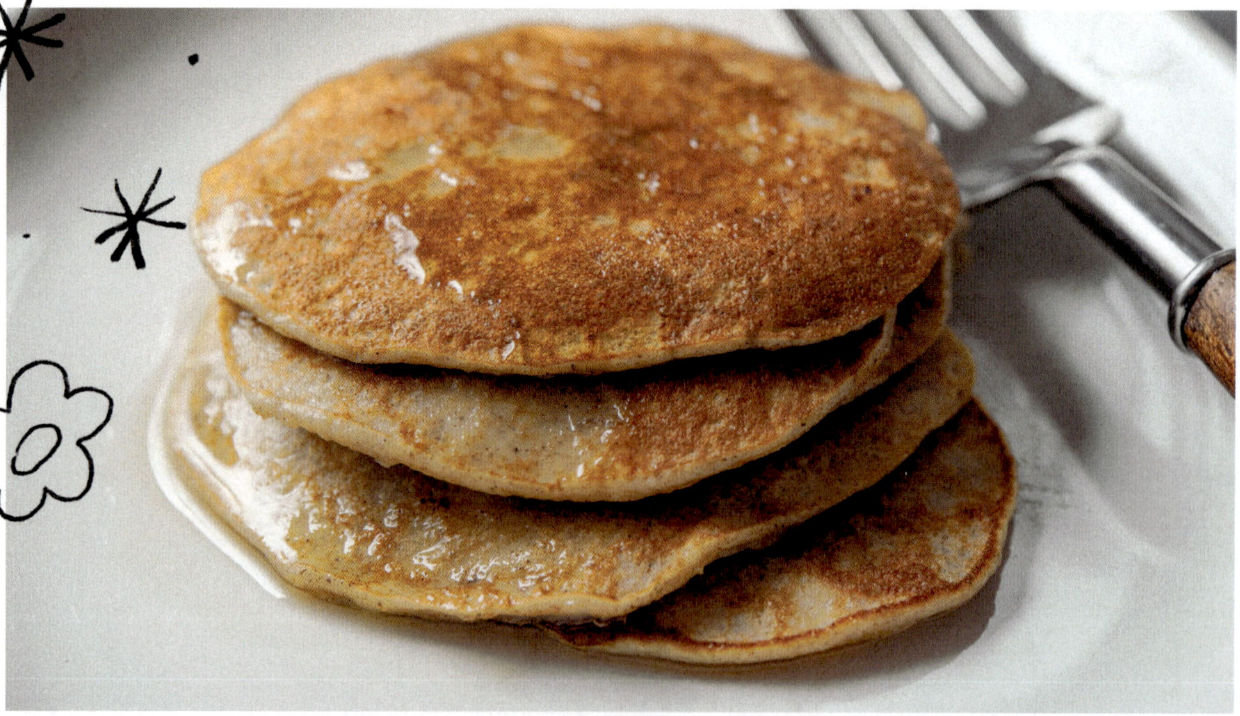

Chef Andrew Johnson

# Blueberry Lemon Ricotta Pancakes

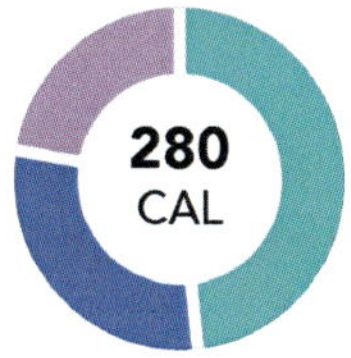


20g Fat
9g Net Carb
12g Protein

**Makes 6 servings:** 1 pancake each ~4", 127 grams

## Ingredients

1 cup almond flour

2 tbsp coconut flour

½ cup golden flaxseed meal

1 tbsp baking powder

½ tsp ground cinnamon

¼ tsp salt

1–2 tbsp granulated sweetener (e.g. allulose)

¾ cup blueberries, fresh or frozen and thawed, divided

3 large eggs

¼ –½ cup milk or dairy-free alternative

¾ cup ricotta cheese

3 tbsp lemon juice (~1 small lemon)

1 tsp lemon rind, grated

½ tsp vanilla extract

1 tbsp butter or avocado oil

Monk fruit sweetened maple syrup (optional)

## Directions

1. Using a large bowl and spoon, combine the almond flour, coconut flour, flaxseed, baking powder, cinnamon, salt, and granulated sweetener. Lightly toss in ¼ cup of the blueberries and gently mix with flour mixture until blueberries are dusted with flour.
2. In a separate bowl, whisk together the eggs, milk of choice, ricotta cheese, lemon juice, lemon rind, and vanilla extract. For a thicker pancake, use just ¼ cup of milk. Combine the wet ingredients with the dry, folding gently. Allow to rest for 5 minutes.
3. Preheat a large non-stick pan over low-medium heat, using butter or avocado oil to grease the pan.
4. Once hot, pour ¼ cup portions of the batter onto the pan and cover immediately.
5. Allow pancakes to cook for 4–6 minutes until the edges brown and bubbles burst on the top of the cake. Flip gently and cook the other side for 2–3 minutes until evenly browned on both sides.
6. Serve immediately and top with monk fruit sweetened maple syrup and the remaining ½ cup of fresh blueberries.

### Kids Can Cook Tips

Kids will have fun measuring all of the ingredients as well as learning how to whisk the eggs. Use a larger bowl with younger kids to help avoid spilling the ingredients. Rubber-bottomed bowls are helpful for that as well.

### Fierce Foods Facts

This flavorful and fun breakfast is loaded with vitamins A and C, which are important for a strong immune system and good skin. It also comes with a nice profile of minerals, including magnesium, calcium, phosphorus, and selenium, important for proper thyroid, bone, and heart function.

Chef Andrew Johnson

# Breakfast Taco Pancake Wraps

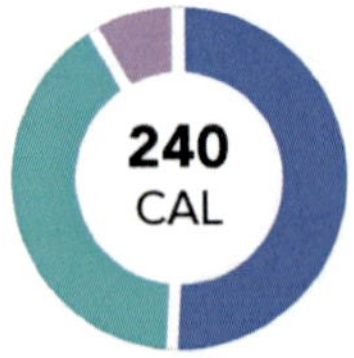


16g Fat
3g Net Carb
20g Protein

**Makes 6 servings:** each ¾ cup, 156 grams

## Ingredients

### Pancake Mix

1 cup protein powder, unflavored

1 cup almond flour

½ cup ground flaxseed

1 tsp baking powder

½ tsp salt

¼ tsp black pepper

¼ tsp garlic powder

¼ tsp chili powder

### For one serving of pancakes

1 egg, beaten

½ cup pancake mix

1 tsp minced chives

1 dollop of butter (or coconut oil) for greasing the pan

## Directions

1. In a large mixing bowl combine: protein powder, almond flour, ground flaxseed, baking powder, and seasonings. You can make multiple batches of this recipe in advance and store it in a mason jar or another sealed container in a cool dry pantry. In a separate mixing bowl whisk the eggs, chives, and pancake mix. Refrigerate batter for at least 15 minutes (up to 24 hours).
2. When you are ready to make the pancakes, place a large griddle or non-stick pan over medium heat, when the pan is hot add the butter or oil. Pour ⅓ cup of pancake batter onto the griddle using a measuring cup or ice cream scoop—depending on the thickness of your batter you may need to smooth out the mixture into even pancake shapes. Cook for approximately 5 minutes until small bubbles appear and the edges are beginning to set.
3. Carefully flip the pancake over and cook on remaining side for 2–3 more minutes until desired golden brown color. Start with 1 test pancake from start to finish and adjust for size and stove heat before attempting multiple pancakes per pan. Serve warm, stuff with delicious breakfast taco fillings, and enjoy.

## Fierce Foods Facts

This recipe is absolutely loaded with protein! According to the protein leverage hypothesis, when we focus on protein (and it's usually hard to get this much in the breakfast meal), we regulate appetite easier, and hopefully blood sugar too. Protein intake (especially nuts and seeds like flax, almond, and hemp that are high in tryptophan), helps to support the production of serotonin, the "feel-good" neurotransmitter in the brain.

4. When meal prepping for that easy grab-and-go breakfast option, you can cook and store these pancakes in the freezer in advance. Fully cook pancakes and let them cool completely. Stack the pancakes with a piece of parchment paper separating each cake to keep them from sticking together. Place the pancakes in a sealed freezer-safe container or Ziploc bags (quart-size for individual portions or gallon size for the entire family), then into the freezer to store.

5. Reheat directly from frozen in the microwave or oven. For the microwave cook on a high setting, uncovered for 20–30 seconds per cake. For the oven, preheat 350°F, place cakes on a parchment-lined sheet pan, and cover tightly with foil. Bake for approximately 10 minutes.

## Kids Can Cook Tips

Kids love pancakes, especially ones they can turn into a wrap so they can eat with their hands. Have kids help measure and mix the ingredients together. Teach younger kids about what to watch for before the pancakes are ready to flip over. Tip: it's when the bubbles are popping!

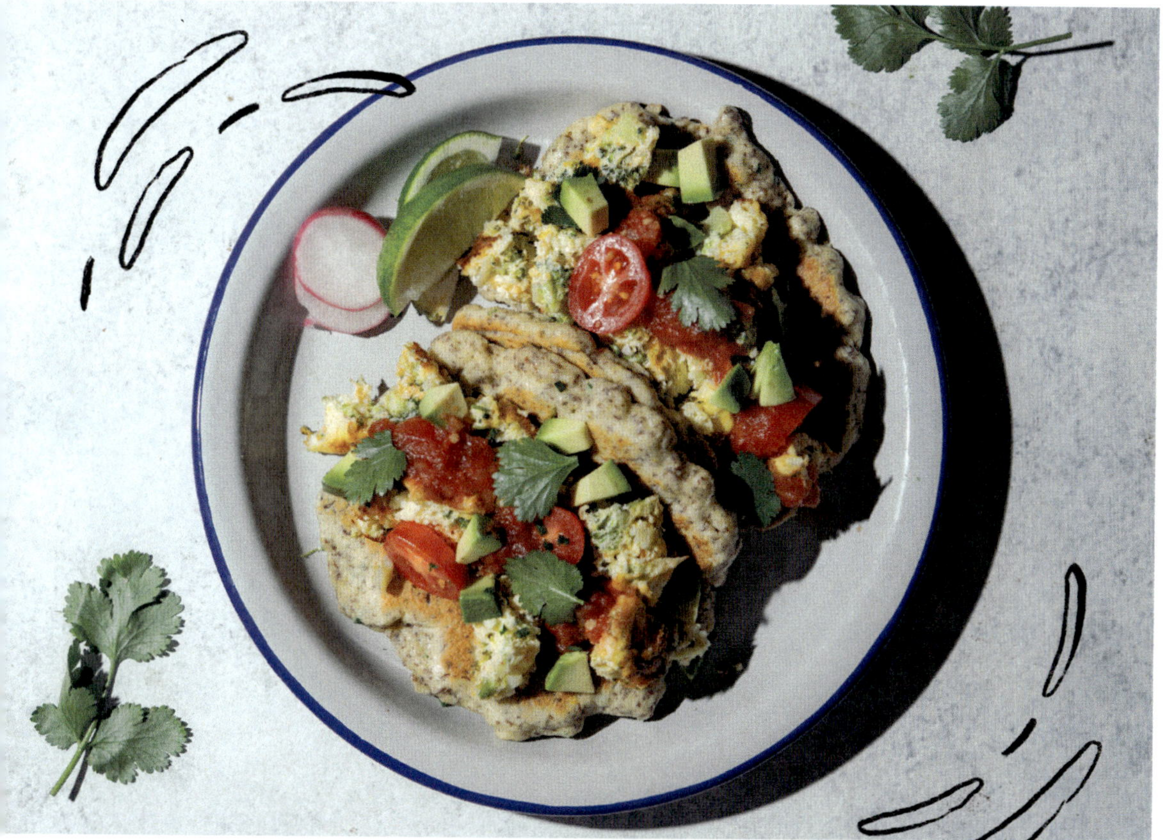

Chef Alexia Hall, RDN

# Carrot Cake Breakfast Bites

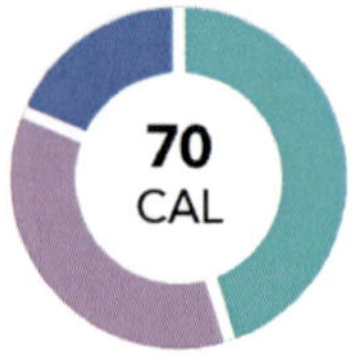


5g Fat
4g Net Carb
2g Protein

**Makes 40 servings:** 1 bite each, 23 grams

## Ingredients

1 cup blanched almond flour

⅓ cup coconut flour

1 cup old-fashioned oats

½ cup ground flaxseed

½ cup buckwheat groats

½ cup pumpkin seeds

⅛ tsp cloves

¼ tsp nutmeg

½ tsp ginger

1 tsp cinnamon

1 cup shredded carrots

¼ cup unsweetened shredded coconut

¼ cup honey or carb-conscious alternative (e.g. Pyure Hunny)

2 tbsp coconut oil

2 large eggs, slightly beaten

## Directions

1. In a blender, food processor, or mixing bowl, mix together the flours, seeds, and spices. Melt the coconut oil, add it to the bowl with honey and egg, and blend well. Fold in shredded carrots and mix once more.
2. Using a 1½" scoop, scoop balls onto a lined cookie sheet, then bake at 350°F for 10 minutes. Cool completely, then store in the freezer until ready to use.

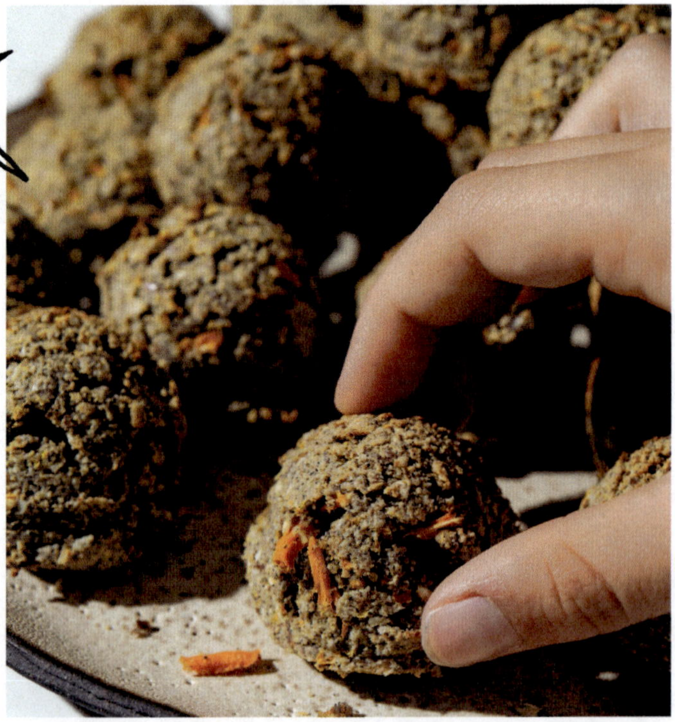

### Fierce Foods Facts

This fun breakfast side has almost 4 grams of fiber, making for a happy gut to start the day! There is plenty of vitamins A and E, thanks to the carrots as well as healthy fat and magnesium from the pumpkin seeds and buckwheat groats. Pair a couple with an egg for a nutrient-dense breakfast!

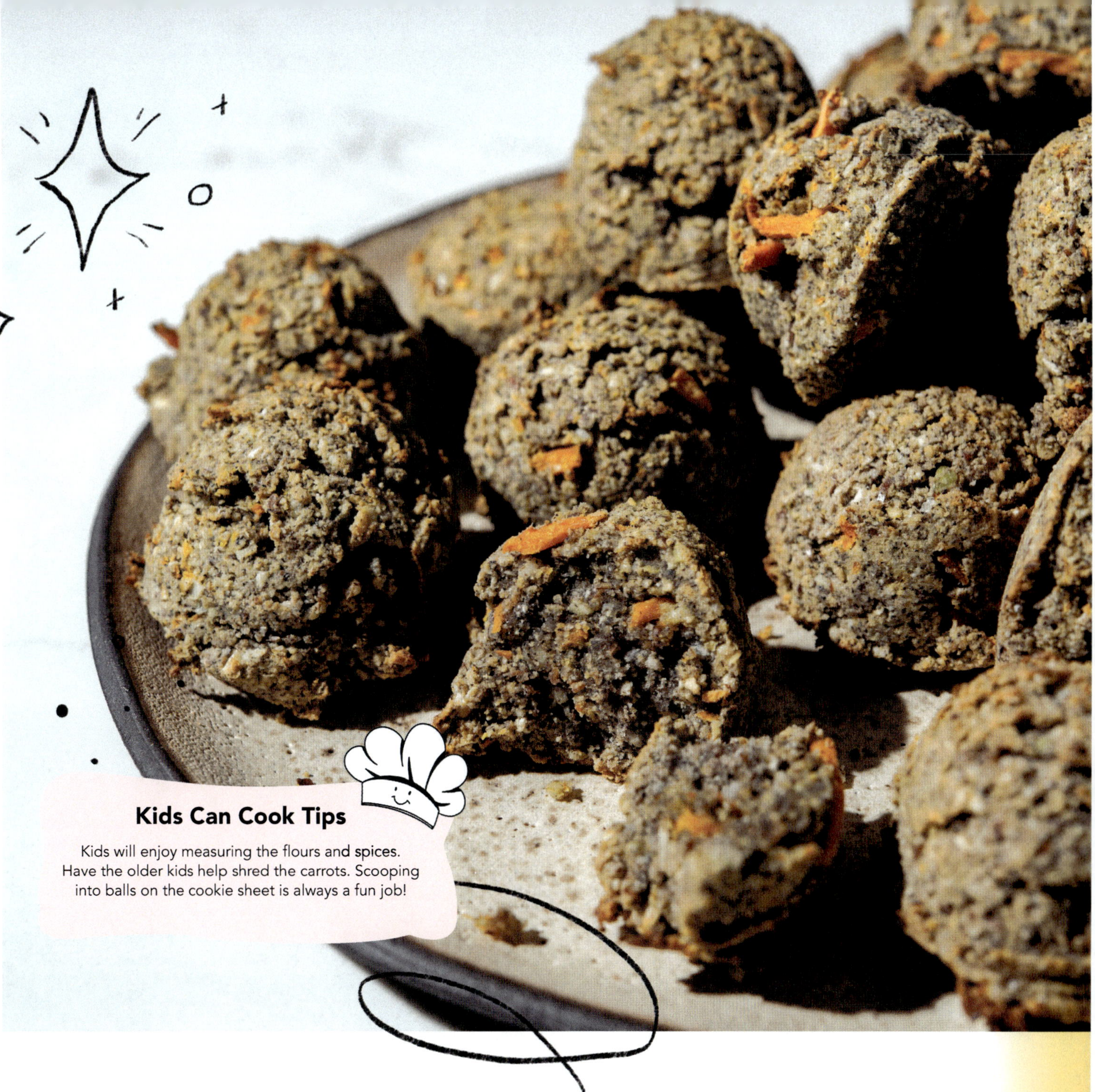

## Kids Can Cook Tips

Kids will enjoy measuring the flours and spices. Have the older kids help shred the carrots. Scooping into balls on the cookie sheet is always a fun job!

Chef Andrew Johnson

# Chia Cauliflower Hashbrowns

**Makes 6 servings:** 2 patties each, 109 grams

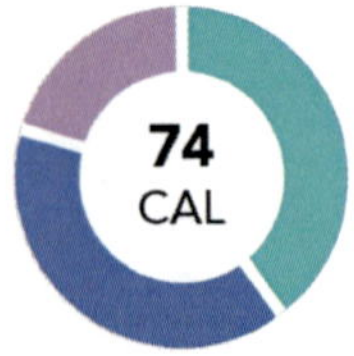


4g **Fat**
2g **Net Carb**
4g **Protein**

## Ingredients

1 medium cauliflower head, riced (approx. 2½ cups)

1 tbsp extra virgin olive oil

1 tbsp chia seeds

3 scallions (green and white parts), minced

2 small handfuls of fresh parsley, minced

2 large organic eggs, lightly beaten

1 tsp sea salt, or to taste

¼ tsp ground black pepper

¼ tsp dried chili powder

¼ tsp dried garlic powder

## Directions

**1.** In a large saucepan add a ½ cup of water and bring to boil over high heat. Add the riced cauliflower, reduce to medium heat and simmer until the cauliflower is tender (about 10–12 minutes). Drain well and let the cauliflower cool to room temperature.

**2.** It's important to let the cauliflower cool to room temperature before combining with the egg mixture—doing so could scramble the eggs before they get to bind with the other ingredients!

**3.** Preheat the oven to 475°F and line 2 large baking sheets with parchment paper.

**4.** In a large bowl add the cauliflower, chia seeds, scallions, parsley, eggs, and spices and stir until well combined. Set aside for 15 minutes (or up to 24 hours in the refrigerator) to allow the chia seeds to expand and set.

**5.** Using a dry ¼-cup measuring cup, drop the mixture onto the prepared baking sheets, then flatten the mixture and round into 12 patties (about 3" in diameter each). Bake the patties for 15–20 minutes, flip over each patty with a spatula, then bake until golden brown (about 8–10 more minutes). Serve warm.

**6.** To serve these as a replacement for potato latkes, serve with a side of full-fat sour cream and unsweetened applesauce. Top each serving with a small dollop of each.

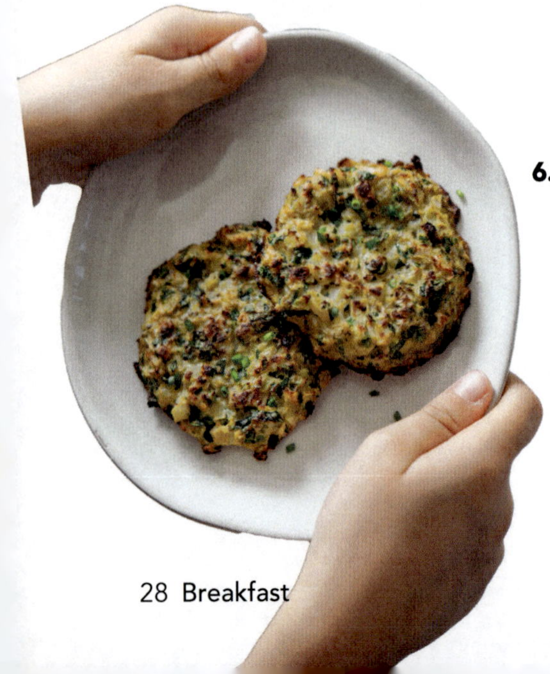

### Kids Can Cook Tips

Kids can help rice the cauliflower, tear the fresh herbs, crack the eggs, and measure the spices. Older kids with knife skills can mince the scallions and help sauté the cauliflower.

Chef Audra DiPadova Wilford

# Strawberry Chia Pudding

**Makes 4 servings:** ½ cup each, 168 grams

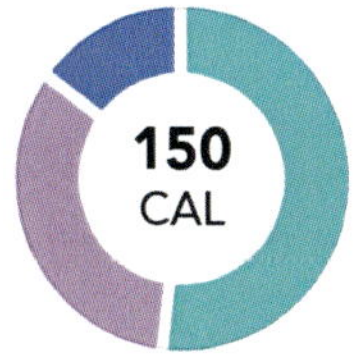


11g Fat
7g Net Carb
3g Protein

## Ingredients

2 cups coconut milk

⅓ cup chia seeds

3 pitted dates or sweetener of choice

(e.g. Lakanto)

1 cup strawberries, sliced

## Directions

1. Add all ingredients to a blender. Blend for approximately 30 seconds or until well combined.
2. Divide into 4 equal servings into sealable half-cup-sized glass jars and refrigerate overnight or for at least 2 hours. Enjoy within 5 days.

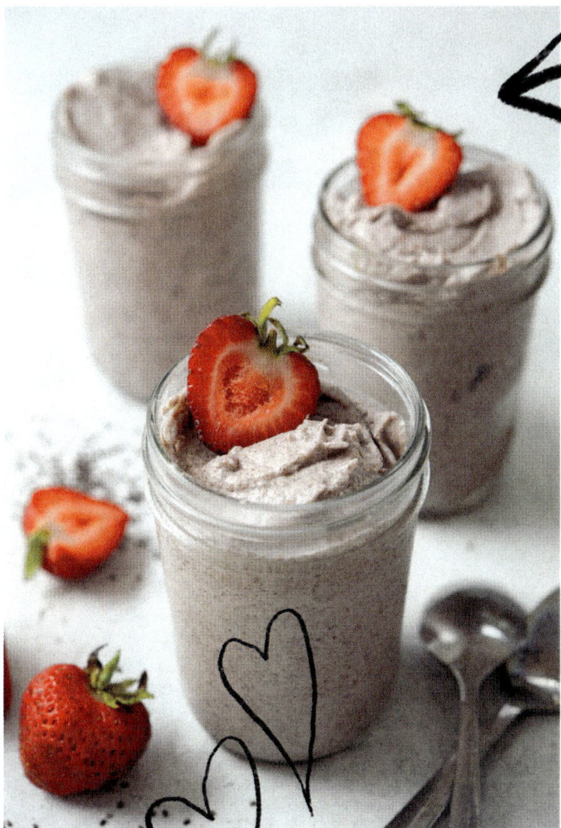

### Fierce Foods Facts

These tiny seeds deliver a mighty punch in a very small package. They are an excellent source of plant-based Omega-3 fatty acids and have high protein and fiber, all of which combine to create an anti-inflammatory, satiating and balanced meal profile. The extra sweetener may be unnecessary with the wonderful sweetness of the strawberries.

## Frittatas

What is an easy no-brainer for breakfast? *Frittatas of course!*

They are the perfect vehicle for a balanced breakfast, one with quality carbohydrates, fat, and protein to provide sustained fuel for an energetic day! Frittatas are easy to make and work well with just about any fresh or frozen vegetable.

It's a good idea to pre-cook sturdier vegetables (such as root vegetables, broccoli, and onions) before adding the eggs, as the raw vegetables will release too much water and won't cook fast enough before the eggs are done.

A good ratio to use is about four eggs to each cup of raw vegetables. Consider sautéing the vegetables in an ovenproof pan and cooking off or draining any excess liquid.

Once tender, add your spices, salt, and pepper. Add the whisked eggs and then finish cooking in the oven, watching closely for the frittata to puff up. Be careful not to overcook. Do not add fresh herbs or tender tomatoes until the dish is out of the oven.

Check out our recipes for Quick Quiches and Greek-Inspired Frittata for some ideas on how to batch cook these breakfast favorites so they are ready-made for those busy weekday mornings!

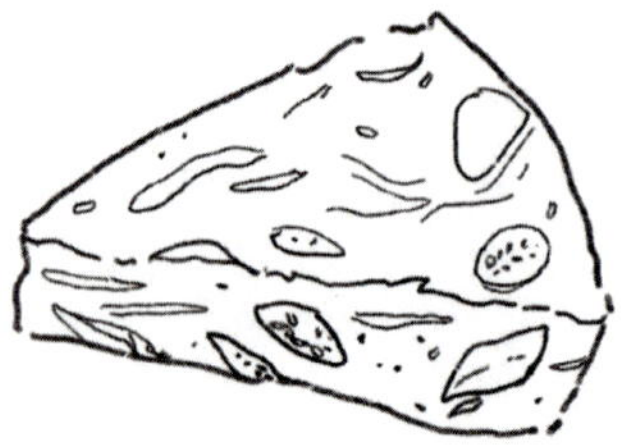

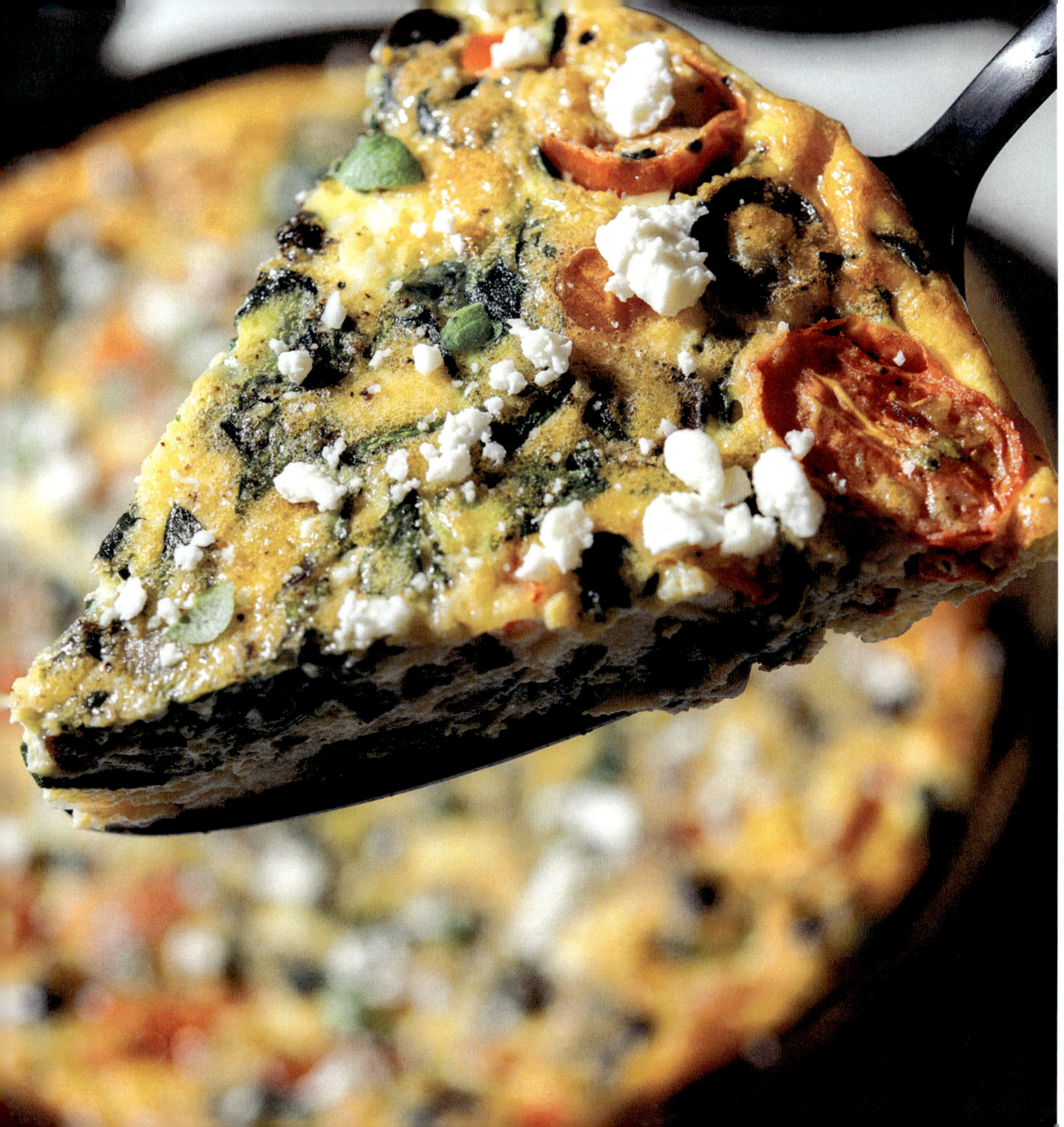

Chef Anne Watson

# Greek-Inspired Frittata

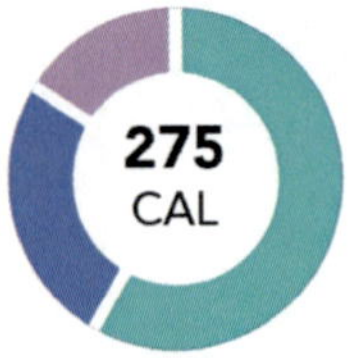


23g **Fat**
6g **Net Carb**
10g **Protein**

**Makes 6 servings:** each ¾ cup, 185 grams

## Ingredients

3 garlic cloves, minced

½ cup red onion, diced

1½ cups baby spinach, roughly chopped

1 cup cherry tomatoes, sliced in half

¼ cup red bell pepper, diced

1 can (2 oz) sliced black or kalamata olives, drained

½ cup crumbled feta cheese, plus extra for garnish

2 tsp chopped fresh oregano, or 1 tsp dried, plus extra for garnish

1 tsp sea salt

½ tsp ground black pepper

6 eggs

1 cup milk

2 tbsp olive oil, plus extra for drizzling

## Directions

1. Preheat the oven to 350°F, then in a large bowl, whisk together eggs and milk. Stir in feta cheese and set aside.
2. In a large oven-proof skillet, heat 2 tablespoons of olive oil over medium-high heat, add the onion, and sauté until soft (3–4 minutes). Add the garlic and spinach, then sauté until fragrant (1 minute). Add in the tomatoes, red bell pepper, olives, oregano, salt, and pepper. Heat through for another 1–2 minutes.
3. Lower to medium heat and pour in the egg mixture and cook for 3–4 minutes just until eggs begin to set. Carefully move the skillet from the stove into the preheated oven and finish cooking for an additional 15–20 minutes.
4. Remove from oven and allow to cool for 5–10 minutes before garnishing with extra oregano, feta, and olive oil.

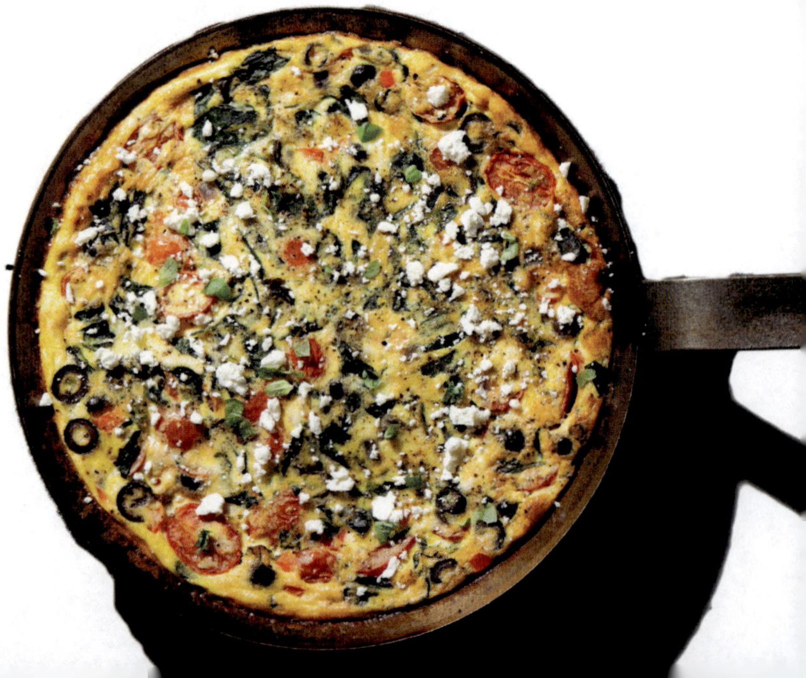

Chef Andrew Johnson

# Frittata Quick Quiches

**Makes 6 servings:** 2 quiches each, 168 grams

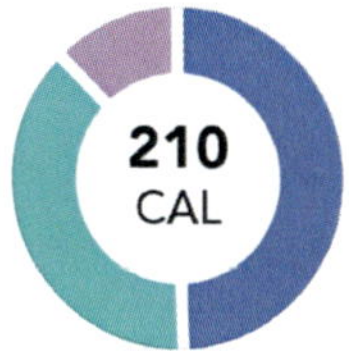


13g Fat
4g Net Carb
17g Protein

## Ingredients

3 slices ham or Canadian bacon, chopped

2 cups broccoli, finely chopped

4 scallions, thinly sliced

12–18 cherry tomatoes, halved

8 large eggs

1 cup cheddar cheese, shredded

½ cup milk

½ tsp salt

½ tsp ground pepper

Smoked paprika to garnish

Olive oil or other oil for greasing pan

### Fierce Foods Facts

Eggs are packed with choline, a vital nutrient for brain health! Studies are growing on the importance of choline to properly support neurotransmitters like dopamine and norepinephrine, which are important for regulating our fight or flight responses! Choline also helps to produce and release acetylcholine, which is heavily involved in memory storage.

## Directions

1. In a large mixing bowl whisk eggs, milk, salt, and pepper. Add in meat, cheese, broccoli, and scallions, and thoroughly mix together. Preheat the oven to 350°F.
2. Liberally coat a 12-cup muffin pan with cooking spray or oil. Divide the egg mixture among the prepared muffin cups. Top each quiche with 2 or 3 tomato halves and sprinkle with smoked paprika.
3. Bake for 25–30 minutes, test doneness by gently shaking the pan to see if the egg is set. Remove from the oven and let cool for a few minutes before removing from the muffin tin. Use a butter knife and carefully ring the muffin cup to allow for the quiche to be removed cleanly from the pan.
4. When meal prepping for that easy grab-and-go breakfast option, you can cook and store these quiches in the refrigerator or freezer in advance. Place quiches in a sealed container or Ziploc bag and refrigerate for up to 3 days or freeze for up to 1 month. To reheat, microwave on high for 20–30 seconds each.

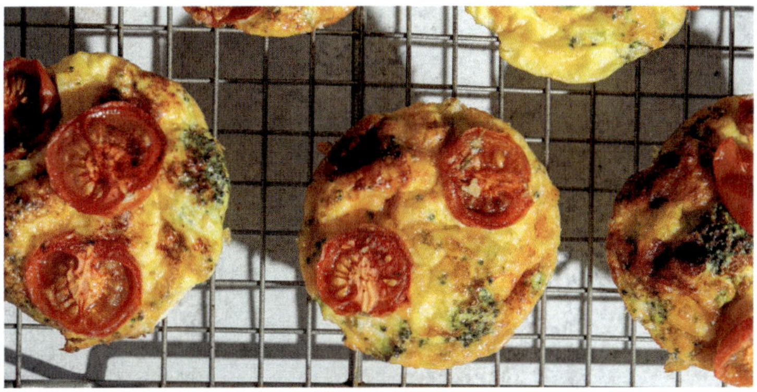

Chef Andrew Johnson

# Overnight Oats

Makes 1 serving: 1½ cups each, grams vary

## Ingredients

**Sweet Variation Base** (52 grams)

½ cup quick oats

1 tbsp chia seeds (increase to 2–3 tbsp for denser consistency) *

1 tbsp unflavored hemp protein powder

1 cup alternative milk (e.g. Not Milk or Ripple Unsweetened)

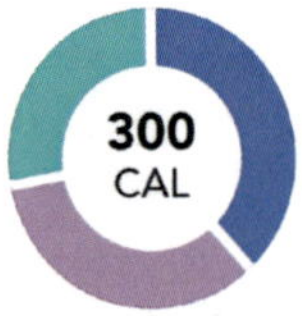


13g **Fat**
16g **Net Carb**
18g **Protein**

**Savory Variation Base** (135 grams)

½ cup quick oats

1 tbsp chia seeds

1 tbsp unflavored hemp protein powder

1 cup alternative milk

1–2 tbsp soy sauce or coconut aminos

A couple drops of sesame oil

A couple drops of Sriracha sauce or sambal (optional)

Salt and pepper to taste

1 egg, poached

1 tbsp cashews, toasted and chopped

½ tsp scallions, finely sliced

sesame seeds

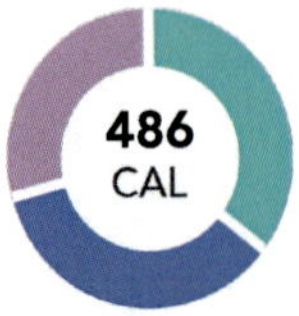


27g **Fat**
22g **Net Carb**
27g **Protein**

**Blueberry Pie** (139 grams)

⅓ cup blueberries

2 tbsp pecans, toasted and chopped

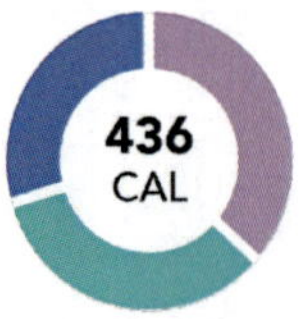


23g **Fat**
25g **Net Carb**
20g **Protein**

*nutrition facts with increased chia

**Zippy Berry** (130 grams)

⅓ cup fresh raspberries

2 tbsp pepitas or sunflower seeds

1 lemon, zested

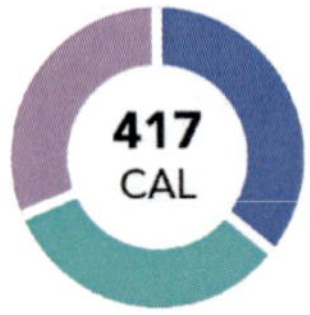


21g **Fat**
20g **Net Carb**
23g **Protein**

**Warm Orchard** (122 grams)

⅓ cup Granny Smith apple, cubed

2 tbsp almonds, toasted and sliced

½ tsp cinnamon

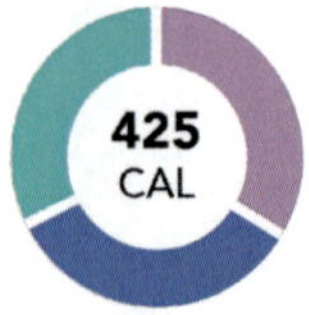


21g **Fat**
22g **Net Carb**
22g **Protein**

**Candy Bar** (96 grams)

1 tbsp Lily's sugar-free milk chocolate chips

1 tbsp peanut, almond, or sunflower butter

1 tbsp unsweetened coconut, shredded

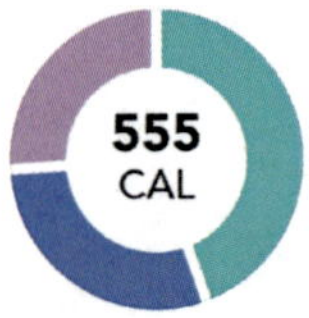


35g **Fat**
20g **Net Carb**
23g **Protein**

**Banana Loaf** (109 grams)

⅓ banana, sliced

1 tbsp unsweetened coconut, shredded

2 tbsp walnuts, toasted and chopped

½ tsp cinnamon

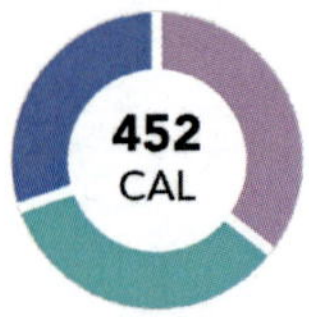


24g **Fat**
25g **Net Carb**
21g **Protein**

## Directions

1. In a pint mason jar (or similar size container with a tight-fitting lid) add oats, chia seeds, hemp protein, and milk. Place the lid on the container and shake until all the ingredients are incorporated. Place in the refrigerator for an hour, overnight, or up to 2 days.
2. Remove from fridge, remove the lid and add topping variations. Serve immediately or place the lid back on and back into the fridge until you are ready to enjoy.
3. May eat cold or warm. To warm, microwave on high for 1 minute, and stir well. Serve within 3 days. We recommended enjoying the savory variation while warm.

### For the poached egg

1. In a small or medium sauté pan, add a ½" of water. Insert silicone muffin cup liners or other stove-safe bowls. Grease muffin cups or bowls with cooking oil spray, and carefully crack eggs into the cups not to break the yolks.
2. Season the tops of the eggs with salt and pepper. Cover the sauté pan (ideally with a glass lid) and heat on high heat. Boil for 5–7 minutes until the egg whites are just set.
3. Remove the pan from heat and quickly remove the egg cups. Let cool slightly and use a spoon or butter knife to release the egg from the sides of the cups.

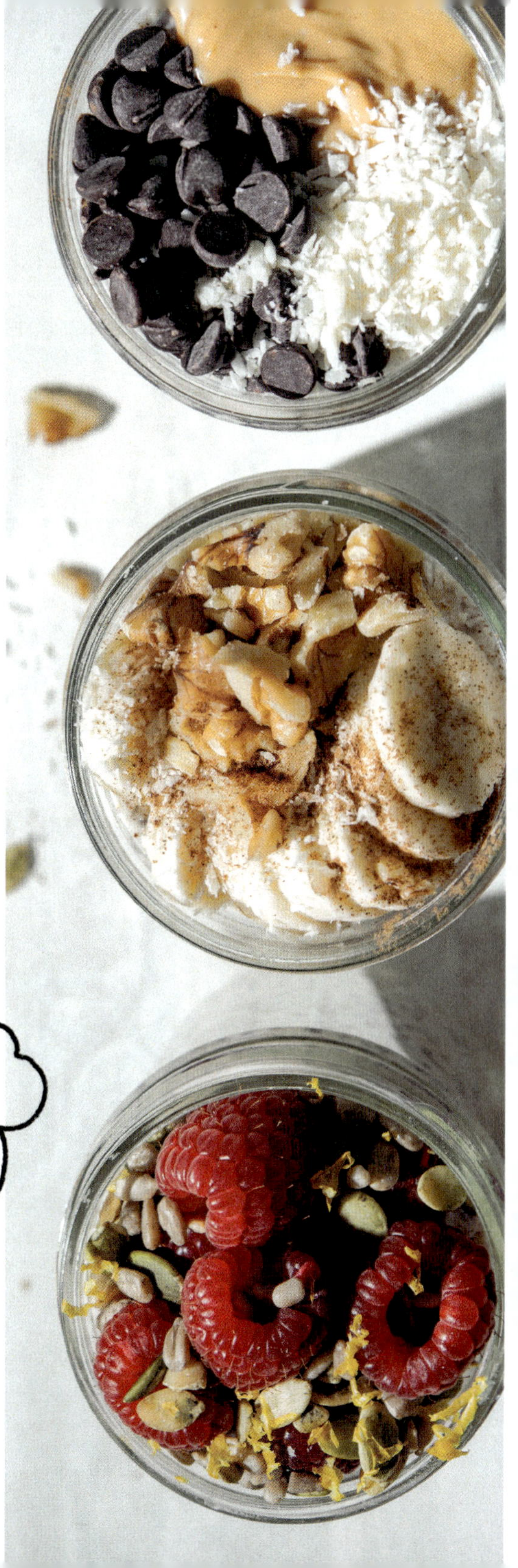

### Kids Can Cook Tip

Give kids more agency over their food choices by letting them choose which variations they might like to have that day for breakfast. Encourage them to come up with new combos and creative recipe names. Encourage them to include a low glycemic fruit, a nut, a seed, and a spice to ensure balance in their new creation.

## Smoothies

A carefully planned and strategically balanced smoothie can be the perfect meal replacement tool when eating is difficult. With our easy 1-2-3-4 plan, you can achieve the right balance of fulfilling high-quality carbohydrates, proteins, and fats that will keep you well-fed and energized!

1. Start with a liquid that is tailored to specific nutrition needs. Need more hydration? Just use water. Feeling low after a sweaty workout? Use unsweetened coconut water for some important electrolytes. Having difficulty getting enough calcium in the day? Use milk or a fortified alternative milk. For a large 4-serving smoothie, about 1 cup of liquid should make blending a breeze.

2. Add a protein. Grass-fed whey protein powder is a great choice to help build muscle and can usually be found unsweetened in a canister. Generally, 1 scoop will provide about 20 grams. Look for one without added extra ingredients. If intolerant to dairy proteins, clean hemp protein powder is a great choice. Just make sure to purchase unsweetened and pure protein powders without added flavors and sweeteners. Another choice might be unsweetened Greek yogurt. Be sure to choose the full-fat varieties to help provide that satiating balance.

3. Fill up most of the remaining blender with non-starchy greens like spinach, bok choy, kale, chard, or broccoli sprouts. These varieties are great to begin a veggie smoothie as they can be milder and taste less bitter than others. Finish with some frozen low-glycemic index fruits such as berries, kiwi, or citrus. Plan on at least a 3:1 ratio of greens to fruit to keep the carbohydrates at a level that won't raise blood sugar.

4. Add 2 tablespoons of healthy fat. Some great choices include half an avocado or a tablespoon of MCT oil or powder. Flaxseed oil is also a great choice as an anti-inflammatory fat, though it can go rancid quickly so be sure to purchase in small containers and store only to the expiration date in the fridge.

Treatments for cancer such as chemotherapy and radiation can often cause changes in both taste and smell. Here are some tips to help make smoothies (and other foods) more appetizing:

**Color matters:** choose foods that will have an appetizing color. If the protein powder and greens create an unappetizing gray-brown, add some bright big blueberries or a small roasted beet to turn it into a more inviting color.

**Rinsing the mouth often** will help to remove strange tastes.

**Some find relief** with tart foods, others with sweets. A quick squeeze of lemon into the mouth or a lingering taste of a sliver of apple may help to alter the sense of taste for just long enough that other foods can be tolerated.

**If the metallic sensation** of metal utensils is problematic, use plastic instead.

**If smells are annoying,** avoid the more robust bitter flavors and utilize lemon, kiwi, or berries to provide a more pleasing fragrance.

**Temperature may make a difference.** Ice cold can sometimes induce headaches so be sure to experiment to find what works best.

See our Breakfast Protein Smoothies recipes for some delicious ways to balance your smoothie!

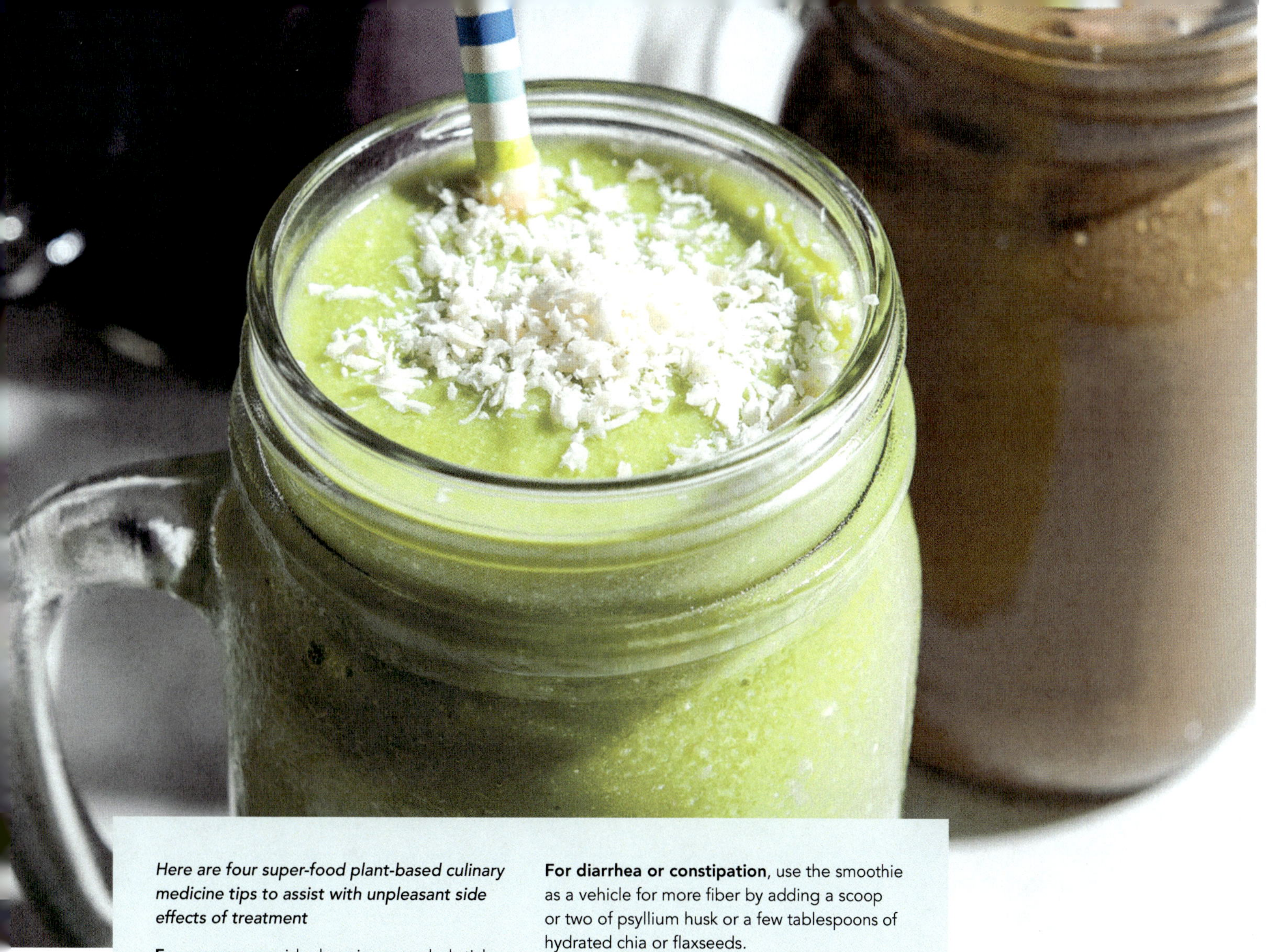

*Here are four super-food plant-based culinary medicine tips to assist with unpleasant side effects of treatment*

**For nausea**, consider keeping a peeled stick of ginger in the freezer. Simply grate a 1-inch piece into a blender full of smoothies and blend well.

**For mouth sores**, consider adding some basil which is known to alleviate this type of pain, or consider coconut "pulling" (gargling with a tea spoon or two of coconut oil before enjoying the smoothie).

**For diarrhea or constipation**, use the smoothie as a vehicle for more fiber by adding a scoop or two of psyllium husk or a few tablespoons of hydrated chia or flaxseeds.

**For anxiety or depression**, consider adding foods rich in Omega-3 like hemp seeds or flaxseeds, magnesium-rich foods like cacao, and selenium-rich foods such as Brazil nuts or sunflower seeds.

Chef Andrew Johnson

# Breakfast Protein Smoothies

**Makes 1 serving:** each 2 cups, grams vary

## Ingredients

### Base Ingredients

1 cup full-fat dairy or alternative milk, fortified with calcium and vitamin D

1 scoop protein powder (e.g. whey or hemp protein),
20 grams protein per scoop

## Directions

Using a high-powered blender, combine protein powder and alternative milk, and blend on high for 30 seconds or until well combined. Add remaining ingredients according to the variation, then blend on high for 60 seconds or until well blended. Divide into pint-sized glass mason jars, and consume immediately or refrigerate for up to 4 days.

**Pro Tip:** Nutrition facts for carbohydrate contents of smoothies. Divide into 2 serving sizes for those who are carbohydrate sensitive or following a modified carbohydrate diet.

**Chocolate Peanut Butter** *(451 grams)*

1 tbsp Lily's sugar-free chocolate chips

½ small frozen banana, sliced
(or ¼ cup cashews if carb-sensitive)

2 tbsp smooth natural peanut butter

3 cups power greens

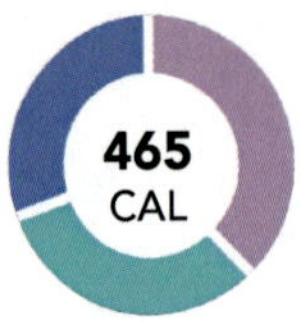


25g Fat
30g Net Carb
24g Protein

**Pumpkin** *(475 grams)*

½ cup pumpkin purée

¼ cup raw cashews

⅛ tsp pumpkin pie spice

3 cups fresh spinach, chopped

+1 drop liquid stevia to taste

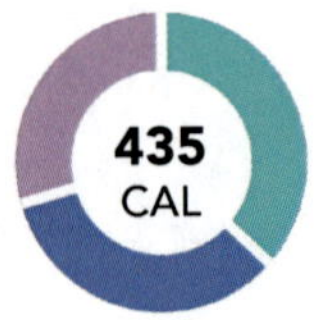


24g Fat
19g Net Carb
22g Protein

**Tropical** *(532 grams)*

3 cups spinach

½ cup frozen mango slices

½ cup frozen papaya

1 tbsp dried unsweetened coconut, shredded

1 tbsp ground flaxseed

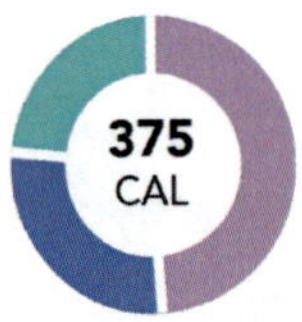


16g Fat
34g Net Carb
19g Protein

**Berrylicious** *(492 grams)*

½ cup frozen blueberries

½ cup frozen strawberries

2 cups spinach

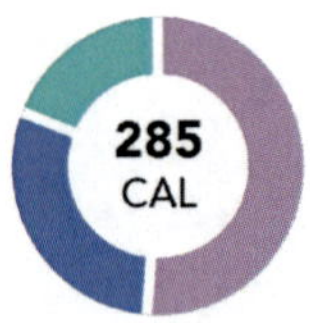


10g Fat
28g Net Carb
16g Protein

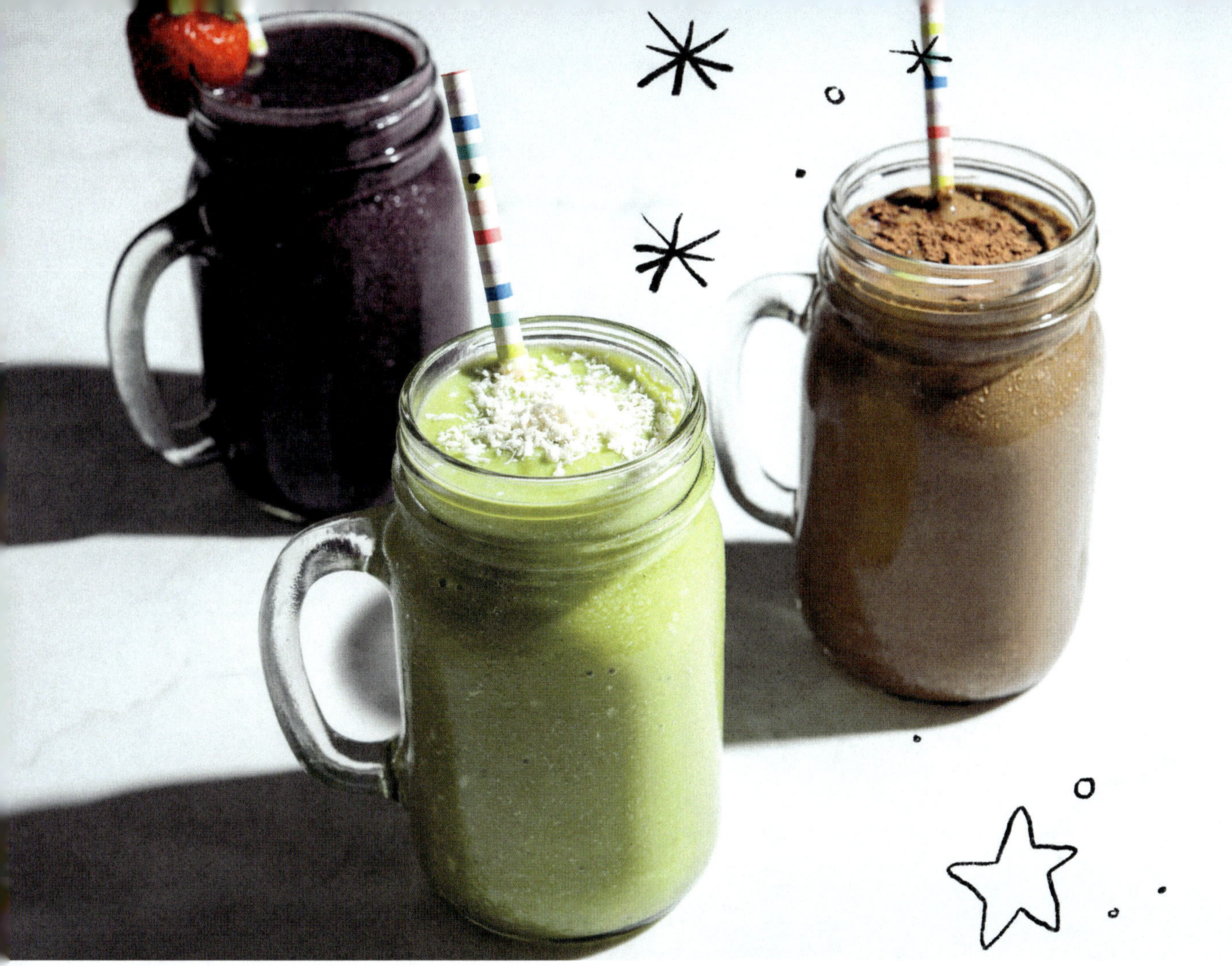

## Fierce Foods Facts

What is a must-have in your smoothie to properly fuel the day? Protein! That and a good balance of quality carbohydrates and healthy fat. Most smoothies are loaded with too much sugar (Some with over 100 grams!), causing first a blood sugar rush, and then a crash later in the day. By combining healthy sources of protein, fat, and quality carbohydrate you can drink your breakfast while fueling your day with a slow and sustained release of energy. A good rule of thumb is to start with 20 grams of protein, add a calcium liquid source, then layer that with a mix of about 75% low glycemic and high protein veggies such as spinach, kale, cauliflower, or bok choy. Fill the remaining 25% of your blender with low-glycemic fruits such as berries, kiwi, citrus, and avocado. Make sure to always retain the fiber in your drinks, ensuring fuel for a happy set of gut bugs too!

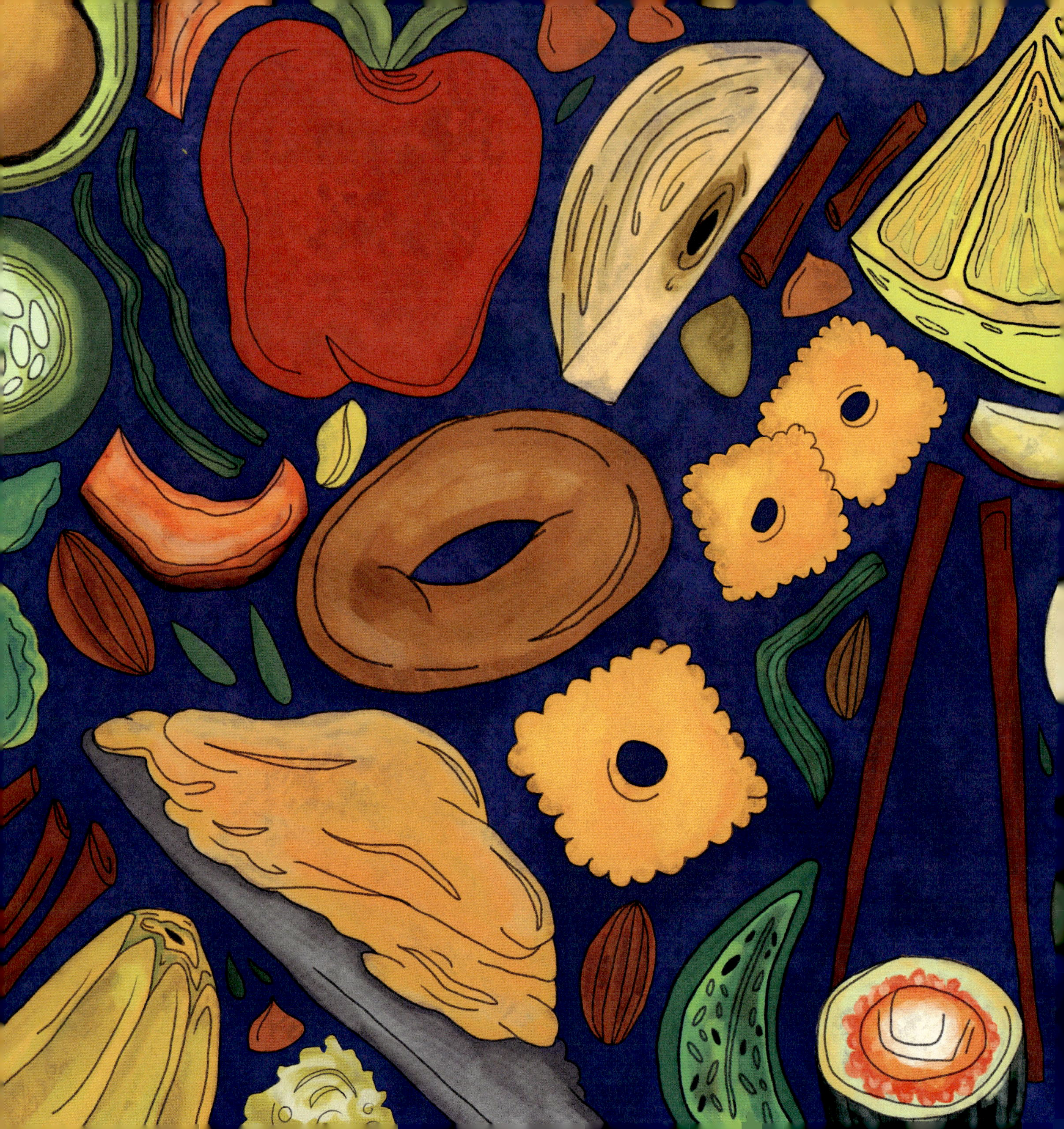

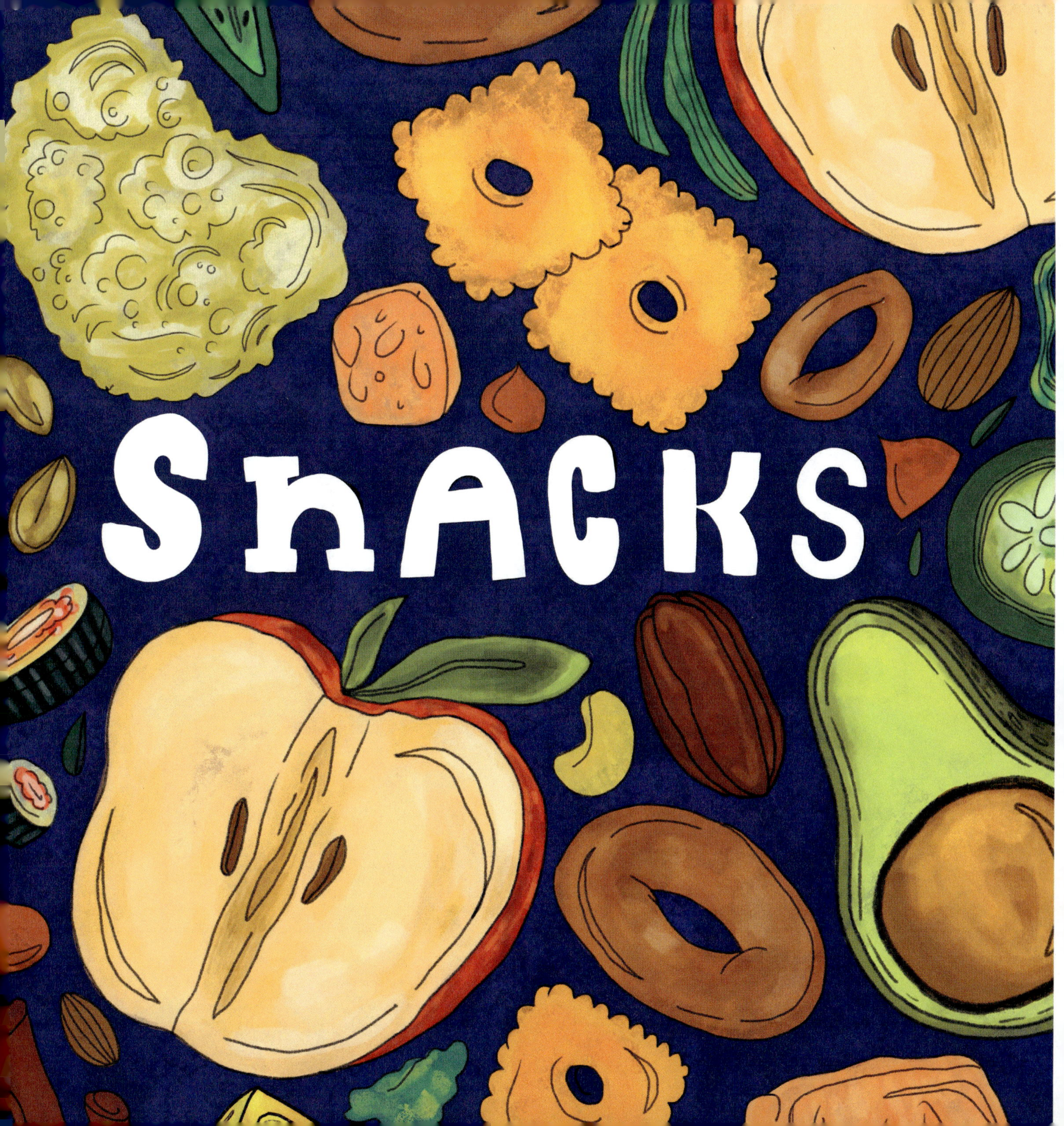
SNACKS

# Snacks



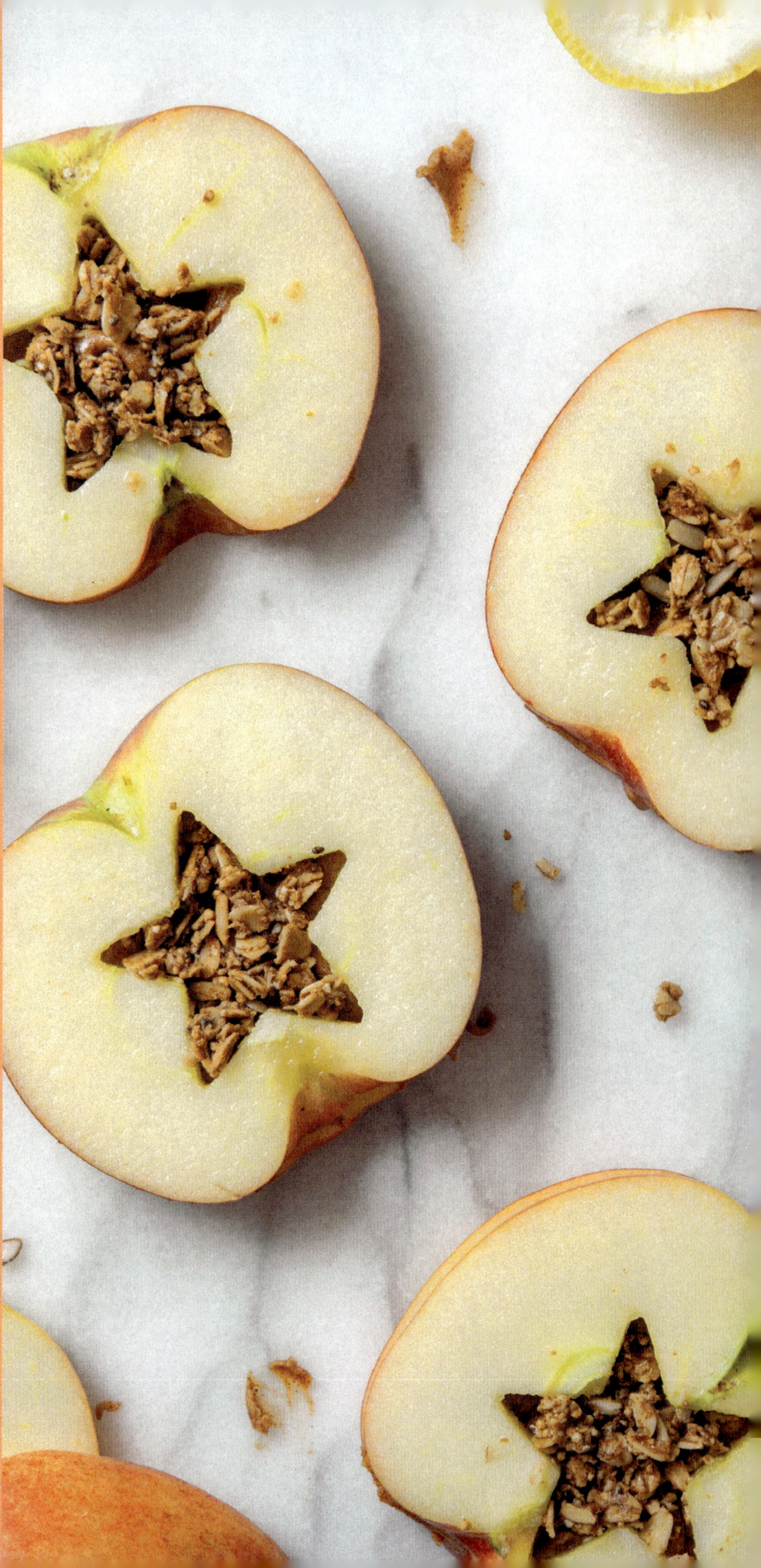

People going through treatment often have greater energy and protein needs than at other times of life. Healthy, nutritious food that is shelf-stable, meaning it can be packed into a bag and held at room temperature for several hours, is of great benefit to the family of the patient undergoing treatment. Hospital food, while convenient, is not often the most nutrient-dense option and generally does not meet the needs of the oncology patient.

Having nutritious food on hand can help sustain energy and patience, allowing the family to reap the benefits of a well-thought-out snack pack.

What does it take to make a healthy snack? Balance of course!

The same macronutrients that make up a healthy breakfast, lunch, or dinner, will also help a snack provide fuel, stabilize blood sugar and help support physical, emotional, and mental fatigue. The other trick is to make the food shelf stable, something that doesn't require refrigeration and is safe to consume for the long hours spent outside of the home. This is easily accomplished with nut mixes, though a bit harder to do with dairy-based dips that will require refrigeration or at least an insulated lunch box with an ice pack.

There are some recipes in this chapter that provide all of the portability you might benefit from with very little prep and others that take a bit more effort but can be batch cooked for a great return on time invested. Hard-boiled eggs are full of protein and healthy fat, are easy to make, or can be purchased ready-made at a store to fit that on-the-go-and-I-need-it-now requirement. Roasted nuts can be batch cooked and stored for weeks, or even purchased in a convenience store if that is what the situation requires. Grain-free granola bars can be made in a large batch and stored in the freezer cut into individual serving sizes where they will last for months. They are also a great vehicle for all kinds of superfoods that can have healing effects on the body.

Take a peek at the recipes for cucumber sushi rolls and the herbed cheese stuffed mini bells for those that require a little more time, though give great rewards in the yum factor! They also offer a chance for creativity and allow kids that hands-on fun when they make their own snacks.

Chef Andrew Johnson

# Apple Donuts

**Makes 12 servings:** ~2 donuts each

**115**
CAL

7g Fat
11g Net Carb
1g Protein

## Ingredients

4 red apples, large

Natural Food Coloring (e.g. Watkins)

1 pkg (8 oz) whipped cream cheese or dairy-free alternative (e.g. Kite Hill almond cream cheese)

**Topping recommendations:** Watkins Sprinkles, cinnamon, assorted nuts and seeds, melted Lily's chocolate chips

## Directions

1. Core each apple while whole, then slice it horizontally and evenly into ¼"-½" slices, taking care to preserve the donut's circular shape with the hole in the center.
2. Using a few drops of natural plant-based food coloring, color the cream cheese into desired shades.
3. Spread 1 tablespoon of cream cheese onto sliced apples, decorate with sprinkles or other optional toppings, then refrigerate for at least 30 minutes to set. Serve immediately.

### Fierce Foods Facts

A little vitamin A, a little vitamin C, a little fiber, and a nice dose of healthy fat help to round out the nutrition in this fun birthday party favorite!

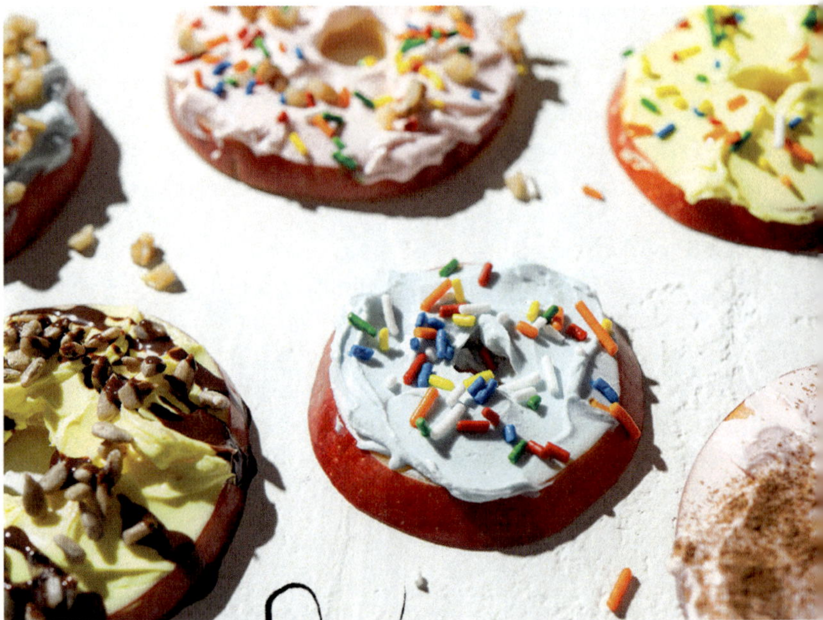

### Kids Can Cook Tips

Make healthy food fun and kids will eat it. Especially food that kids can decorate themselves!

Chef Alexia Hall, RDN

# Avocado Toast with Pepita Dip

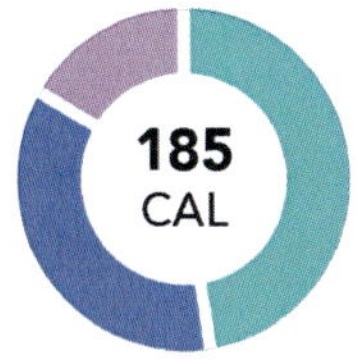


12g Fat
4g Net Carb
9g Protein

**Makes 8 servings:** each ~2 tablespoons dip and 1 slice bread, 89 grams

## Ingredients

2 large avocados, pitted and sliced (approx. 2 cups)

1 cup cilantro, minced, lightly packed

1 large jalapeño, seeded and minced (approx. 2 tbsp)

2 cloves garlic, minced

1 tsp sea salt

Freshly ground black pepper to taste

½ cup pepitas (pumpkin seeds), toasted or sprouted

1 large lime, juiced and separated (approx. 3 tsp)

8 slices of bread (e.g. Carbonaut)

## Directions

1. To make the pepita dip, combine the avocado, cilantro, jalapeño, garlic, salt, and pepper in a food processor or blender and blend to desired consistency. Add the pepitas and blend until chopped. Add 2 teaspoons of the lime juice, and pulse a few more times. May add more to desired taste.
2. Toast your bread slices, spread 2 tablespoons of the dip on top, then top with some more pepitas. You can also serve it as a dip for chopped vegetables or add it to your favorite wrap or salad.
3. To store, use the remaining teaspoon of lime juice to sprinkle over the dip so it doesn't turn brown, and cover tightly in the refrigerator. Use within 3 days.

### Fierce Foods Facts

Each serving provides 9 grams of fiber, almost half the day's serving for a teenager or a third for an adult. This recipe also provides mono-unsaturated heart-healthy fats from the avocado along with vitamin C and vitamin K. Blood sugar balancing ratios of carbohydrates, protein, and fat make this a great snack or meal for any time use.

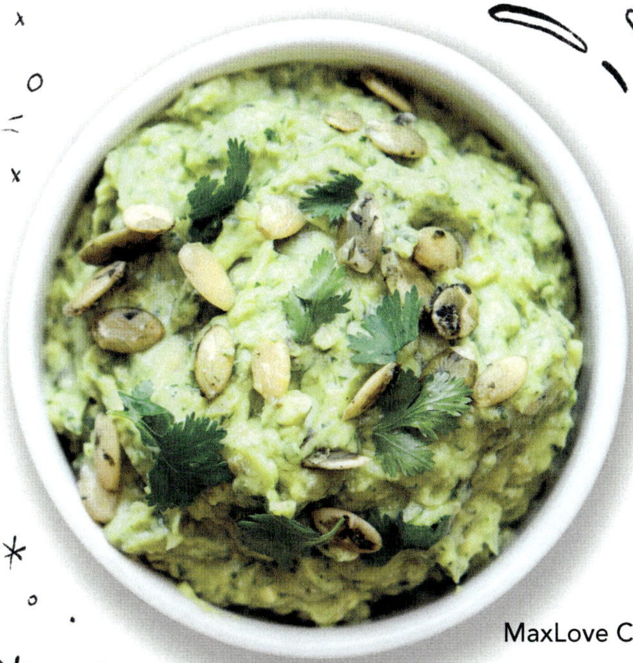

Chef Alexia Hall, RDN

# School Lunch Apple Almond Butter Sandwich

**Makes 4 servings:** 1 sandwich each, 140 grams

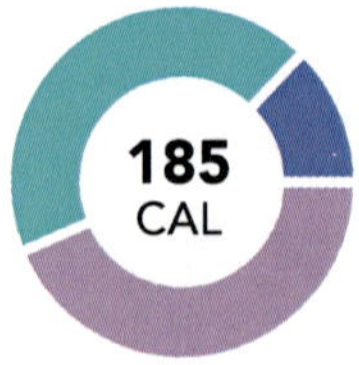


10g Fat
17g Net Carb
5g Protein

## Ingredients

2 red apples, sliced into ¼" rings

4 tbsp almond butter

4 tbsp granola

1 tsp lemon juice

## Directions

1. Wash apples, then slice into ¼" rings. Using a 1" cookie cutter (we used stars but any shape may be used), cut out the center of the apple slices that still have seeds in them.
2. Spread 1 tablespoon of almond butter on 1 apple slice that does not have seeds in the middle. Top with 1 tablespoon of granola, then sandwich with an apple slice that has its center seeds and core removed. Enjoy immediately or spritz lightly with lemon juice to avoid the browning. Use within 1–3 days.

### Fierce Foods Facts

This balanced protein and carbohydrate snack is perfect for fighting off the mid-afternoon low energy crisis. It is loaded with heart-healthy anti-inflammatory vitamin E thanks to the almond butter. It also has almost 5 grams of fiber to help support a healthy microbiome.

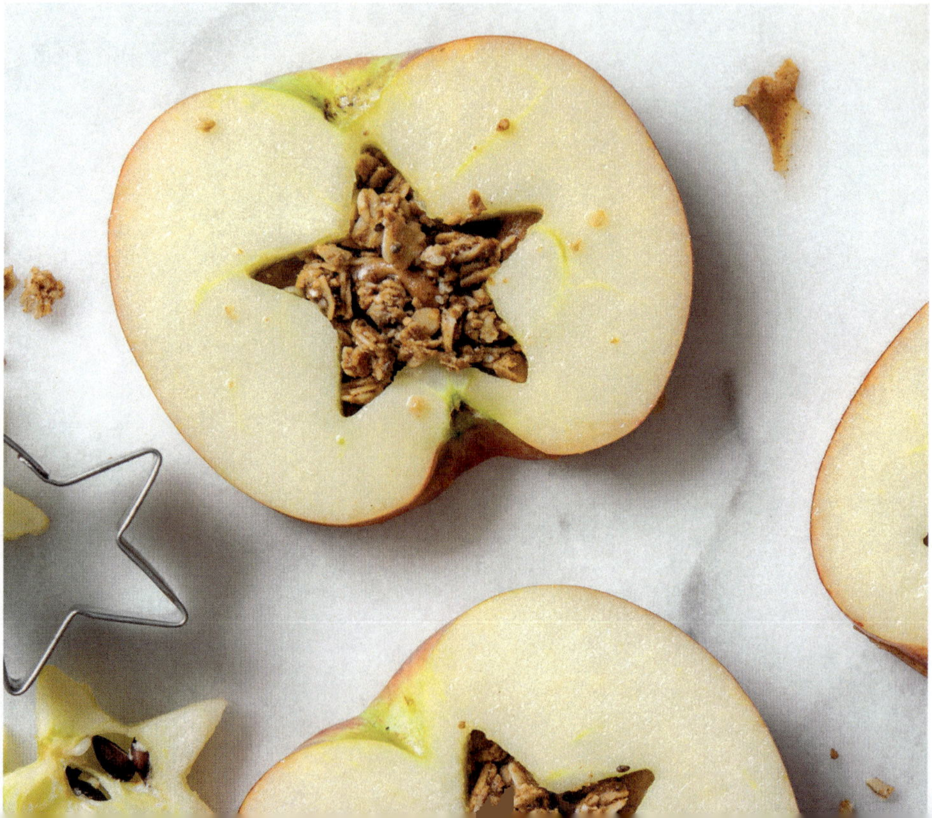

Chef Cathy McKnight

# Cheese Crisps

**Makes 8 servings:** each ~¼ cup, 27 grams

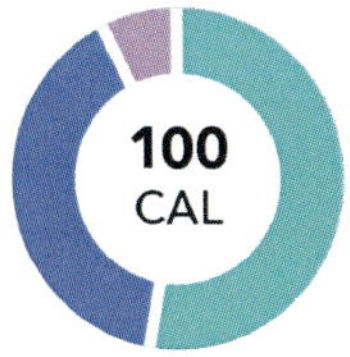


8g Fat
1g Net Carb
6g Protein

## Ingredients

2 cups cheddar or parmesan cheese, shredded

2 tbsp of seasoning (e.g. Italian or chili lime), optional

### Fierce Foods Facts

This is a delicious way to get those calcium needs each day! Each serving provides 200 mg of this bone-building and heart-supporting mineral.

## Directions

1. Preheat the oven to 400°F. On a baking sheet pan lined with parchment or a silicone baking mat, make 1-tablespoon piles of cheese at least 2" apart and sprinkle with seasoning.
2. Bake for 10–12 minutes, then remove from the oven and allow to cool. For fun shapes, work quickly after removing from the oven and lay each crisp on a rolling pin to create canned potato chip shapes, or use the round handle of a spoon and a pair of tongs to roll up the cheese crisp into poof shapes.
3. Enjoy immediately or on the same day.

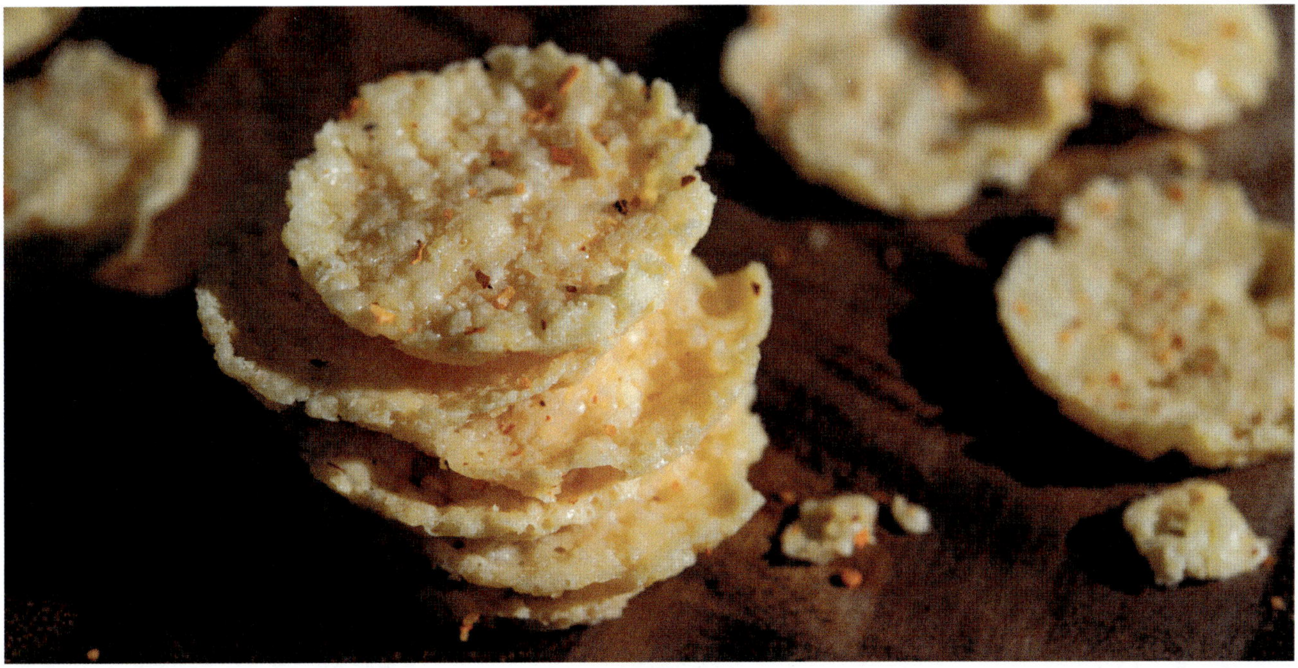

Chef Audra DiPadova Wilford

# Grain-Free Cheese Crackers

Makes 4 servings (~24 crackers): 6 crackers each, 44 grams

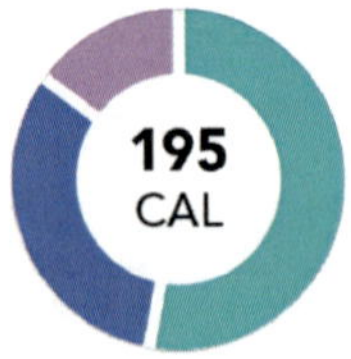


15g **Fat**
4g **Net Carb**
9g **Protein**

## Ingredients

1 cup parmesan cheese, grated

1 cup macadamia flour, cashew flour, or almond flour

Cold water, as needed

1 tsp sea salt

Sea salt flakes (optional)

### Kids Can Cook Tips

Kids will have fun measuring the ingredients into the food processor and helping to decide whether or not the dough is "wet" enough. The biggest fun will be in rolling it out and cutting it into fun shapes. Add a cookie cutter or two and let the creativity bloom!

## Directions

1. Preheat the oven to 350°F. Add the cheese and nut flour (or sunflower seed flour) to a food processor or mixing bowl with 1 teaspoon of sea salt. Pulse or stir until combined and evenly distributed. Optional: for a "whole grain" texture, add chia seeds and hemp hearts. Slowly add cold water, teaspoon by teaspoon, until mixture forms a hard dough. Do not overwater—the dough should not be very wet.
2. Place the dough onto parchment paper and place another layer of parchment paper on top to roll it out. Flatten the dough to the desired thickness, cut with a cookie cutter, and place on a silicone mat or a cookie sheet. Top off with sea salt flakes if desired
3. Bake for about 12–15 minutes until browned and crispy. Cool on a rack, then enjoy with a fatty dip or homemade guacamole.
4. Store completely cooled in a sealed container at room temperature for up to 5 days, or freeze for up to 6 months.
5. To make nut-free, simply replace the nut flour with sunflower seed flour or pumpkin seed flour.

## Fierce Foods Facts

This low glycemic flavorful cracker packs a wonderful amount of protein, thanks to the nuts and the cheese. Also loaded with immune-supporting vitamin E and bone-supporting minerals like calcium, phosphorus, and magnesium, this sure-to-please snack has got it all!

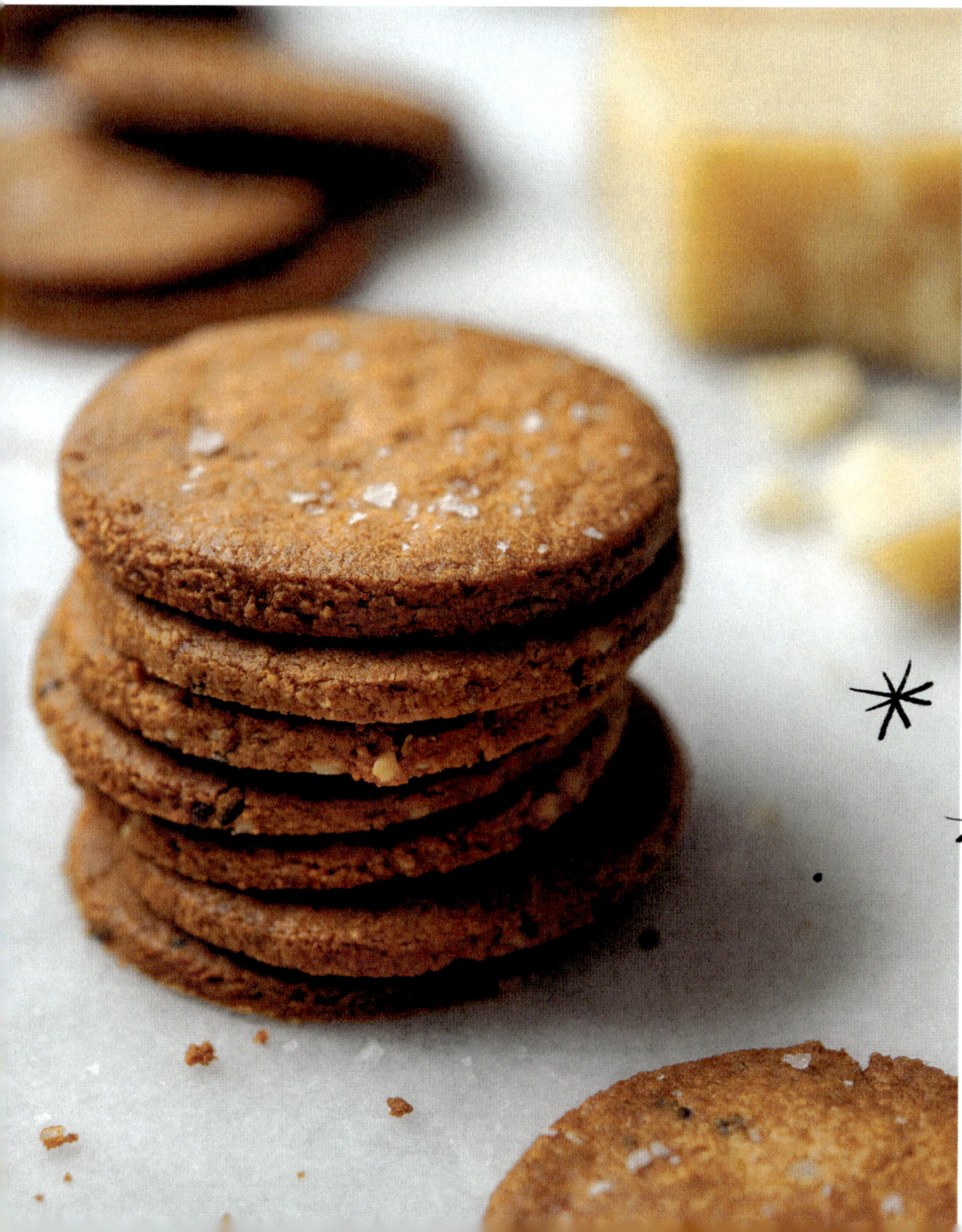

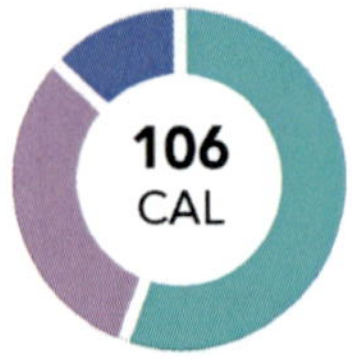


9g Fat
5g Net Carb
2g Protein

Willett Children's Hospital

# Chocolate Date Energy Bites

**Makes 5 servings:** 3 balls each, ~57 grams

## Ingredients

1 cup pecan halves

½ cup Medjool dates, pitted, gently packed (~80 grams)

⅓ cup + 2 tsp unsweetened cocoa powder

2 tbsp sunflower butter

½ tsp vanilla extract

½ cup unsweetened coconut flakes

⅛ tsp salt

## Directions

1. Using a food processor, grind the pecan halves until finely chopped. Add the dates to the food processor and blend.
2. Add the cocoa powder, sunflower butter, vanilla extract, ¼ cup shredded coconut flakes, and salt to the pecan and date mixture in the food processor. Blend until well processed and the mixture begins to resemble a dough.
3. Roll the mixture into 15 balls (1½" each). Once all the balls are formed, roll them into the remaining ¼ cup of shredded coconut flakes and serve.
4. They will store well in a sealed container in the refrigerator for up to 1 week, or freeze for up to 6 months.

### Fierce Foods Facts

These delicious energy balls are a great source of fiber and provide a low glycemic nutrient-dense carbohydrate in a balanced format with healthy protein and fat.

### Kids Can Cook Tips

Kids will have fun measuring the ingredients and forming and rolling the balls!

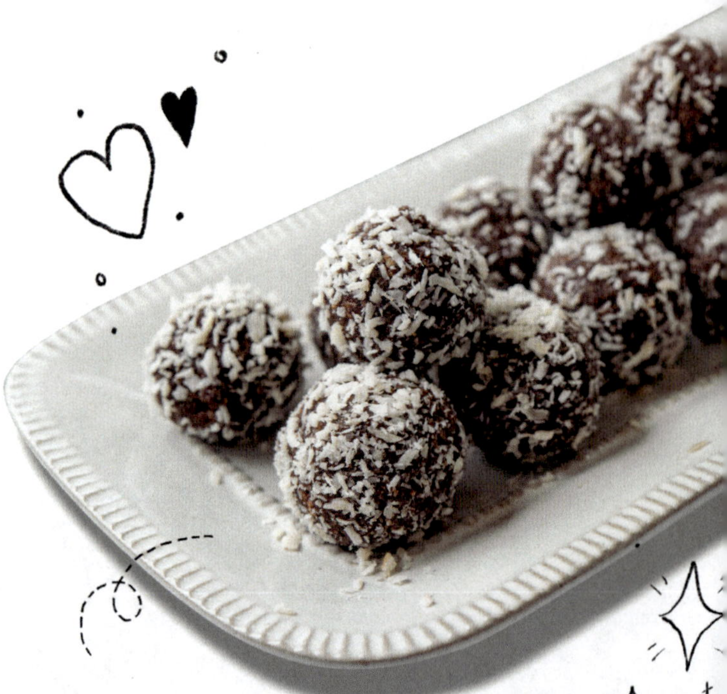

Chef Andrew Johnson

# Grain-Free Seed Granola Bars

**Makes 12 servings:** each 1 bar, 70 grams

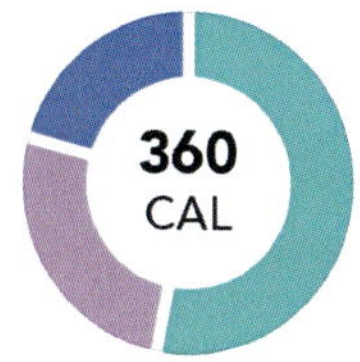


29g **Fat**
14g **Net Carb***
11g **Protein**

* (4 grams without dried fruit and substituting Lakanto for honey)

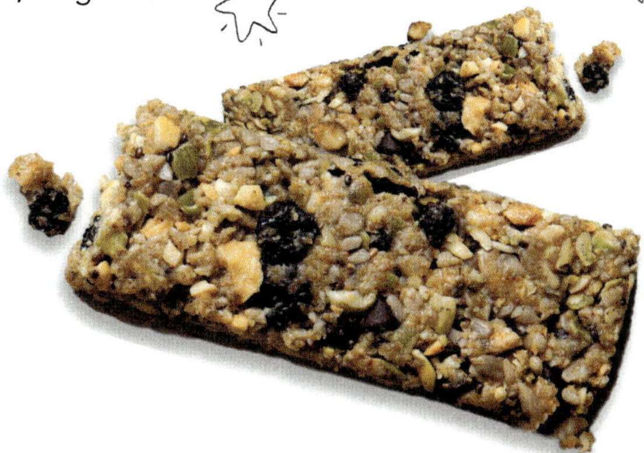

## Ingredients

1 cup sunflower seeds

1 cup pumpkin seeds

1 cup cashews, toasted

½ cup flaxseeds

½ cup dried fruit

¼ cup unsweetened coconut, shredded

2 tbsp cacao nibs or chocolate chips

3 tbsp coconut oil or unsalted butter, melted

⅓ cup almond butter

⅓ cup honey

1 tsp vanilla extract

½ tsp cinnamon

½ tsp sea salt

### Individual Portion

1½ tbsp sunflower seeds

1½ tbsp pumpkin seeds

1½ tbsp cashews

1½ tsp flaxseeds

1½ tsp dried fruit

1 tsp coconut, shredded

1 tsp coconut oil

1 tbsp almond butter

1 tsp honey

2 drops vanilla extract

⅛ tsp cinnamon

⅛ tsp sea salt

## Directions

1. Place sunflower seeds, pumpkin seeds, flaxseeds, and cashews inside a food processor. If using large pieces of dried fruit you can also add them to the processor at this time or chop them by hand. Pulse ingredients for a short time. You aren't trying to get them super tiny, larger chunks are okay. Add the coconut, chopped dried fruit, and chocolate chips to the mixture.

2. Using a separate bowl and fork, blend the coconut oil, almond butter, honey, vanilla, cinnamon, and sea salt. Then, add the mixture from the food processor into the wet mixture and combine by hand.

3. Scoop the mixture out onto a flat surface lined with parchment paper. Press firmly and evenly to make a flat square in your desired thickness, then cut out desired shapes with cookie cutters. Store in the refrigerator or freezer.

4. Alternatively, kids can each make an individual portion. Place the following into a plastic bag and allow kids to "squish" the bag to combine the ingredients and cut into desired shapes.

Chef Andrew Johnson

# Hard Boiled Eggs

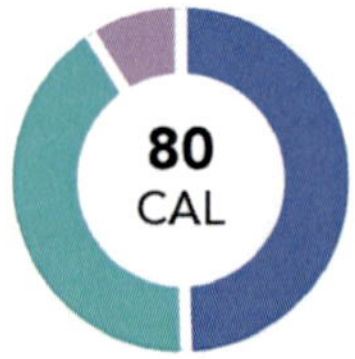


5g Fat
1g Net Carb
6g Protein

**Makes 12 servings:** 1 egg each, 50 grams

## Ingredients

12 eggs, large

1 gal water

1 tsp sea salt

1 tbsp white vinegar

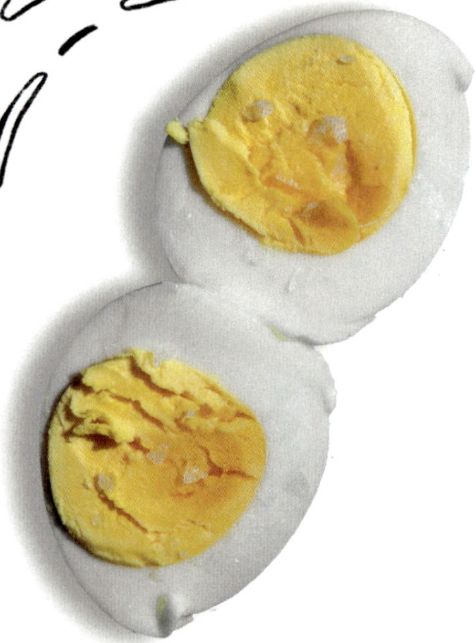

## Method

1. Making the perfect hard boiled eggs is an easy kitchen skill once you know the tricks. First, identify how many eggs you want to hard boil. Find a sauce pot that will hold all of your eggs in a single layer on the bottom of the pot with as little extra room as possible for the eggs to bang around.

2. To the pot, add cold water and cover eggs by 1" or up to the first joint of your fingertip. Place the pot on the stove uncovered on high heat and bring to a boil. To the pot add about 1 teaspoon to 1 tablespoon of sea salt—the brine should taste like seawater. Add a splash of white vinegar.

3. When the bubbles of the boil reach ¼" in size, set a timer.
   - For "jammy" egg yolks (best for eating whole or for egg salad) set the timer for 6–7 minutes.
   - For deviled eggs, set the timer for 8–10 minutes.

4. Once the time has gone off, immediately remove the pot from the flame, turn the stove off, and carefully pour out the water without disturbing the eggs. Then add ice to the pot and cover the hot eggs entirely.

5. Once the eggs are cool they are ready to be peeled. To peel the eggs, gently smack the egg repeatedly against the counter or cutting board starting with the roundest point (the bottom) and then all around the side of the egg towards the top. Carefully start peeling the egg at the bottom, it has an air pocket that will make an easy place to start. Plus, the added salt and vinegar will make the peeling step a breeze.

6. Once hard boiled, before or after peeling, store them in the refrigerator for up to 7 days.

Chef Alexia Hall, RDN

# Mini Bells Stuffed with Herbed Goat Cheese

**Makes 8 servings:** 4 stuffed mini peppers each, 74 grams

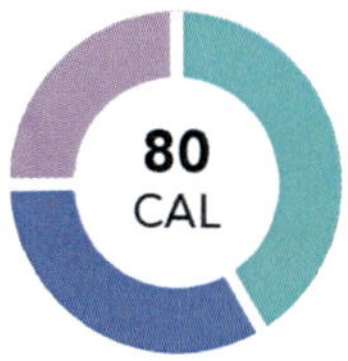


5g Fat
3g Net Carb
4g Protein

## Ingredients

5 oz log goat cheese

1 tbsp olive oil

1 tbsp milk

¼ tsp salt

¼ tsp ground black or white pepper

1 tbsp lemon zest

1 tbsp fresh oregano

1 tsp fresh garlic cloves

1 pkg mini tri-colored bell peppers (approx. 32 peppers)

## Directions

1. Place the goat cheese, olive oil, lemon zest, oregano, salt, pepper, and granulated garlic in a small plastic bag. Seal the bag, and knead the mixture until soft, smooth, and well incorporated.
2. Snip off a small corner of the bag. Slice ¼" off the top of the mini peppers (including the stem) and clean out the seeds, leaving small cone shape. Using the bagged goat cheese, pipe the mixture into the cavity of the mini pepper.
3. Enjoy immediately or refrigerate for up to 3 days.

### Fierce Foods Facts

This fun and colorful snack provides excellent balance with a beautiful array of vitamins and minerals. It's wonderful for strong bones and muscles, and is pretty fun to make too!

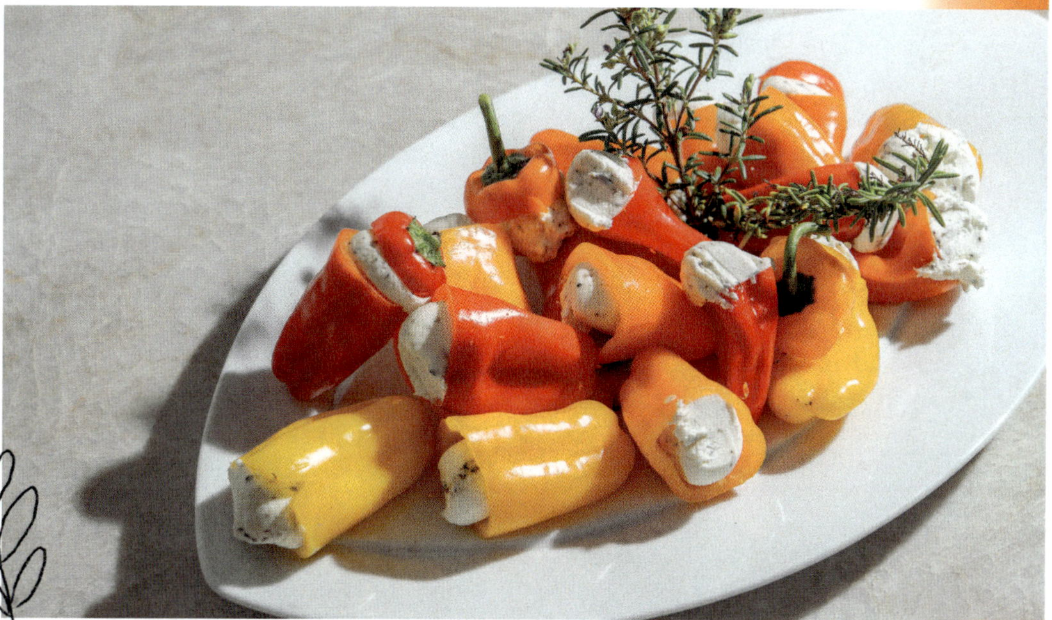

Chef Andrew Johnson

# California Cucumber Sushi Rolls

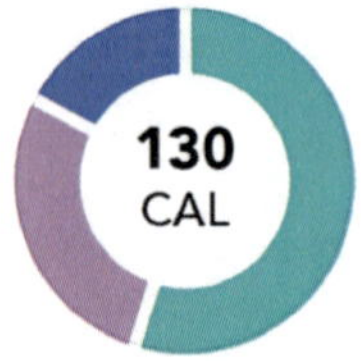


10g Fat
5g Net Carb
3g Protein

**Makes 8 servings:** each ~2 rolls, 170 grams with dip

## Ingredients

**Roll**

2 cucumbers, medium to large

1½ cup cauliflower rice, cooked and drained

¼ cup cream cheese

1 avocado, sliced

1 red bell pepper, julienned

2 carrots, julienned

1 tbsp sesame seeds, toasted

1 tsp soy sauce, ponzu, or coconut aminos

**Spicy Mayo Dipping Sauce**

4 tbsp mayonnaise

1 tbsp Sriracha sauce

½ lemon, juiced

### Kids Can Cook Tips

This kid-friendly dish is perfect for a lunchbox. Younger kids can help scoop out the center of the cucumbers.

## Directions

1. In a large mixing bowl add cooked and thoroughly drained cauliflower rice, cream cheese, soy sauce, and sesame seeds, then mix until fully incorporated and refrigerate until needed.
2. Cut each cucumber in half (there should be 1 end left on each half) and scoop out the seedy center and flesh with a spoon, melon baller, or long thin knife (save the seedy center flesh for other recipes like tzatziki). This will result in creating a long, hollow tube with ~¼" thick walls of flesh remaining all the way around.
3. Spoon in a small amount of cauliflower rice mixture, then press it to one side of the tube using a butter knife. On top of the cauliflower mixture add a couple of slices of avocado, a couple of slices of pepper, and a couple of slices of carrot. Then add more cauliflower rice to fill the cucumber tube. Press in the rice mixture until it has filled all of the space inside the tube and is packed full, suspending the other veggies in the middle.
4. With a sharp knife, slice off the end of the cucumber to expose the veggies inside, with a small spoon or clean finger gently press the mixture towards the opposite end to ensure the tube is packed full with no air gaps. You can add a bit more filling if you notice a void. Then cut the cucumber into ½" thick disks.
5. For the dipping sauce, evenly combine mayonnaise, Sriracha, and lemon juice. You can also consider adding protein such as salmon, shrimp, chicken, or tofu.
6. For a more traditional sushi experience serve with pickled ginger, soy sauce, wasabi, and chopsticks.

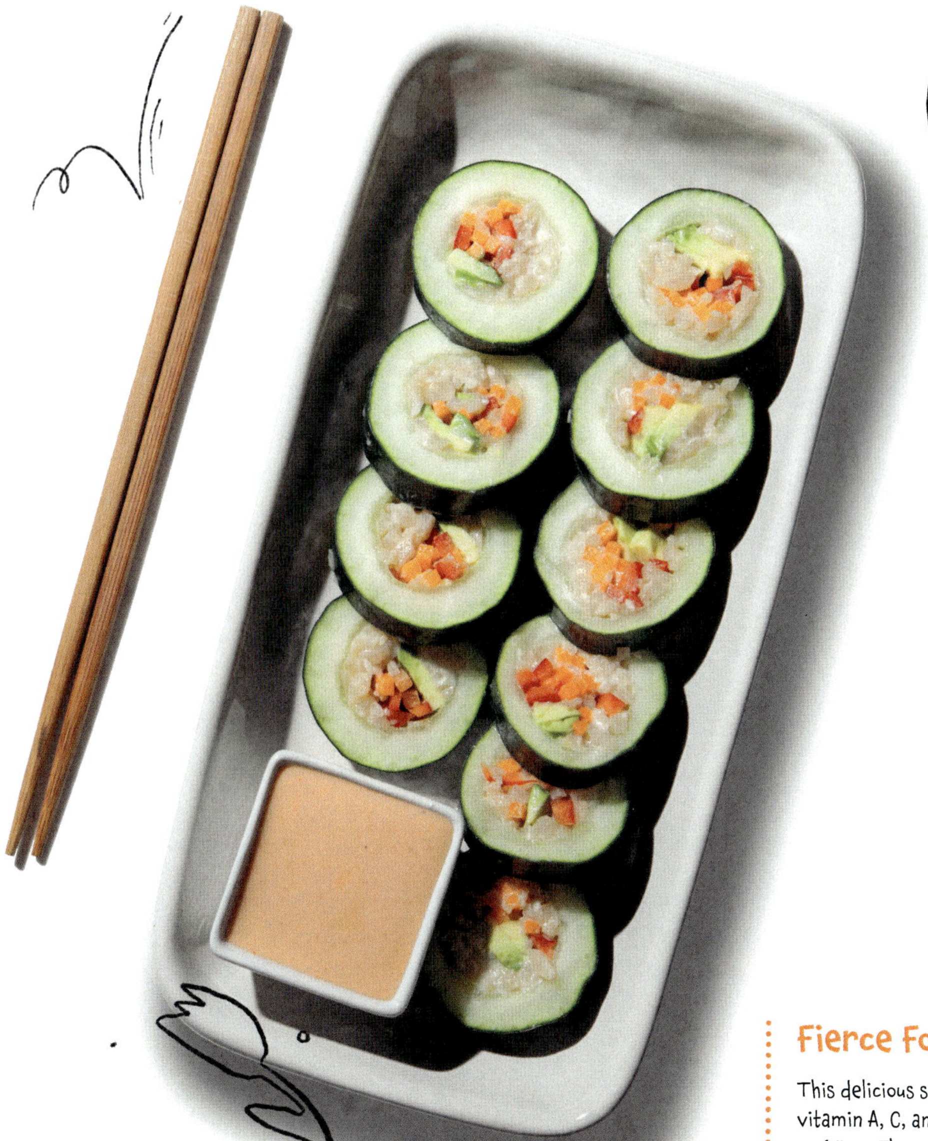

## Fierce Foods Facts

This delicious snack has a wonderful amount of vitamin A, C, and K thanks to all of the delicious veggies. The added fiber from the cauliflower rice helps to make this dish nutrient-dense and a high-quality carbohydrate choice!

Chef Andrew Johnson

# Low-Carb Quesadilla

**Makes 8 servings:** 1 filled tortilla each, 130 grams

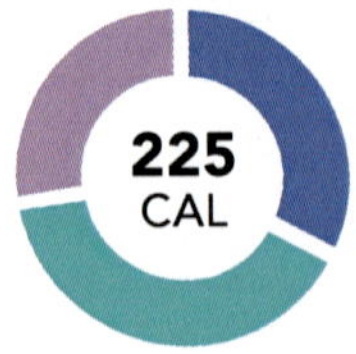


14g Fat
11g Net Carb
13g Protein

## Ingredients

8 low-carb tortillas, ~8"-10" each

2 cup Monterey Jack or cheddar cheese, shredded

½ cup cilantro, chopped

2 cup cauliflower, roasted and chopped fine **(refer to Roasted Cauliflower recipe)**

2 cups shredded roasted chicken,* turkey, or ribs

1 cup corn (canned and drained or frozen and thawed)

¼ cup pickled jalapeño

½ tsp smoked paprika

½ tsp garlic powder

½ tsp chili powder

½ cup sour cream

½ cup salsa

** Consider using a rotisserie chicken to shorten prep time*

## Directions

1. In a medium or large mixing bowl add chopped cauliflower, corn, jalapeños, cilantro, and spices, and mix well. Lay the tortillas flat on a clean surface or cutting board, then sprinkle one side with about an ounce of cheese, top with ¼ cup of filling, and top with another ounce of cheese. Fold in half and repeat.
2. It's easy to make a dozen or more quesadillas in advance and store them in the fridge ready to be cooked. To cook, preheat a large nonstick pan over medium-low heat. Place 2 quesadillas in the pan with the folded edges together, and press down with another heavy pot. Cook for 3–5 minutes until the underside is super golden brown and crispy. Carefully flip and cook for another 3–5 minutes until crispy.
3. Transfer to a cutting board, and cut in half, then serve immediately with a dollop of sour cream, your favorite salsa, and a couple of cilantro leaves.

**Pro Tip:** Adding 2 ounces of shredded meat to each quesadilla will increase protein to 28 grams per serving.

### Fierce Foods Facts

This recipe provides 10 grams of fiber, half of most people's daily goal. Quesadillas are a fun food and this recipe provides a nice amount of vitamins A, C, and K as well as almost 30% of the day's recommended calcium! Add protein for a beautifully balanced meal or hearty snack.

### Kids Can Cook Tips

Kids will enjoy layering the cheese and toppings on the tortilla and helping to watch until it is ready to turn. Have them try customizing their own quesadilla by choosing and designing their own toppings.

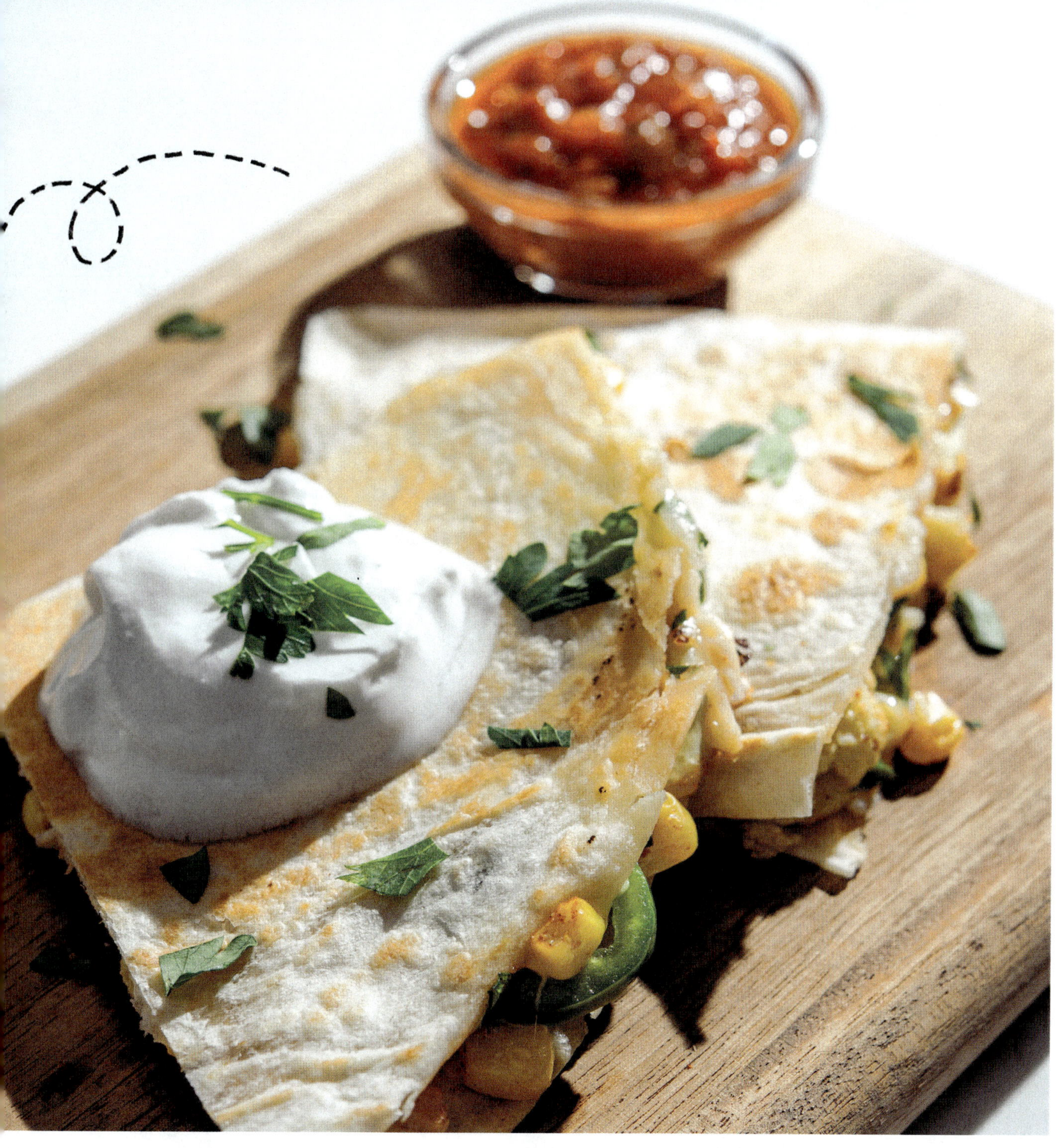

Chef Andrew Johnson

# Spiced Seed and Nut Clusters

**Makes 6 servings:** each ~¼ cup, 59 grams

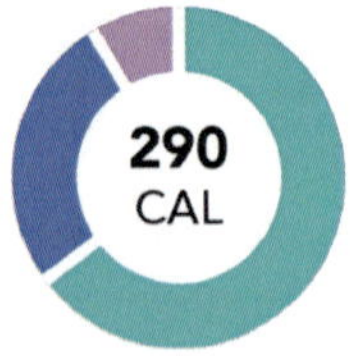


25g Fat
3g Net Carb
10g Protein

## Ingredients

1 cup of raw nuts (e.g. pistachios and peanuts)

½ cup raw pepitas

½ cup raw sunflower seeds

2 tbsp butter or vegan butter

¼ cup brown alternative sweetener (e.g. Lakanto Gold)

½ tsp vanilla extract

¼ tsp ground cinnamon

⅛ tsp chili powder

Sea or kosher salt to taste

## Directions

1. Add nuts and seeds to a large sauté pan over medium heat, and cook for approximately 10 minutes until golden. Remove the nuts and seeds from the pan and return the pan to the stove. Add in the butter and sweetener, then stir and cook until the butter browns and the sweetener is fully dissolved and starting to caramelize.
2. Turn off the stove and toss the nuts and seeds into the pan, then add the spices and vanilla extract, and toss until everything is evenly coated. Line a sheet pan with a silicone mat or parchment. Transfer the nut and seed mixture to the lined baking sheet and spread it out with a rubber spatula into a ½" thick sheet. Push all of the stray nuts and seeds into the middle to form 1 mass of nut clusters so they all stick together, keeping the nuts bunched up and close so they stick together as it cools.
3. Place the sheet pan flat in the refrigerator for at least an hour. Enjoy after chilling or store in an airtight container in the fridge or freezer.
4. Alternatively, you can use this recipe to make a brittle by doubling the volume of sweetener and butter.

### Fierce Foods Facts

Just a quarter cup of this healthy snack mix will deliver over 20% of many B vitamins as well as almost 50% of the daily vitamin E. But even more important are the abundant variety of minerals. Just a ¼ cup serving provides a great supply of copper, magnesium, iron, phosphorus, selenium, and zinc, which are important for bones, thyroid, blood, and energy supply!

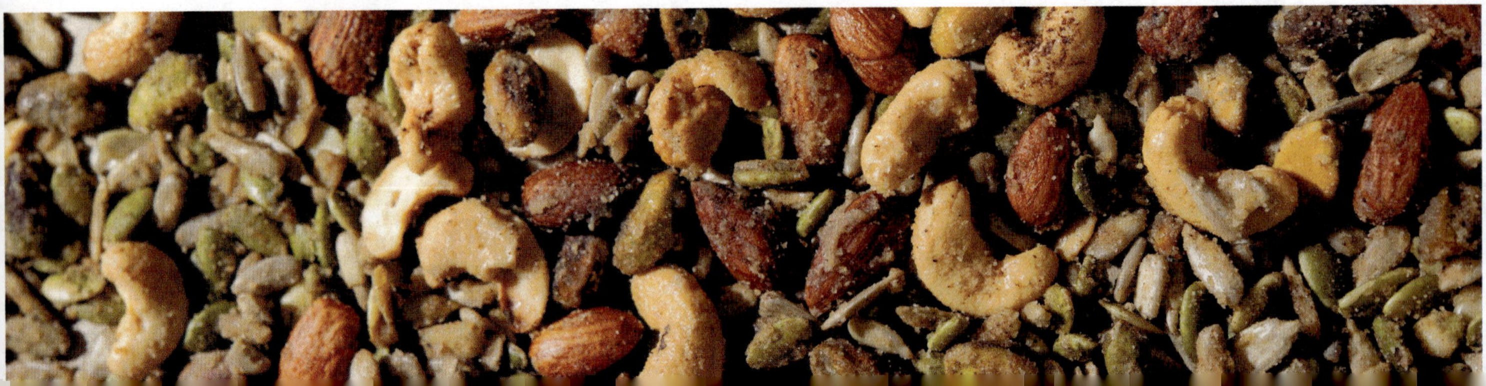

Chef Andrew Johnson

# Zucchini Fries

**Makes 8 servings:** each ~2/3 cup, 144 grams

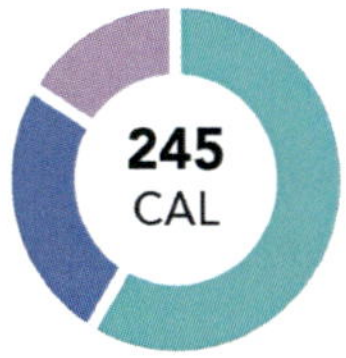


19g **Fat**
5g **Net Carb**
8g **Protein**

## Ingredients

4 medium zucchini, julienned into ¾" sticks

⅓ cup mayonnaise

¼ cup Dijon mustard

2 cups coarse ground flaxseed or crushed pork rinds

½ cup parmesan cheese, grated

## Directions

1. Preheat the oven to 425°F. In a large mixing bowl add the zucchini sticks, mayonnaise, and mustard, then toss to evenly coat. Add the flaxseed or pork rinds and parmesan cheese, then toss to evenly coat.
2. On a parchment-lined 18"x13" sheet pan, lay out the zucchini fries in a single layer, spaced out so they are touching as little as possible. Bake for 15–20 minutes until golden brown.

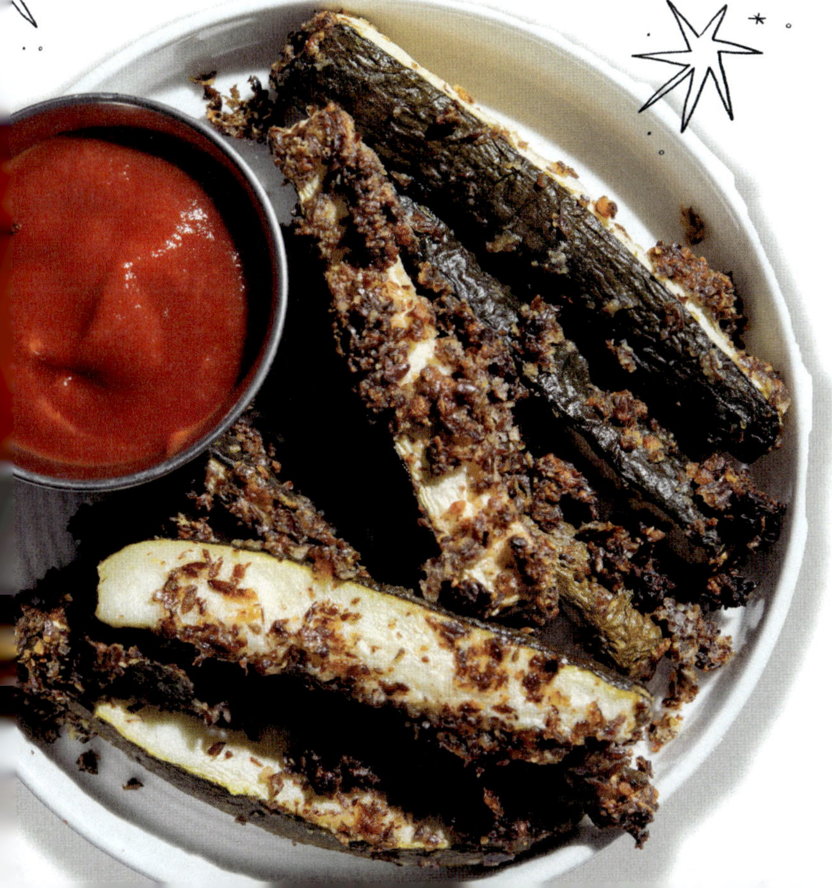

### Fierce Foods Facts

This is a great kid-friendly way to use up your bumper crop of zucchini this year! This recipe remake offers a low carbohydrate option with 7 grams of fiber to happily fuel a healthy microbiome. The flax provides some anti-inflammatory Omega-3 fat, while the zucchini adds some immune supporting vitamin C.

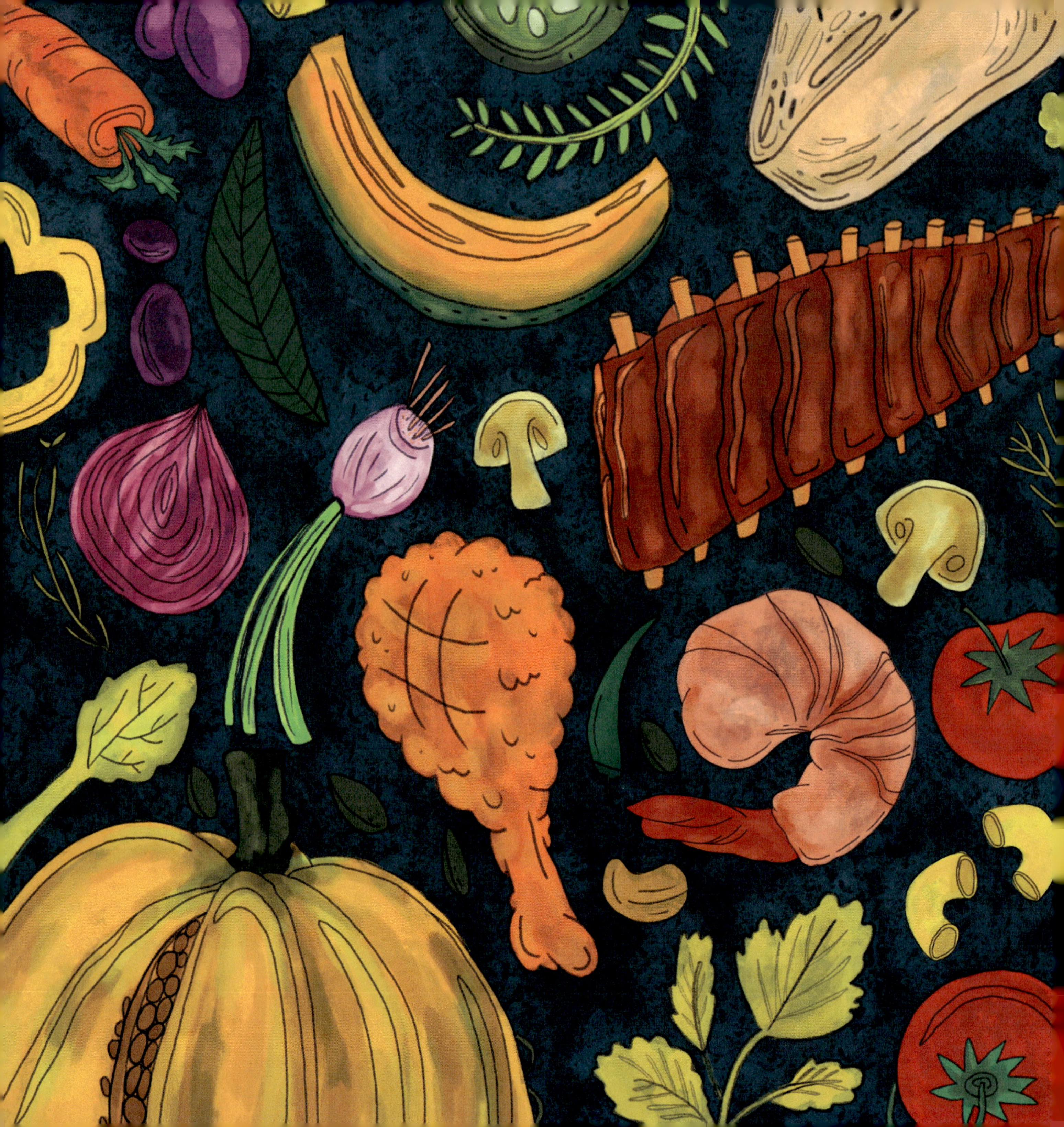

# MAIN

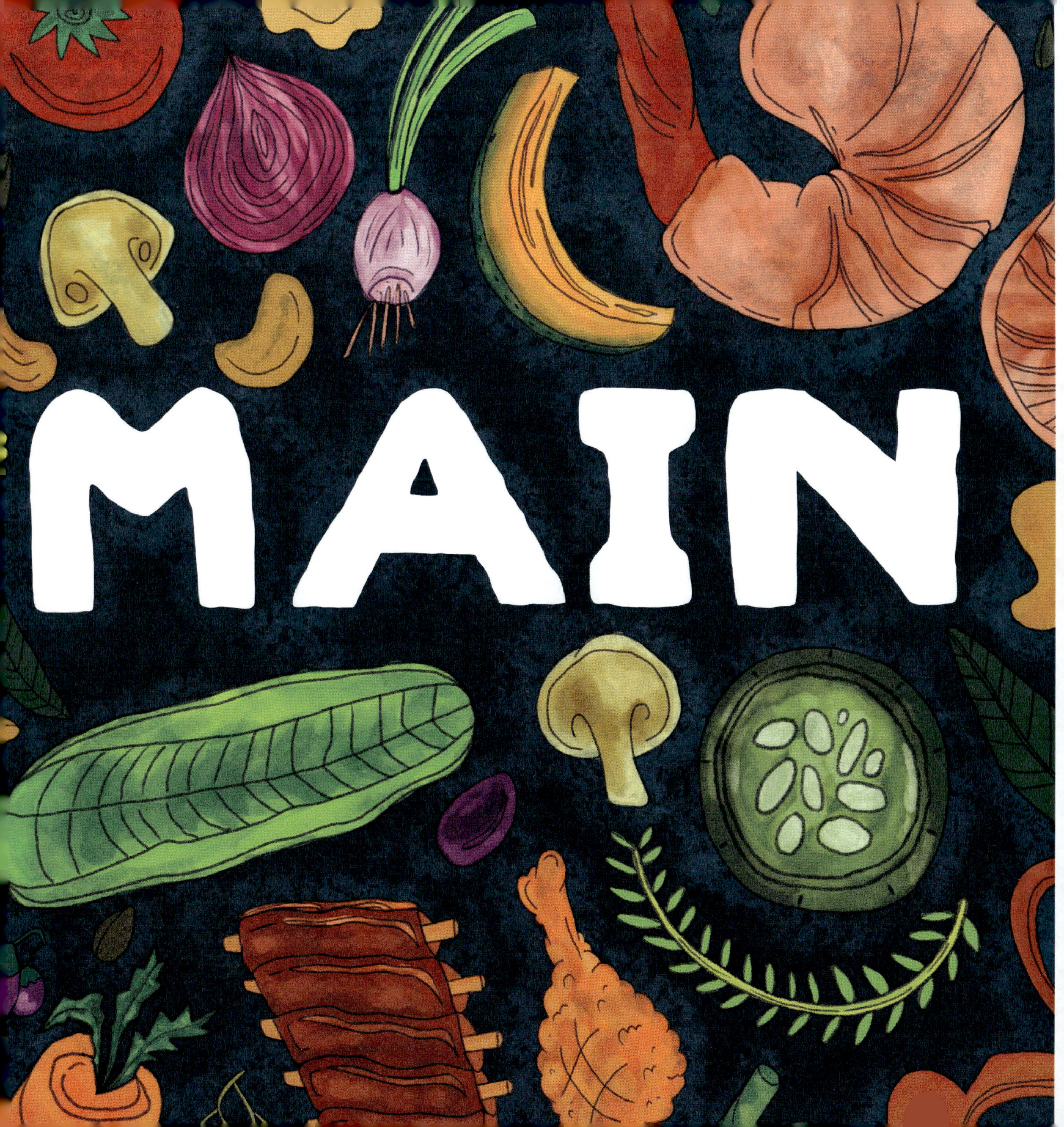

# Main



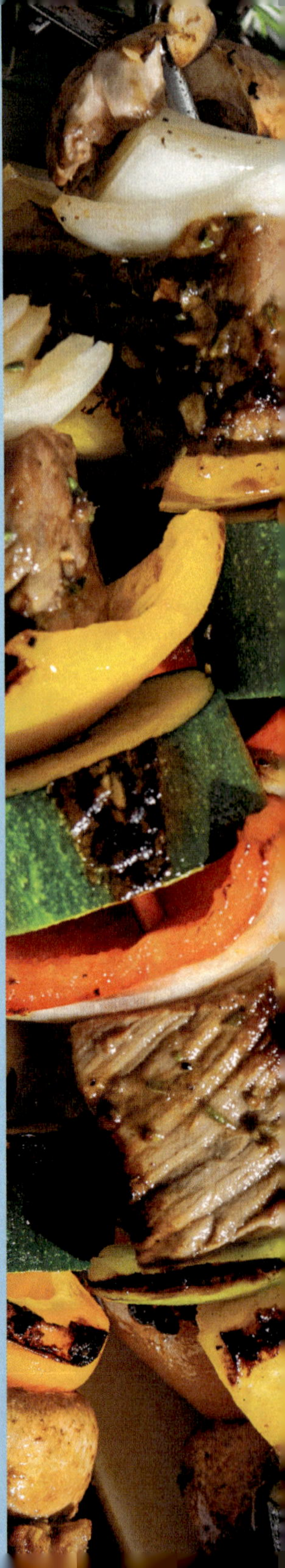

Dinnertime just got a little simpler! Many of this chapter's recipes work for batch cooking, easy weeknight dinners, and dishes that can be remade easily into different flavors to ward off any "leftover blues." Having ready-made nutrient-dense foods on hand is a powerful tool for families to have access to when impacted by the rigors and side effects created by undergoing cancer treatment.

A balance of healthy carbohydrates, proteins, and fats is important at each meal, though dinner often provides opportunities for consuming more protein than other meals.

One of the main uses of protein in our diet is to support the growth of adequate muscle, but protein also has many other important jobs. It's used to produce many components of the immune system (especially those critical white blood cells), hormones, (the chemical messengers), and the neurotransmitters that the brain uses to issue commands and keep the body running smoothly. Making sure we get enough protein will also help keep our thought processes in focus, as adequate protein will support good physical, mental and emotional health.

Proteins are made from smaller parts called amino acids. There are 20 of these little molecules in foods, and 13 of them are considered essential, meaning we have to get them from food and cannot make them ourselves. Animal protein contains all 13 of the essential amino acids and are called complete proteins for that reason. Anything from an animal, including chicken, steak, fish, milk, cheese, and eggs, is considered a complete protein. Four ounces of animal protein (which is about the size of a deck of cards) will provide about 30 grams of protein.

There is also protein contained in plants, though very few have all 13 amino acids, so they are not considered complete. A 4-ounce portion of plant protein will likely have far less than 30 grams. Animal proteins may also be utilized in a more efficient way in the body due to their chemical structure. For example, whey protein derived from dairy is considered more effective at making new muscle than other sources.

How much protein each person requires is dependent on many things including age, muscle mass, level of stress, and specific health conditions. However, everyone requires nutrient-dense protein in order to thrive.

We are sure you will find some new family favorites in this collection to meet that need!

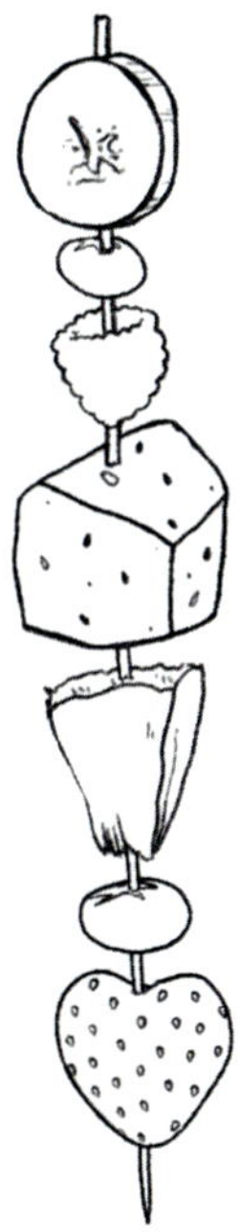

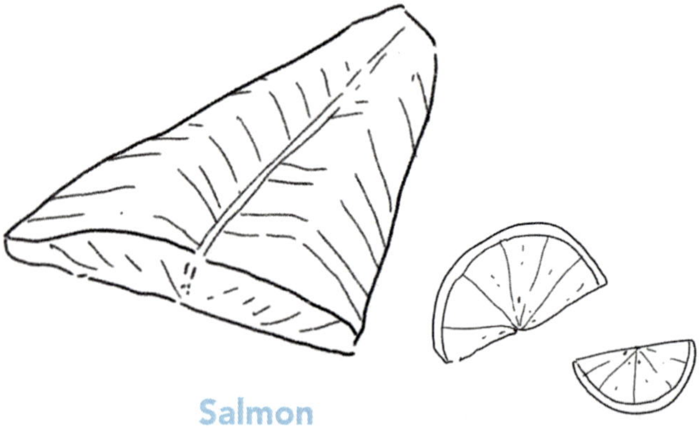

## Salmon

Salmon should be high on everyone's dinner list, and for good reason! Salmon is loaded with anti-inflammatory Omega 3 fats. In fact, the average 4-ounce piece of wild salmon contains about 3,100 mg of the good stuff, a lot higher than many supplements!

It is important to note that wild salmon contains far more nutrients than the farmed variety as what animals are fed matters. When salmon are allowed to eat in their natural habitat, they lay down a higher density of quality fat, vitamins, and minerals. When force-fed grain, the difference quickly becomes apparent for nutrients that are lacking. A 4-ounce piece of wild salmon has almost 400 international units of Vitamin D, an immune-supporting superstar vitamin, which is almost 100% of a child's daily need!

Salmon is loaded with vitamin B12, a nutrient important for supporting brain health, neurological function, and new cell division. Salmon is also high in both selenium and iodine, minerals that are needed to support thyroid function.

Salmon can be intimidating for some due to both the price as well as the perceived difficulty of cooking. Set yourself up for success by looking for sales at your local markets to help bring the price per serving down to something reasonable, asking your local butcher to point out the fish that has already been cleaned and the bones removed, and checking out the frozen section for even more economical, properly-portioned and appropriately-cleaned servings.

A salmon entree doesn't have to be an upstream battle! Turn the page to view several quick, easy, and delicious recipes for some fail-proof ways to bump up the nutrition of your next family dinner.

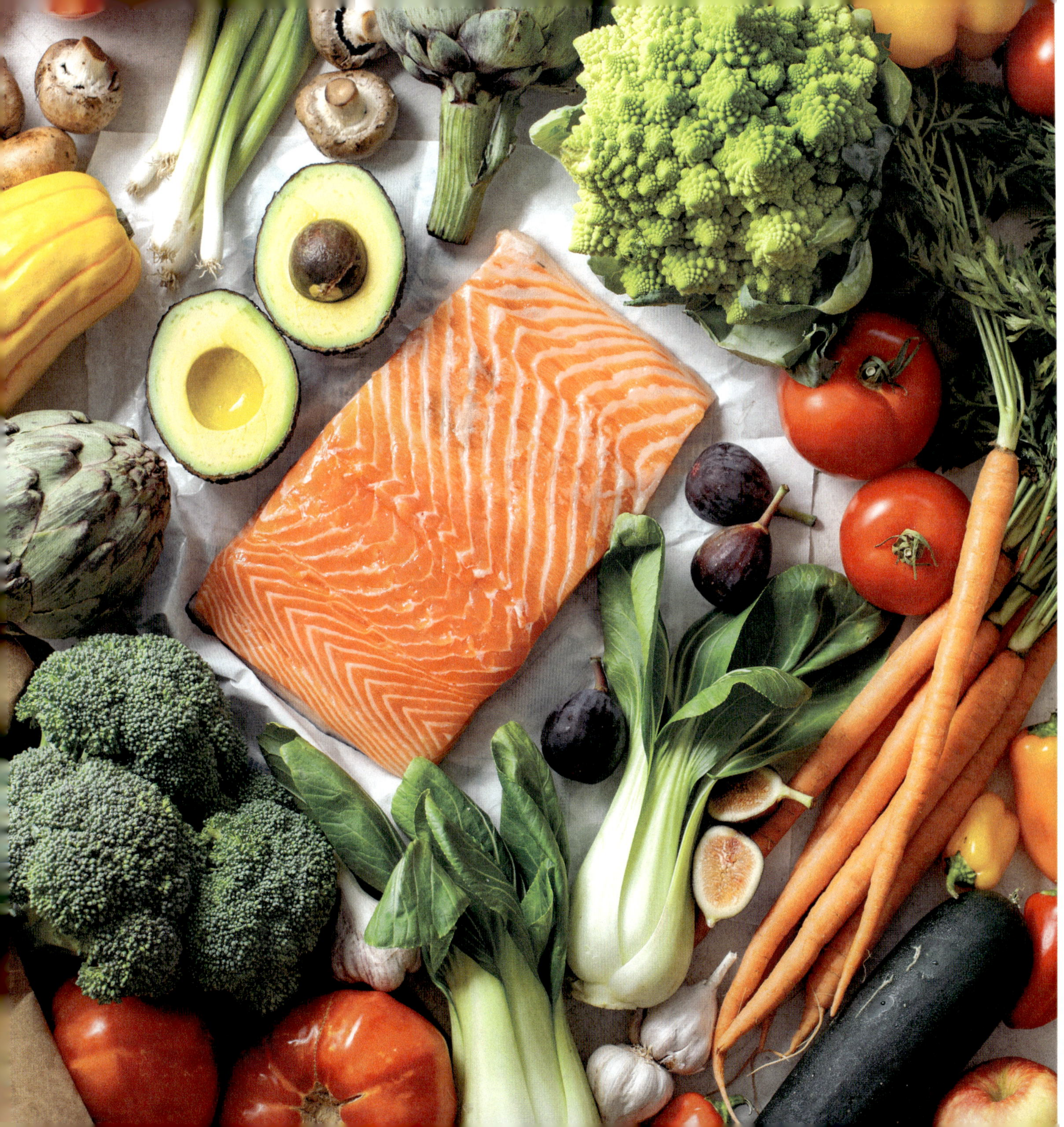

Chef Alexia Hall, RDN

# Easy Baked Salmon

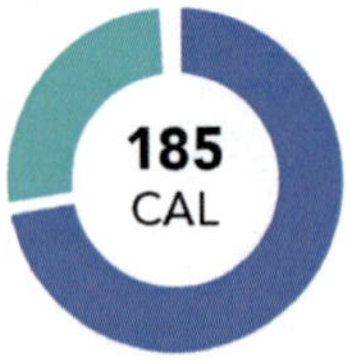


9g Fat
0g Net Carb
25g Protein

**Makes 4 servings:** each ~4-ounces, grams vary

## Ingredients

1 lb salmon fillet

**Basic** (122 grams)

2 tbsp olive oil

½ tsp garlic powder

½ tsp salt

¼ tsp pepper

## Directions

1. Mix marinade ingredients together according to the flavors desired. Place the fillet in a snug-fitting glass dish, then pour the marinade over to coat. Marinade fillet skin side up in the refrigerator for 4–6 hours.
2. Preheat the oven to 450°F. Place salmon skin side down on an oven-safe baking dish (preferably a stone but any pan will do). Do not use tin foil as this will steam the salmon instead of roasting it. Bake for 5 minutes, then reduce the temperature to 350°F without removing the salmon from the oven. Cook another 10 minutes.
3. Remove from the oven, and use a spatula to easily slide the salmon skin off. Serve with cauliflower rice and steamed vegetables.

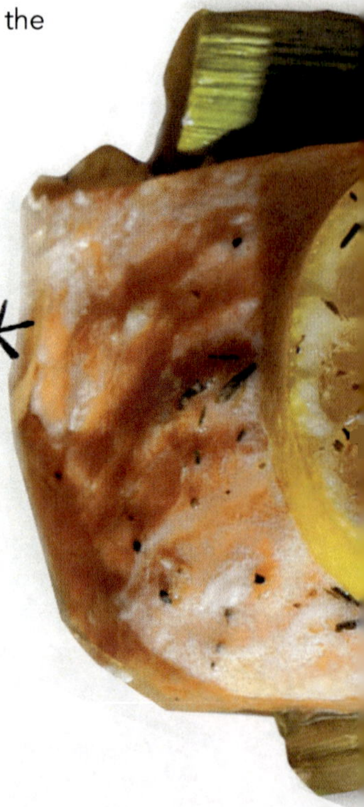

**Lemon Garlic** (144 grams)

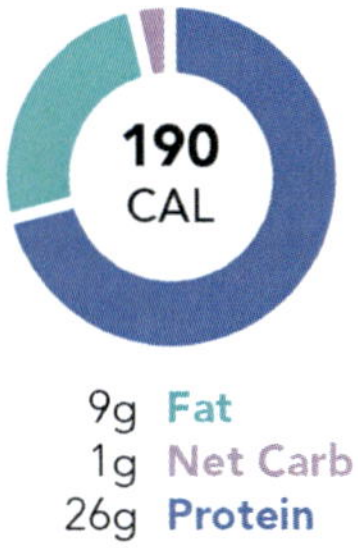


2 tbsp olive oil

1 large lemon, sliced thin with seeds removed

2 cloves garlic, minced

½ tsp sea salt

¼ tsp pepper

**Asian-Inspired** (150 grams)

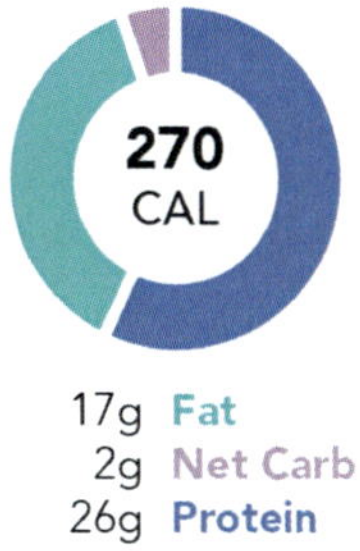


2 tbsp peanut oil

1 tbsp sesame oil

1 tsp chili oil

2 tbsp soy sauce, tamari, or coconut aminos

1 tbsp balsamic vinegar

2 tbsp green onion, thinly sliced

1 tbsp brown sugar or Pyure Hunny

2 cloves garlic minced

½ tsp ground ginger

⅛ tsp salt

⅛ tsp freshly ground black pepper

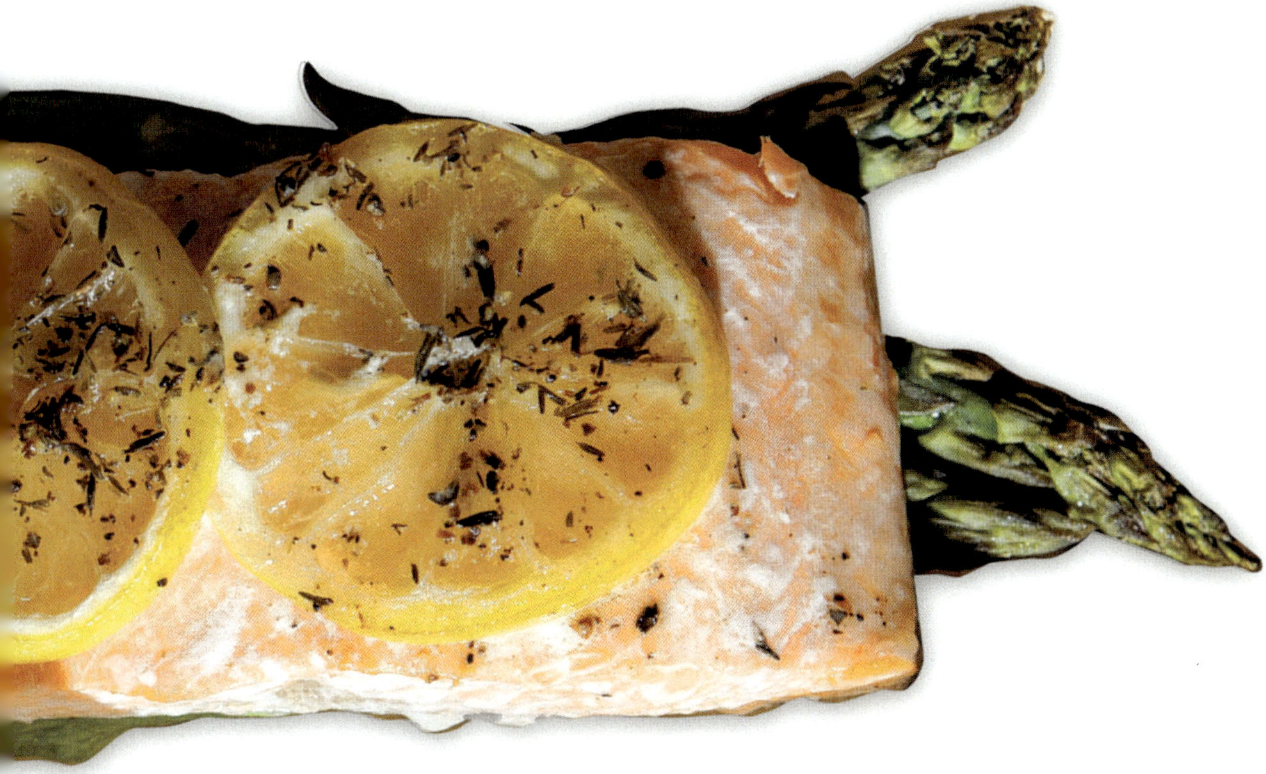

Chef Andrew Johnson

# Fish en Papillote

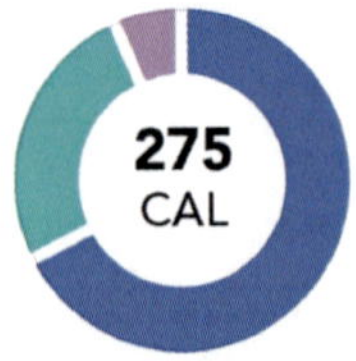


13g Fat
3g Net Carb
34g Protein

**Makes 8 servings:** each ~1 ¼ cups, 178 grams

## Ingredients

2½ lb salmon (or alternative), skin removed, cut into 6 filets (6 oz each)

1 large Vidalia onion, sliced into ¼" thick rounds

1 bunch asparagus, stems trimmed (approx. 1 cup)

2 lemons, sliced thin into rounds

1 bunch fresh thyme (approx. 2 tbsp)

6 tsp unsalted butter

Salt to taste

Lemon pepper to taste

Olive oil, grapeseed oil, or avocado oil

*Will also need:*
6 pieces of parchment paper, each 12"x16"

## Directions

1. Preheat the oven to 400°F, then fold each 12"x16" piece of parchment paper in half like a greeting card. On a sheet tray, lay out all of the ingredients (minus the lemon and thyme), and season with kosher salt and lemon pepper.
2. Open the parchment cards up and directly against the middle crease layer: the sliced onion, 4–6 asparagus spears, salmon, 2–3 lemon slices, 1 teaspoon of butter, and a sprig of thyme. Fold the top of the parchment back to meet the other side and, starting at the top corner, fold and crease a triangle and repeat with longer triangles around the outside of the packet to seal in the meal. Once you arrive at the bottom end, fold the last piece under and then over, tucking it in to lock the origami fish packet. Repeat with all of the other packets.
3. On 2 sheet pans, place the fish packets and lightly coat the outside with oil to keep them from burning. Place the sheet pans with fish packets in the oven and bake for 20 minutes. Remove from the oven and, using kitchen shears, cut open the top of each packet and carefully remove the contents and assemble them on a plate for dinner, or you could place each packet directly on the plate and have everyone open their own packet and enjoy right from the packet.

### Kids Can Cook Tips

Kids will have a blast folding the parchment and layering all of the "parts" of this fun meal!

## Fierce Foods Facts

This is the perfect easy recipe that comes out right every time. It's loaded with anti-inflammatory Omega-3 fats that supply the brain with DHA, excellent for improving the brain's ability to learn. DHA is essential for the proper growth and functional development of growing infants. It is also one of the few natural sources of vitamin D and a single serving provides all that is needed to supply the daily requirement.

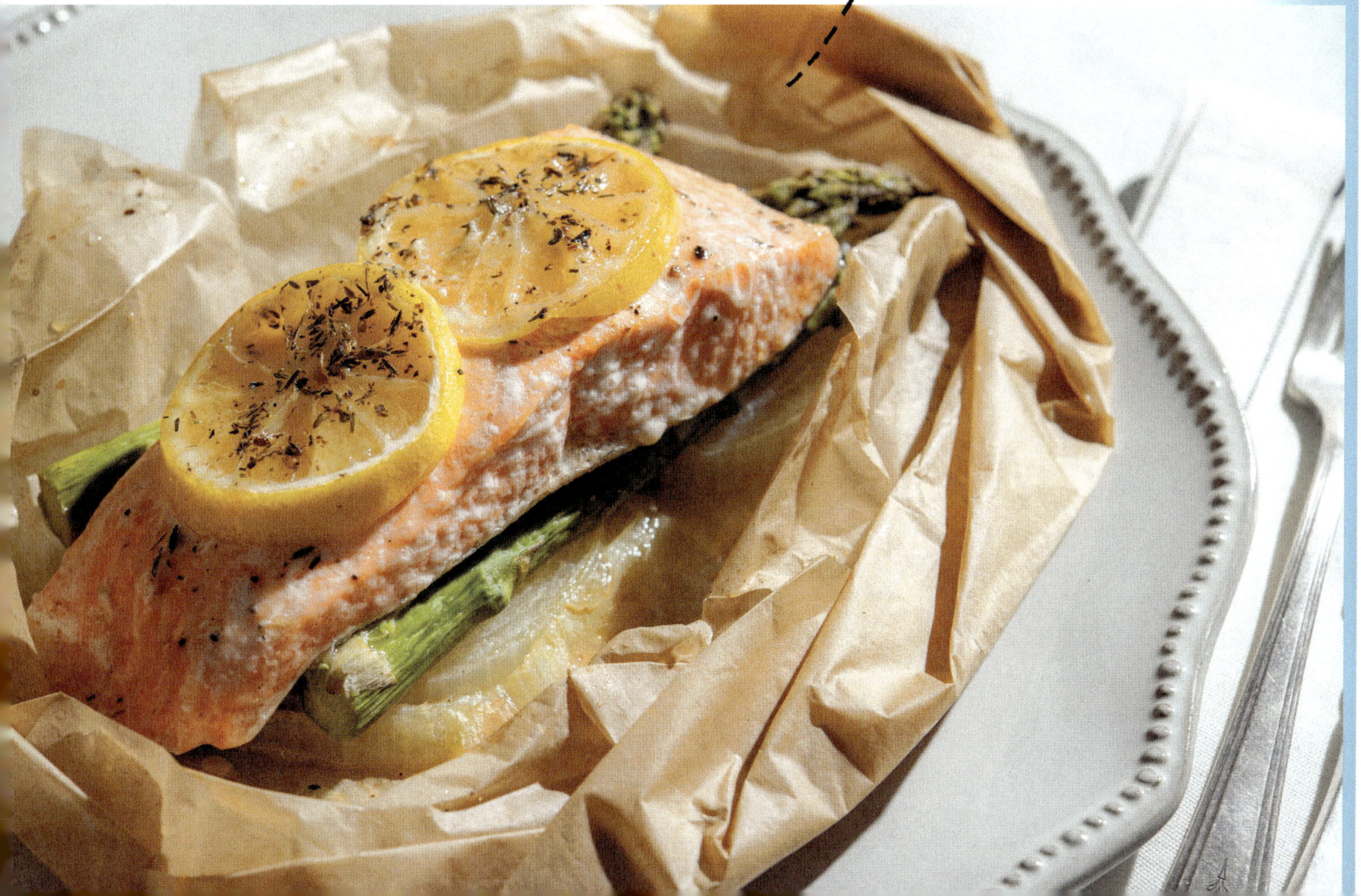

Chef Andrew Johnson

# Salmon with Power Greens and Tahini Dressing

**Makes 4 servings:** each 4 ounces salmon and 2 cups veggies, 363 grams

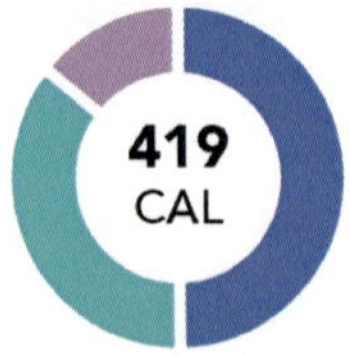


25g Fat
9g Net Carb
34g Protein

### Ingredients

5 oz mixed baby greens: arugula, spinach, kale, and/or Swiss chard

1 cup cherry tomatoes, halved

2 cups cucumber, diced

1 medium avocado, skin and pit removed, diced or sliced

¼ cup flat-leaf parsley, stems removed and roughly chopped

1 oz red onion, thinly shaved

1 lb salmon fillet, skinless, cut into 4 portions

1 tbsp olive oil

2 cloves garlic, minced

½ tsp salt

1 tsp lemon pepper seasoning

**Tahini Dressing**

3 tbsp unsalted tahini

1 clove garlic, peeled and minced

1–3 tbsp lemon juice to taste

½ tsp sea or kosher salt

¼ tsp coriander powder

¼ tsp black pepper

Water to thin dressing to desired consistency

### Directions

1. Preheat the oven to 400°F degrees. Rinse the salmon fillet and pat dry with a paper towel. On a parchment-lined sheet pan assemble salmon presentation side up (the presentation side is the side opposite of the bloodline).
2. In a small bowl, mix the minced garlic and olive oil. Brush or pour the garlic oil evenly over the salmon and then season with salt and lemon pepper. Roast the salmon in the oven for 9–12 minutes, then remove from the oven and cool slightly.
3. While the salmon is cooking, whisk together or blend the dressing ingredients in a blender or food processor, adding water as needed to thin it to your desired consistency. In a large mixing bowl add greens, tomatoes, cucumber, and parsley. Lightly drizzle with dressing and toss to coat evenly.
4. Divide the salad into 4 serving bowls. Cut the avocado and coat in lemon juice to keep it from browning, then gently top each salad with avocado and shaved red onion. Place 4 equal portions of the cooled salmon atop the salad in each bowl, drizzle the top of the salmon with dressing, then finish with salt and pepper to taste.

**Fierce Foods Facts**

This dinner is packed with protein, Omega-3s, and so many other important vitamins and minerals. It covers almost 50% of every B Vitamin, nearly 42% of vitamin A, 74% of vitamin C, and gives a powerful 98% of the RDA of vitamin D—all so incredibly important to support anti-cancer nutrition.

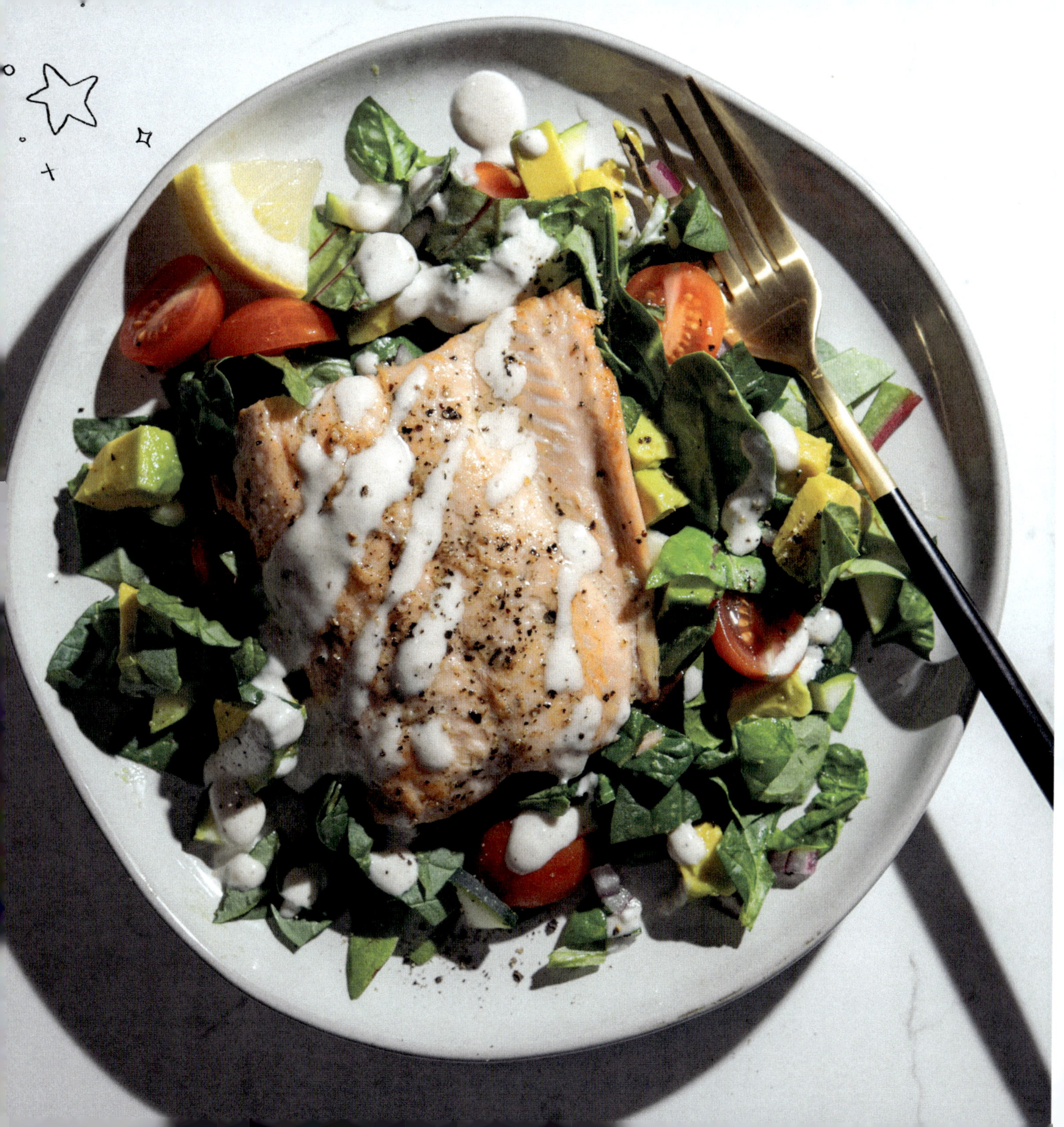

Chef Andrew Johnson

# California Salmon Spring Rolls

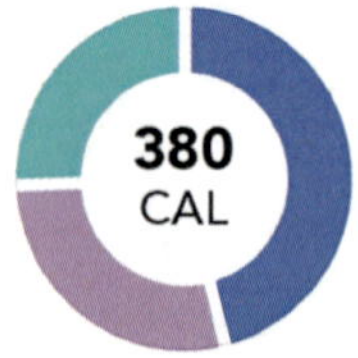


18g Fat
20g Net Carb
33g Protein

**Makes 4 servings:** 2 rolls each, ~229 grams

## Ingredients

8 sheets of Dynasty 22-cm rice paper

1 cup baby spinach

1 avocado, thinly sliced

½ cup cucumber, julienned

½ cup carrot, julienned

16 oz **Easy Baked Salmon**

Drizzle of **Sugar-Free Teriyaki Sauce**

2 tbsp sesame seeds, toasted

## Directions

1. In a large mixing bowl, fill half with warm or hot water. Submerge a sheet of rice paper in the hot water for 10–15 seconds. Place the wet rice paper flat on a clean cutting board.
2. In the middle of the paper, layer ingredients horizontally in the following order: a sprinkle of sesame seeds, a handful of spinach leaves (remove the stems or position the stems towards the middle so not to rip the paper when rolling), a slice of avocado, a couple of pieces of cucumber, a couple of pieces of carrot, 2 ounces of roasted salmon, a drizzle of teriyaki sauce.
3. Picture the rice paper as a clock: fold the 6 o'clock side over the contents in the middle and tuck it in. Then begin to gently roll, fold in the 3 o'clock side and then the 9 o'clock side, and finish continuing rolling into a complete spring roll. Enjoy cold.

**Carb-conscious options:**
Use nori wraps or lettuce wraps to reduce the net carbs from 20 grams to 6 grams.

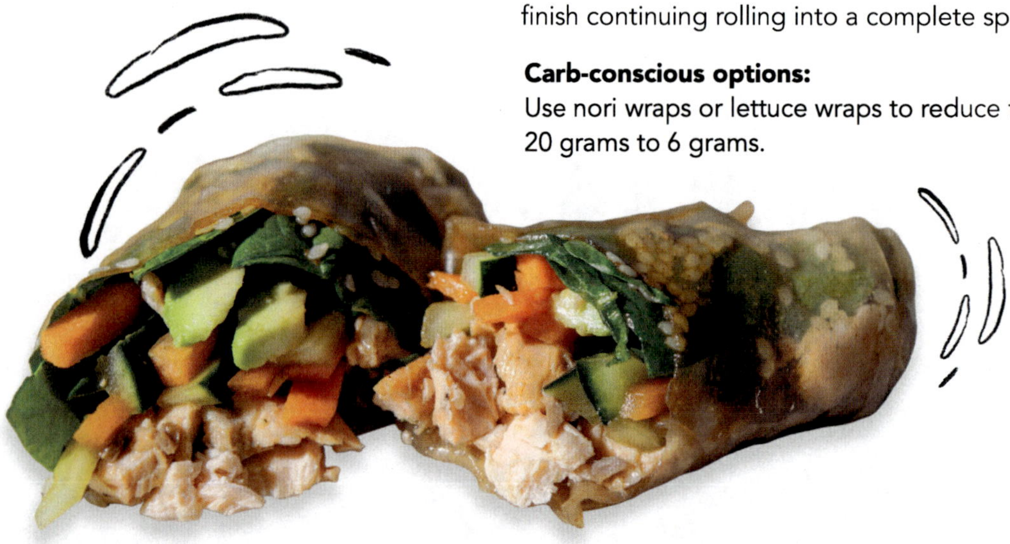

Chef Andrew Johnson

# Slow Cooker Chicken Tikka Masala

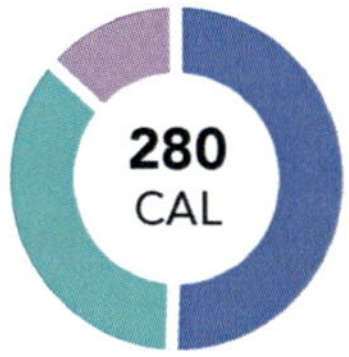


17g **Fat**
6g **Net Carb**
24g **Protein**

**Makes 8 servings:** each ~¾ cup, 200 grams

## Ingredients

2 lb boneless, skinless chicken thighs, cut into 1" cubes

1 cup yellow or white onion, finely chopped

1 can (14 oz) tomato purée, preferably San Marzano style

2 tbsp coconut oil

3–4 cloves garlic, minced

1 tbsp ginger, minced or grated

1 can (14 oz) full-fat unsweetened coconut milk

1–2 tbsp Sambal Oelek or chili paste (optional)

2 tsp ground cumin

2 tsp ground coriander

1–1½ tsp salt

1 tsp ground black pepper

1 tsp ground paprika

1 tsp ground turmeric

¼ tsp ground cinnamon

⅛ tsp ground cardamom

A pinch ground nutmeg

A pinch ground clove

## Directions

**1.** In a medium sauté pan on medium-high heat, add oil, onions, chicken then garlic, ginger, and chili paste. Cook for 5–6 minutes to soften and get some color, stirring frequently.

**2.** Pour the sauté pan contents into a 6-quart slow cooker, scraping the pan to ensure you get all of the oil and pan bits. Add all of the spices and coconut milk into the slow cooker bowl and stir to evenly coat the chicken.

**3.** Cook tikka masala on high for 5 hours or low for 8 hours. Serve over long grain rice or cauliflower rice and garnish with cilantro leaves.

### Fierce Foods Facts

Throw this warm and flavorful dish in the crockpot in the morning and come home from a long day with comfort food for dinner easily made. This recipe has a nice amount of immune-supporting nutrients including vitamin A. Pair with cauliflower rice for a well-rounded, low-carbohydrate dinner.

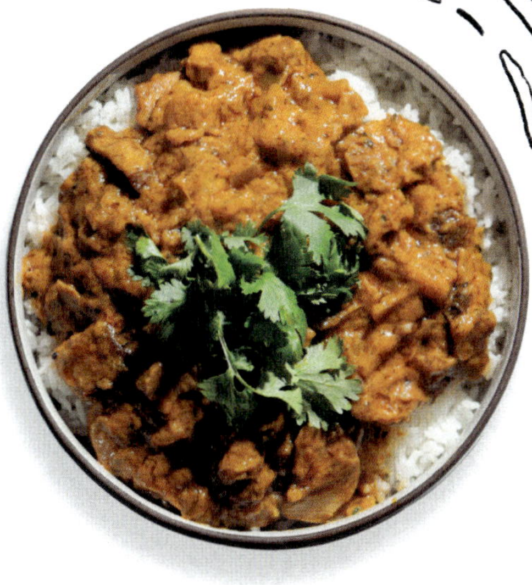

Chef Andrew Johnson

# Portobello Mushroom Pizza

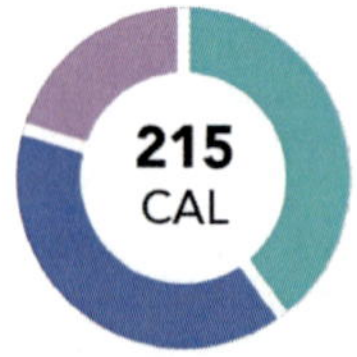


14g Fat
7g Net Carb
14g Protein

**Makes 4 servings:** 1 each, 176 grams

## Ingredients

4 portobello mushrooms, stems and gills removed

1 tbsp olive oil, divided

1 tsp oregano

½ tsp garlic powder

1 tsp parsley

¼ tsp salt

1 dash ground black pepper

1 dash chili flakes (optional)

½ cup pizza or pesto sauce, divided

1 cup shredded mozzarella or dairy-free alternative, divided

½ cup shredded parmesan or dairy-free alternative, divided

¼ fresh basil, sliced thin

### Topping recommendations

Bell pepper, diced red onion, diced spinach, fresh, chopped cherry tomatoes

## Directions

1. Preheat the oven to 400°F. Place mushrooms stem side up on a baking sheet. Lightly drizzle olive oil on the base of the mushroom and spread evenly with the back of a spoon or your fingers.
2. In a small bowl, combine oregano, garlic powder, parsley, salt, and pepper. Sprinkle 1 teaspoon of spice mixture evenly over each mushroom. Fill each mushroom with 2 tablespoons pizza sauce, then chopped vegetables of choice.
3. Sprinkle ¼ cup shredded mozzarella cheese over each pizza, covering vegetables. Bake for 10 minutes or until mushrooms are tender and cheese is melted. Remove from oven, top with fresh sliced basil, and serve immediately.

**Carb-conscious options:**
Use **Basil Pesto Cream Sauce** in place of pizza sauce to reduce net carbohydrates to 5 grams per serving. Do not use cherry tomatoes.

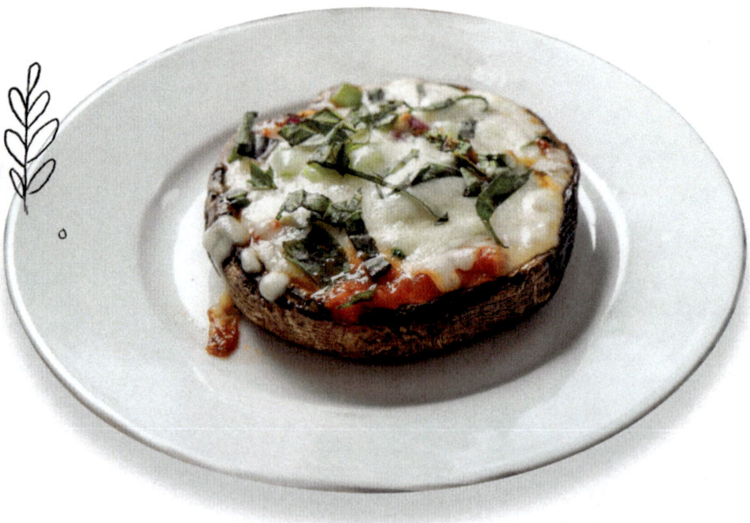

### Fierce Foods Facts

This recipe has your B vitamins covered along with some vitamins A, E, and K! The cheeses and the dark green leafy vegetables provide calcium, phosphorus, and zinc, which are helpful for building strong bones.

Chef Alexia Hall, RDN

# School Lunch Collard Green Wrap

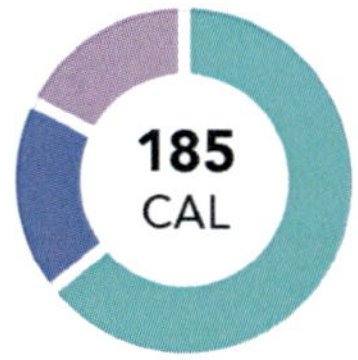


16g **Fat**
4g **Net Carb**
4g **Protein**

**Makes 4 servings:** each ~2 wraps each, ~150 grams

## Ingredients

4 collard green leaves, washed and center stems removed

½ cup **Basil Pesto Cream Sauce**

2 medium cucumbers, sliced lengthwise

1 cup fresh spinach leaves, sliced

1 cup fresh tomato, sliced

1 avocado, sliced

1 pkg (4 oz), micro-greens, fresh

basil leaves (optional)

## Directions

1. Prepare each collard green by carefully removing the center stem. Spread the pesto cream sauce across the middle of the leaf, then layer the cucumber, spinach leaves, tomato slices, avocado slices, micro-greens, and the basil.
2. Fold the wrap tightly, as you would a burrito, tucking in all of the veggies with the first roll and then rolling firmly to the end. Cut in half and serve.

### Fierce Foods Facts

This mineral-packed lunch provides calcium, iron, magnesium, manganese, and selenium, all in one convenient wrap! It also comes in at a whopping 160% of the daily vitamin K. All of this works together to support strong blood, heart, and bones!

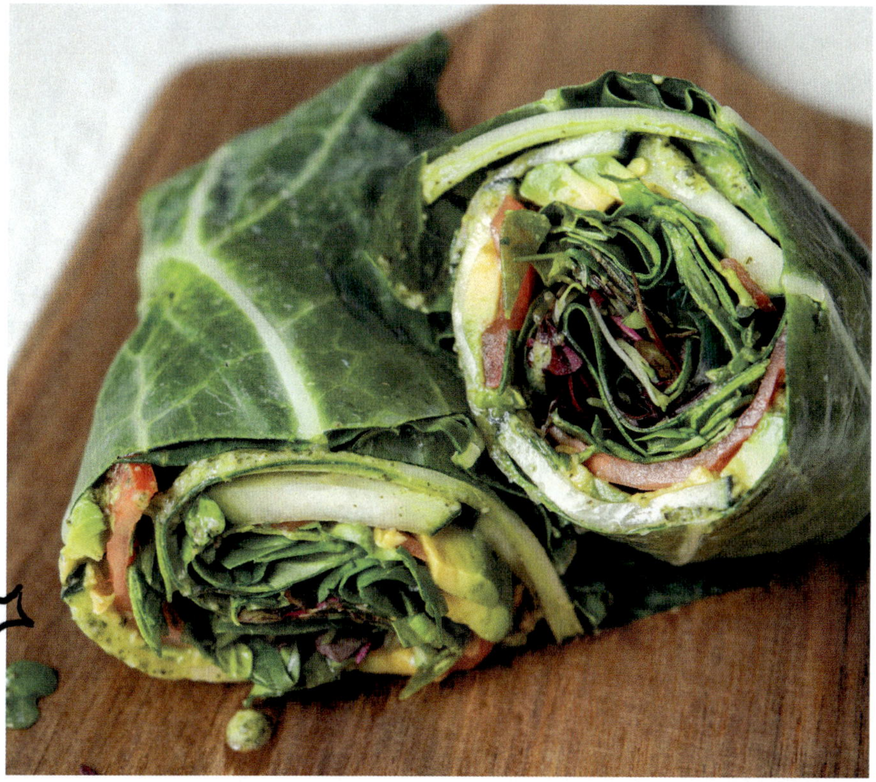

Chef Andrew Johnson

# Southern Barbecue Ribs

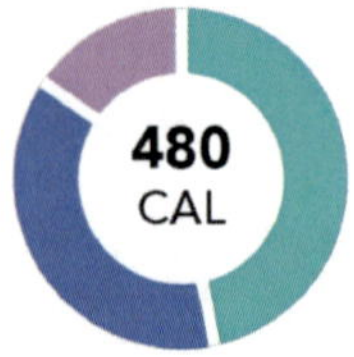


35g Fat
11g Net Carb
28g Protein

**Makes 8 servings:** each ~4 ounces, 178 grams

## Ingredients

2 racks baby back pork ribs (approx. 2 lb each)

½ cup Dijon mustard

1 tbsp salt

1 tbsp black pepper

2 tbsp smoked paprika

2 tbsp garlic powder

2 cups barbecue sauce*

1 cup water, chicken, or beef stock

* See recipe for **Sugar-Free Peach Habanero Barbecue Sauce**

## Directions

1. Preheat the oven to 300°F. On a cutting board or sheet pan, lay out the racks of ribs. Peel the membrane off of the bottom side with the bones (optional but will produce best results). Flip the racks back over onto the top or meat side and evenly coat the entire top side with Dijon mustard and a liberal coating of the spices.
2. For the oven method, place the ribs in a large roasting pan, cover tightly with foil, then bake in the oven for 3–4 hours.
3. In the Instant Pot bowl, add the wire rack and a cup of water, chicken, or beef stock. Lay the racks into the bowl standing on end with the meat side facing the wall of the bowl, bending the racks to mimic the curve of the bowl. Attach the lid and cook on high pressure for 25 minutes. Once done allow 10–15 minutes to pressure release naturally.
4. To finish the ribs, preheat the grill to medium-high heat. Remove them from the oven and coat the top side with barbecue sauce. Place the racks on the grill for 10–15 minutes, then flip and cook until the barbecue sauce has caramelized to your liking. To caramelize both sides of the ribs, coat the under side of the ribs with sauce then flip until caramelized.
5. Remove from the grill, let rest for 1–2 minutes and slice the ribs for plating.

## Fierce Foods Facts

This tangy take on Southern barbecue ribs provides a flavorful and fun celebration of summer's harvest. Filled with satiating protein, pair this with the ranch dip and vegetables for a balanced lunch of protein and quality carbs along with some bone-building calcium.

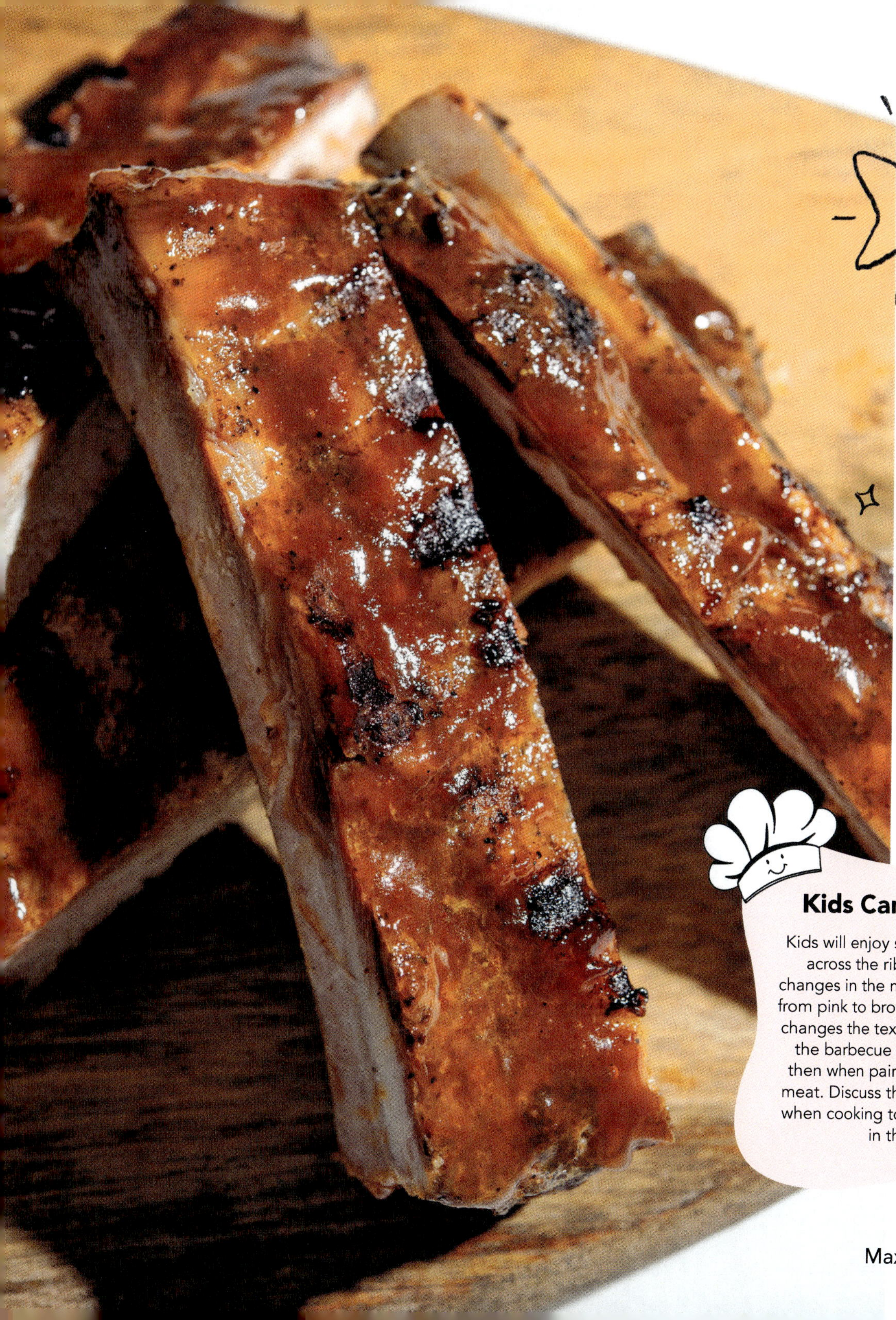

### Kids Can Cook Tips

Kids will enjoy sprinkling the spices across the ribs. Talk about the changes in the meat color as it cooks from pink to brown and how the heat changes the texture. Have kids taste the barbecue sauce by itself and then when paired with the cooked meat. Discuss the need for moisture when cooking to prevent toughness in the meat.

Chef Andrew Johnson

# Low-Carb Meatballs

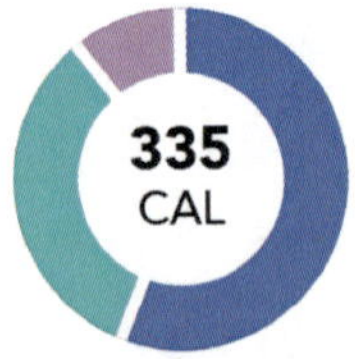


20g Fat
6g Net Carb
34g Protein

**Makes 8 servings:** each ~3 meatballs, 151 grams

## Ingredients

2 lb turkey, ground 80/20 to 93/7

½ bunch parsley, finely chopped

½ yellow or white onion, small diced

2 eggs

⅓ cup sunflower seeds

⅓ cup chia seeds

1 tsp salt

1 tsp black pepper

Olive oil to drizzle

## Directions

1. Preheat oven to 350°F. In a large mixing bowl, add all of the ingredients and mix well. Refrigerate for 30 minutes or overnight to allow the chia seeds to set.
2. Line a sheet pan with parchment and scoop or ball by hand 2-ounce balls onto a sheet pan. Drizzle olive oil over the meatballs, then bake for 15 minutes.

### Fierce Foods Facts

This flavorful meatball represents almost every B Vitamin there is and almost all of the daily required B12, helpful for creating new cells and important for brain function. The seeds also offer anti-inflammatory vitamin E and a healthy dose of Omega-3 type fats. The parsley also lends all of the day's supply of vitamin K—great for strong bones and supporting appropriate blood clotting.

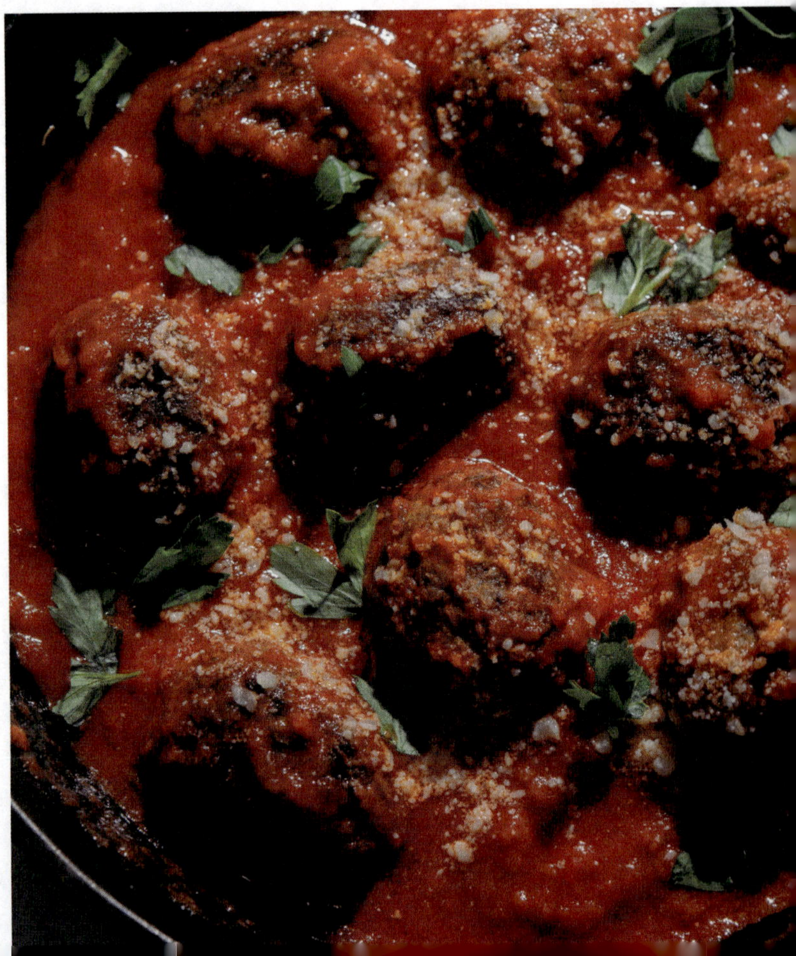

Chef Andrew Johnson

# Modern Sloppy Joes

**Makes 6 servings:** each ~1 cup, 214 grams

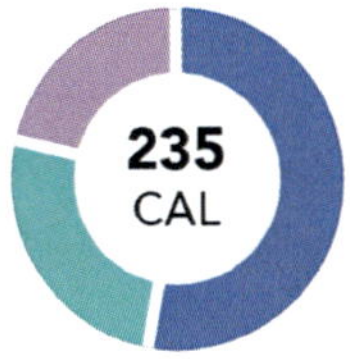


11g **Fat**
9g **Net Carb**
23g **Protein**

## Ingredients

1 tbsp extra virgin olive oil

1 lb lean ground beef, turkey, chicken, or pork

1 cup carrots, finely chopped

1 cup red bell pepper, finely chopped

1 cup yellow onion, finely chopped

1 clove garlic, minced

1 tbsp fresh thyme (or 1 tsp dried)

1 tbsp fresh oregano (or 1 tsp dried)

1 tbsp smoked paprika

2 tbsp Dijon mustard

1 tbsp Worcestershire sauce

1 cup tomato sauce

¼ cup barbecue sauce (e.g. Sweet Baby Ray's no sugar added)

## Directions

1. Set your Instant Pot to sauté and add olive oil. Add the ground meat, allowing to brown. Break up the meat as it cooks and approximately halfway to brown, add the rest of the ingredients.
2. Seal on the Instant Pot lid and turn on high pressure for 10 minutes.
3. Serve on your favorite roll, over a baked potato or yam, or even in a taco shell or lettuce wrap. It also pairs really well with some quick pickles.

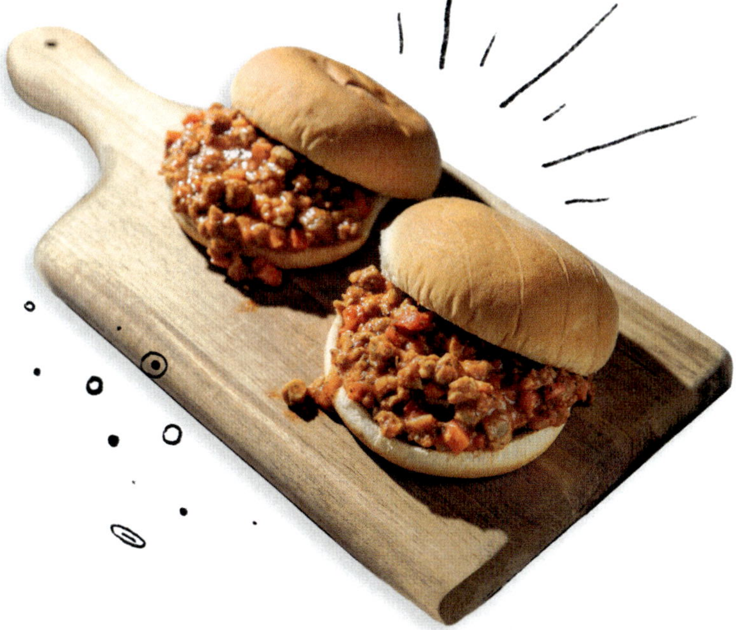

### Fierce Foods Facts

This quick weeknight favorite comes packed with protein, vitamins A and C, and over 100% of brain-building vitamin B12. This recipe is also packed with almost 50% of the daily need for zinc, which is critical for preventing depression and anxiety according to recent studies.

Chef Alexia Hall, RDN

# Steak and Veggie Kabobs

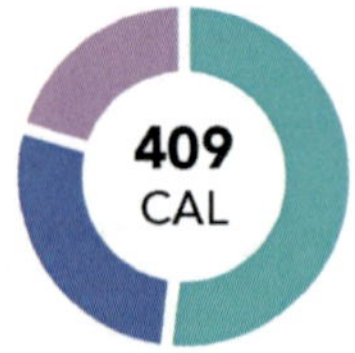


34g Fat
13g Net Carb
18g Protein

**Makes 6 servings:** each ~12 ounces, 353 grams

## Ingredients

1 lb ribeye or NY strip steak

1½ tsp sea salt

½ tsp freshly ground black pepper

6 thick rosemary branches (10"–12"), or 4 bamboo skewers (12"), soaked in water for at least 1 hour

3 orange, yellow, and/or red bell peppers, rinsed, seeds and inner membrane removed

1 red onion, peeled and sliced into ½" chunks

1 lb Baby Bella mushrooms, rinsed, stems removed

½ cup pineapple, sliced into ½" chunks

1 zucchini, sliced into ½" chunks

### Marinade

¼ cup balsamic vinegar

⅓ cup olive oil

⅓ cup soy sauce

1 whole lemon juiced

2 tbsp Dijon mustard

4 cloves garlic

1 tsp lemon pepper

1 tsp oregano

1 tbsp fresh rosemary, chopped

1 tbsp fresh lemon verbena, chopped

2 tsp fresh thyme, chopped

1 tsp salt

## Directions

1. Using a large, nonreactive bowl, combine all ingredients for the marinade, and set aside.
2. Slice the red onion and bell peppers into eighths and the pineapple and beef into 1" chunks. Season the beef with ½ teaspoon of sea salt and black pepper. Skewer a piece of pineapple followed by a piece of steak on the rosemary branch, followed by a red onion, another piece of steak, red pepper, zucchini, and mushrooms. Continue in the same manner until all skewers are threaded, leaving 1" on either end.
3. Separate the marinade into evenly split portions. Baste the kabobs with half of the marinade recipe and chill in the refrigerator for 2–4 hours, up to overnight. Use the remaining marinade to baste the skewers as they cook.
4. Heat a grill to medium-high and lightly oil the grill grates. Grill the kebabs, basting with the remaining marinade as they cook, for about 3 minutes. Turn and cook for another 3 minutes, basting before turning over to cook on the first side again. Continue to cook on the first side for another 2–3 minutes before turning over and cooking for a final 2–3 minutes. Season the kebabs with the remaining teaspoon of salt. Enjoy immediately.

### Fierce Foods Facts

Vitamin-C-packed peppers add a bright splash of fresh flavor and a crispy texture to the marinated meat. They also carry antioxidants that help fight cancer. Flavonoids contained in citrus also help neutralize the carcinogens that occur when carbohydrates are charred on the grill.

### Kids Can Cook Tips

Younger kids can measure the ingredients for the marinade, help to juice the lemon, and clean and tear the fresh herbs. Older kids with knife skills can assist with chopping vegetables.

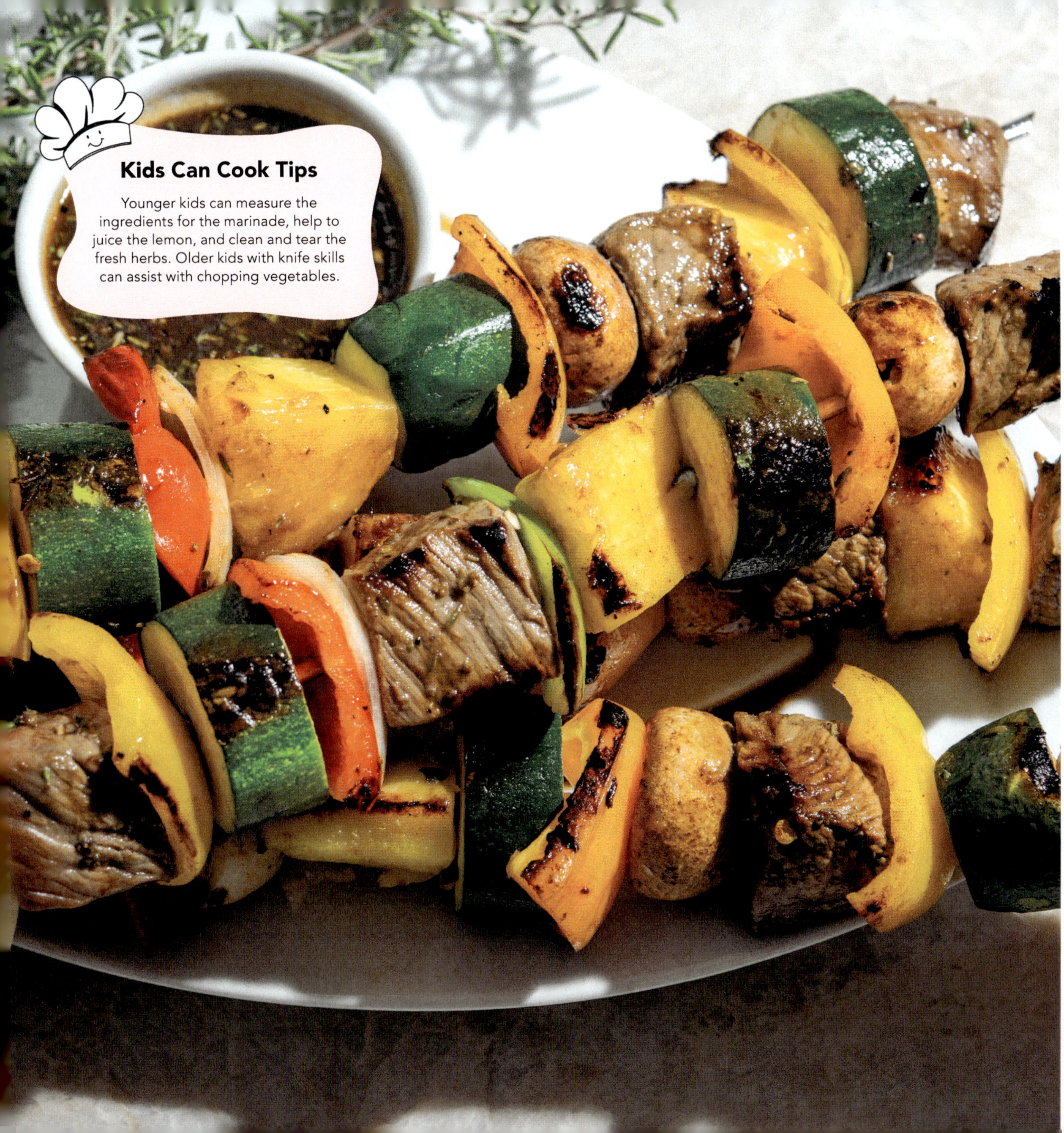

Chef Cathy McKnight

# Beef Taco Salad

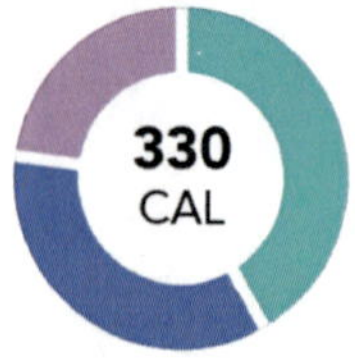


23g **Fat**
12g **Net Carb**
19g **Protein**

**Makes 10 servings:** each ~1 cup, 239 grams

## Ingredients

2 tbsp extra virgin olive oil

2 medium onions, diced

2 cloves garlic, crushed

1 pound ground beef

1 tsp ground cumin

1 tsp salt

1 tsp black pepper

2 tsp chili powder

1 bunch fresh epazote, or 1 tsp dried

8 oz cherry tomatoes

1 head iceberg lettuce, shredded

2 cups shredded cheddar cheese

1 cup sour cream

1 medium jicama, peeled and julienned

6 oz black olives, sliced

2 green jalapeños, diced

1 bunch cilantro, chopped

## Directions

1. Using a large sauté pan, heat the olive oil and add the onion and garlic. Add in the beef and stir to break up clumps. Add in the cumin, salt, pepper, and chili powder, then add the dried epazote (if using fresh epazote, incorporate it at the end with the cilantro).
2. Cook until the beef is cooked through and no longer pink, then add in the cherry tomatoes. Remove from heat and set aside.
3. Using a platter or individual plates, layer the salad in this order: lettuce as the base, beef, cheese, sour cream, jicama, olives, and jalapeño. Sprinkle cilantro (and fresh epazote) over the top of the salad and serve immediately.

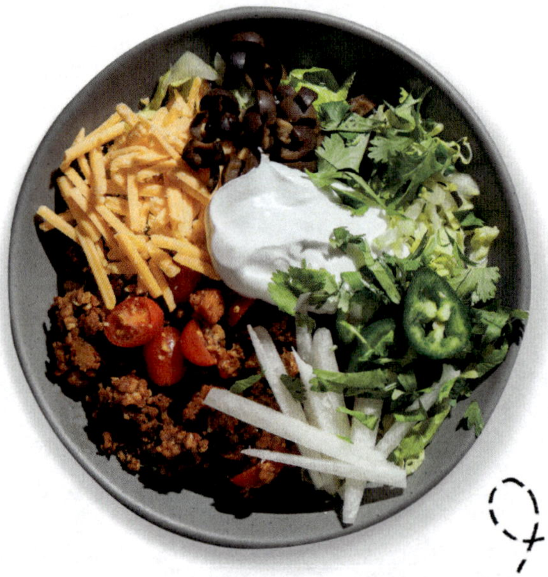

### Fierce Foods Facts

This easy-to-make, crowd-pleasing dinner is packed with satiating protein. This dish provides 25% of daily calcium needs, helpful for strong bones as well as a strong heartbeat! This is a great source of animal-based iron which is essential for healthy blood cells. It also contains 40% of the daily needed vitamin C and almost 30% of the daily zinc—a **super** combination for healthy skin.

Chef Andrew Johnson

# Easy Pan Chicken Fajitas

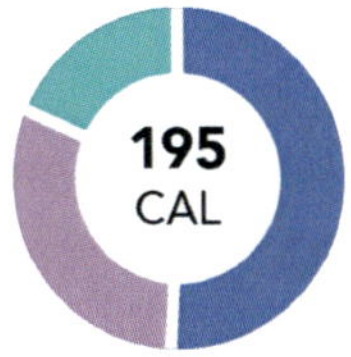


7g Fat
12g Net Carb
20g Protein

**Makes 10 servings:** each 1 cup, ~236 grams

## Ingredients

2 lb chicken thighs, boneless/skinless, sliced into strips

16 oz corn kernels, frozen

1 large Vidalia onion, sliced

1 red bell pepper, sliced

1 orange bell pepper, sliced

1 yellow bell pepper, sliced

1 pint cherry tomatoes

1 lime, wedged

2 cloves garlic, minced

2 tbsp Tajin seasoning

1 tbsp smoked paprika

2 tbsp oil (olive or avocado)

Salt and pepper to taste

**Garnish recommendations**

Chopped cilantro or scallions

## Directions

1. Preheat the oven to 400°F, then line a sheet pan with parchment paper. On the sheet pan, pour the corn in a mound towards the middle of the pan. In a large mixing bowl add sliced chicken, sliced peppers, garlic, oil, and spices, then toss to evenly coat.

2. Pour the contents on top of the corn, then add the tomatoes and lime wedges into the pan in a random pattern. Place the sheet pan into the oven and bake for 25–30 minutes. Turn the oven to broil for a few minutes to get a little char/color on the top. Remove from the oven and with tongs, squeeze the lime wedges all over the pan. Garnish with chopped cilantro or scallions and serve with your favorite tortillas.

### Fierce Foods Facts

This easy recipe provides plenty of protein for a clean weeknight meal. Save the leftovers for multiple uses including soups and salads! It is loaded with immune-supporting Vitamins A and C, thanks to the bell peppers and onions. The dark meat in the chicken is also loaded with iron compared to the traditional white meat breasts, helpful for strong red blood cells!

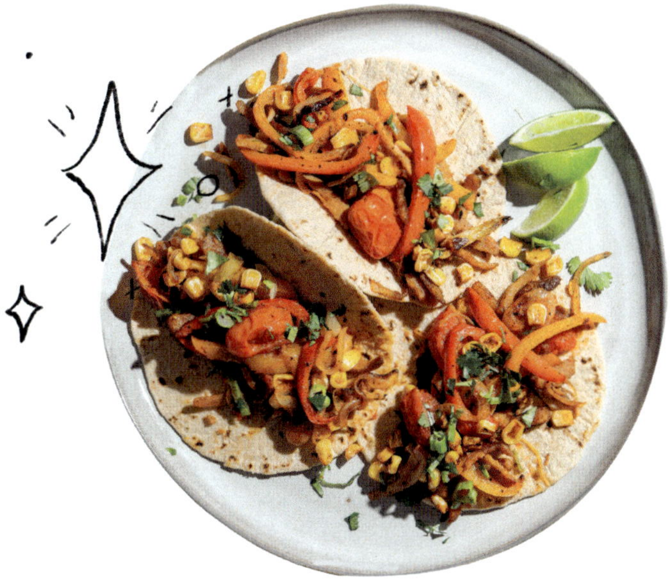

Chef Azmin Ghahreman

# Baked Chicken with Marinade

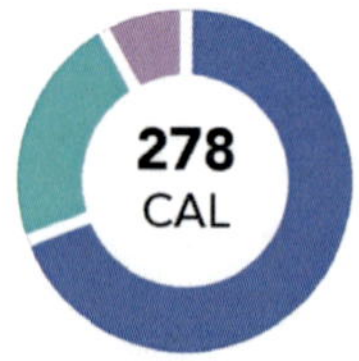


12g **Fat**
4g **Net Carb**
38g **Protein**

**Makes 6 servings:** each ~1 cup, 226 grams

## Ingredients

### Original

2½–3 lb chicken, consider spatchcocked, or any other bone-in (e.g. wings, legs, or breasts)

¼ cup olive oil

1 tbsp garlic, peeled and minced

½ tsp dried, crushed oregano

1 tbsp fresh mint, chopped

1 tbsp fresh basil, chopped

¼ tsp black pepper, freshly ground

½ tbsp kosher salt

1 lemon, zested and juiced

½ yellow onion, peeled and grated

1 pinch chili flakes

2 pinches mild smoked paprika

1 cup milk

### Keto Garlic

¼ cup Sambal Oelek chili paste

1 orange, juiced

⅛ cup melted butter, ghee, or olive oil

⅛ cup Lakanto brown monk fruit sweetener

⅛ cup honey

1 tsp smoked paprika

1 tsp salt

1 tsp black pepper

### Buttermilk

2 cups buttermilk

¼ cup olive oil

2 cloves garlic, minced

¼ tsp black pepper

### Lemon

¼ cup olive oil

1 lemon, juiced

½ tsp salt

¼ tsp black pepper

## Directions

1. If you desire a spatchcocked chicken, your butcher can prepare this for you or you can prepare it yourself with the following directions. At the joint, cut off the tips of the wings. Rest the chicken upright, and split its back down the center from neck to tail, cutting alongside one side of the spine. Lay the chicken down and cut along the other side of the spine so you can remove it. Next, break the breastbone so the chicken lays flat in a butterfly position.

2. For the original marinade, put the grated yellow onion in a large bowl, then add the minced garlic, lemon juice, and lemon zest. Add in the rest of the dry ingredients, mixing as you add, then pour in the olive oil and milk and whisk the mixture together. Next, add the herbs and make sure everything is fully incorporated.

3. If using a spatchcocked chicken, place the chicken into the bowl and massage the marinade into the meat. Alternatively, if using separated chicken parts, consider pouring marinade into a large gallon-sized Ziploc bag and place chicken parts inside, sealing to prevent leaks.
4. Cover and refrigerate for 24 hours. After your chicken has marinated, preheat your oven, and prepare a large, hot cast iron pan with smoking hot olive oil. Sear the chicken (breast-side-down first if using spatchcocked) until it is beautifully brown.
5. Note that there are two baking options. For the first option, bake the chicken at 425°F for 40 minutes. For the second option, bake the chicken at 420°F for 15 minutes, then finish it off at 375°F for 25 minutes.

### Kids Can Cook Tips

Kids can help tear the fresh herbs, zest the lemon, and measure the other ingredients. Older kids with knife skills can help mince the garlic and the onion.

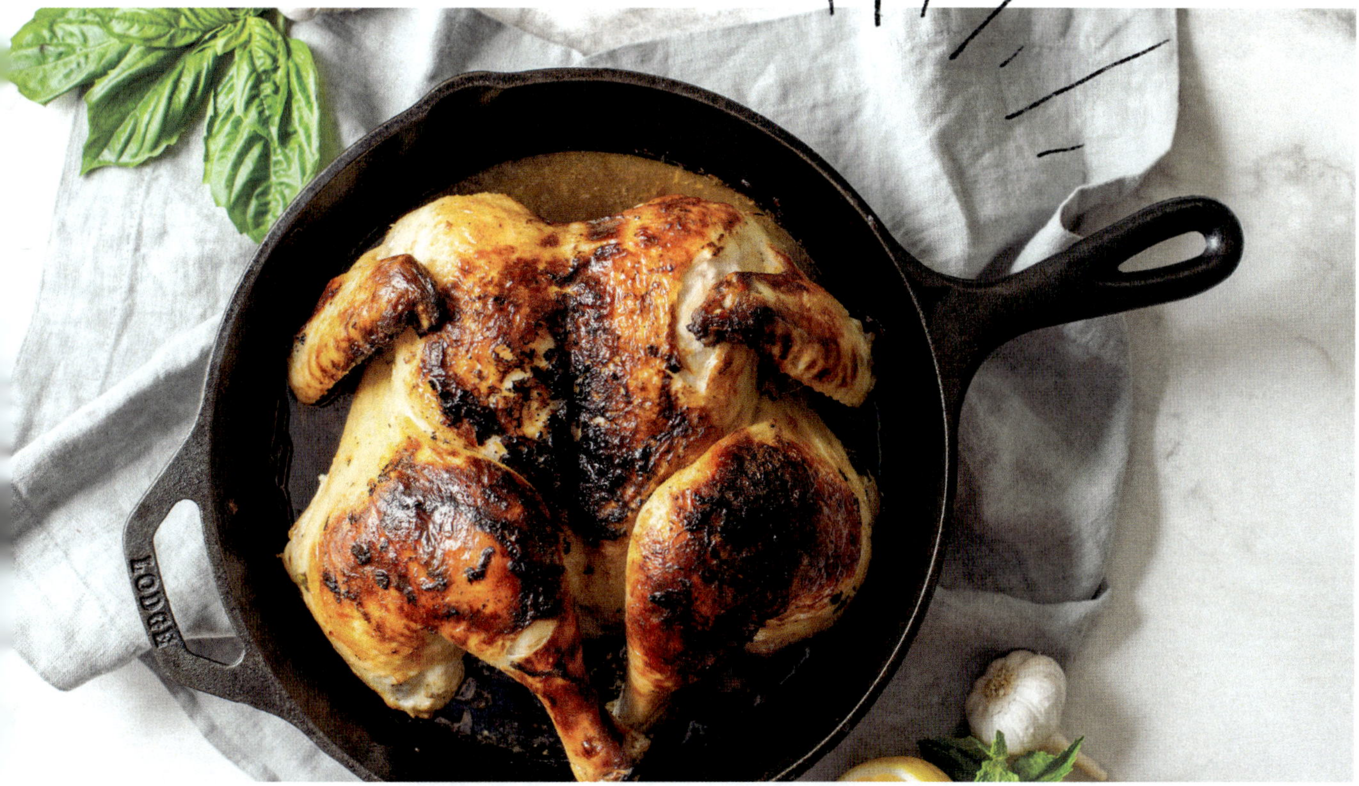

Chef Alexia Hall, RDN

# Chicken Taco Bar

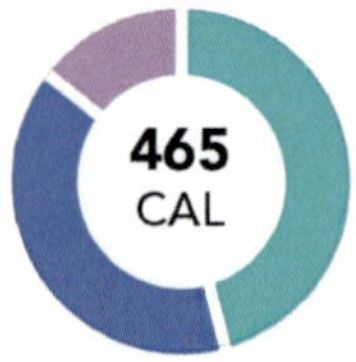


30g Fat
9g Net Carb
26g Protein

**Makes 12 servings:** about ¾ cup in 2 tortillas, 215 grams

## Ingredients

2 lb chicken breast

1 jar (16 oz) green (verde) or mild red enchilada sauce

16 oz cheddar cheese, grated

5 oz shredded lettuce (or mixed greens)

1 pt salsa

¼ cup jalapeños, sliced

¼ cup pepitas, toasted

1 pt sour cream

8 oz cherry tomatoes

16 tortillas, keto or other low-carbohydrate option

## Directions

1. Place chicken breasts in a large crockpot and pour enchilada sauce over them. Cook on low for 8 hours or on high for 4 hours, as needed. Stir vigorously to shred.
2. You can set up a taco bar by providing multiple toppings in small bowls and allowing guests to create their own.
3. For dairy-free options, consider Forager cashew-based sour cream and VioLife shredded non-dairy cheddar or jack cheese.

### Fierce Foods Facts

This healthy and nutritionally balanced taco bar comes loaded with lots of B vitamins to help sustain good energy for those party-goers! It also has a nice amount of just about every mineral to help sustain healthy bones, teeth, skin, and hair!

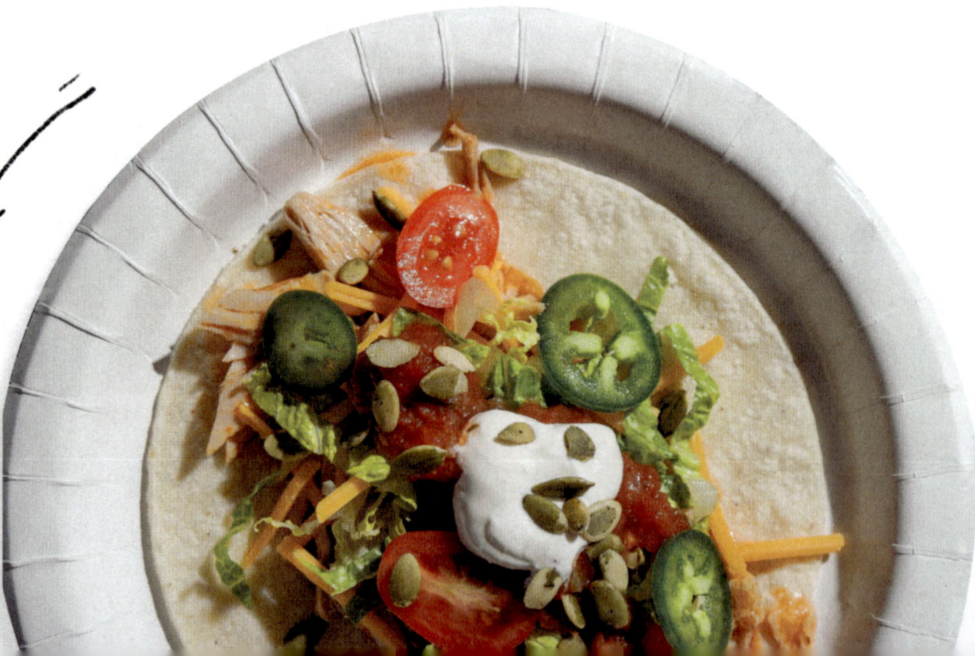

Chef Andrew Johnson

# Zucchini Ravioli

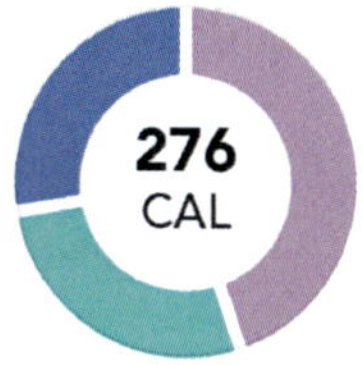


14g Fat
23g Net Carb
14g Protein

Makes 6 servings: ~ 2 ravioli each, 378 grams

## Ingredients

4 large zucchini, thinly sliced lengthwise

1 cup whole-milk ricotta

1 cup shredded mozzarella cheese, divided

¼ cup shredded parmesan cheese

1 qt Bolognese sauce

1 whole egg

1 tbsp fresh oregano, finely chopped

¼ tsp ground cinnamon

kosher salt and pepper to taste

### Fierce Foods Facts

The zucchini swap for the traditional white flour version is helpful for those who are carbohydrate sensitive. Using the zucchini also provides more fiber, vitamin A, and vitamin C while providing 65% less overall carbohydrate grams.

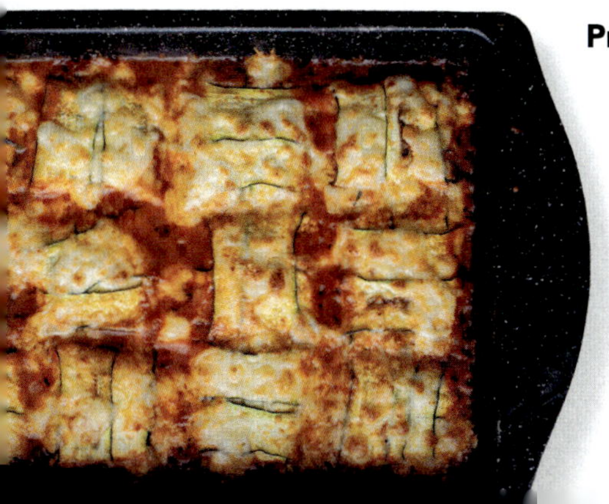

## Directions

1. Preheat oven to 450°F. With a vegetable peeler or mandoline, slice zucchini lengthwise into thin ribbons. On a baking sheet, lay the zucchini ribbons flat and sprinkle them with kosher salt. Let the zucchini sit for 20 minutes (this will allow the salt to draw out the water and make the ribbons more pliable), then pat dry.
2. In a large mixing bowl, thoroughly mix ricotta, ½ cup mozzarella, egg, oregano, cinnamon, salt, and pepper.
3. In a 9"x13" baking dish, spoon in the Bolognese sauce.
4. Lay out 2 zucchini ribbons vertically and slightly overlapping, then on top of those ribbons, lay 2 more horizontally, making a cross shape. Spoon 1½ tablespoons of the cheese filling onto the center of the cross, then tightly fold the zucchini ribbons over the cheese mixture in an alternating fashion, ending with a square bundle. Carefully flip over the zucchini raviolis and place it down in the sauce. Repeat this until you have filled the pan, 4 rows of 3 ravioli (a total of 12 ravioli).
5. Place the baking dish in the oven and bake for 20–25 minutes. Remove the dish and top with parmesan and remaining mozzarella, then bake for another 5–10 minutes until the cheese is bubbly and golden brown.

**Pro Tip:** Add another ¼ cup of mozzarella for an extra-gooey topping.

## Soups & Stews

Mom's Minestrone is a family heirloom recipe that has been made hundreds of times bringing sustenance and comfort to friends and other family members who have been challenged by illness or stressful situations. It has also been used in joyful situations, equally received as a welcome expression of love and care.

It is made in a large batch recipe, easily divided into individual servings, and frozen,perfect for showering a loved one. This recipe has been carefully honed over time to include nutritious vegetables and low glycemic additions such as riced cauliflower.

The Pumpkin Lentil Chili is also a fun family favorite and even won a prize at a recent neighborhood chili competition! Vinnie's Pozole takes a heritage recipe and converts it into a low glycemic version, perfect for retaining that comfort factor, while still achieving desired health and wellness goals. Soups and stews are a great way to consume more vegetables and proteins in an easily digested format. As the vegetables cook in flavorful and healthy bone broths, they release vitamins and minerals that are not drained off and stay in the soup to provide many health benefits. Sprinkling fresh chopped herbs over the top of the warm soup helps to maximize nutrient content as well. Since soups and stews have a high liquid-to-solid ratio, they are also a great way to stay hydrated.

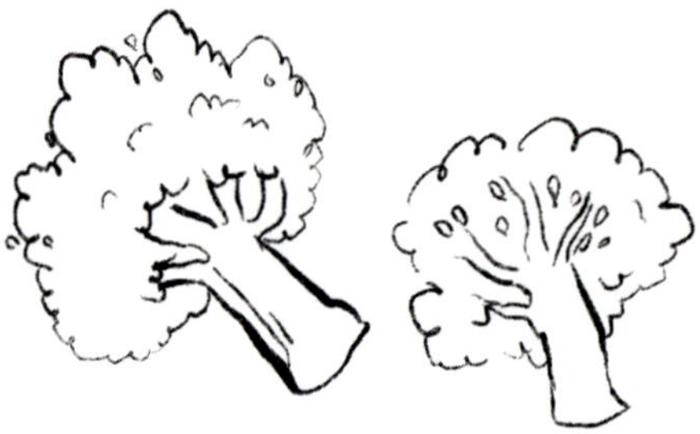

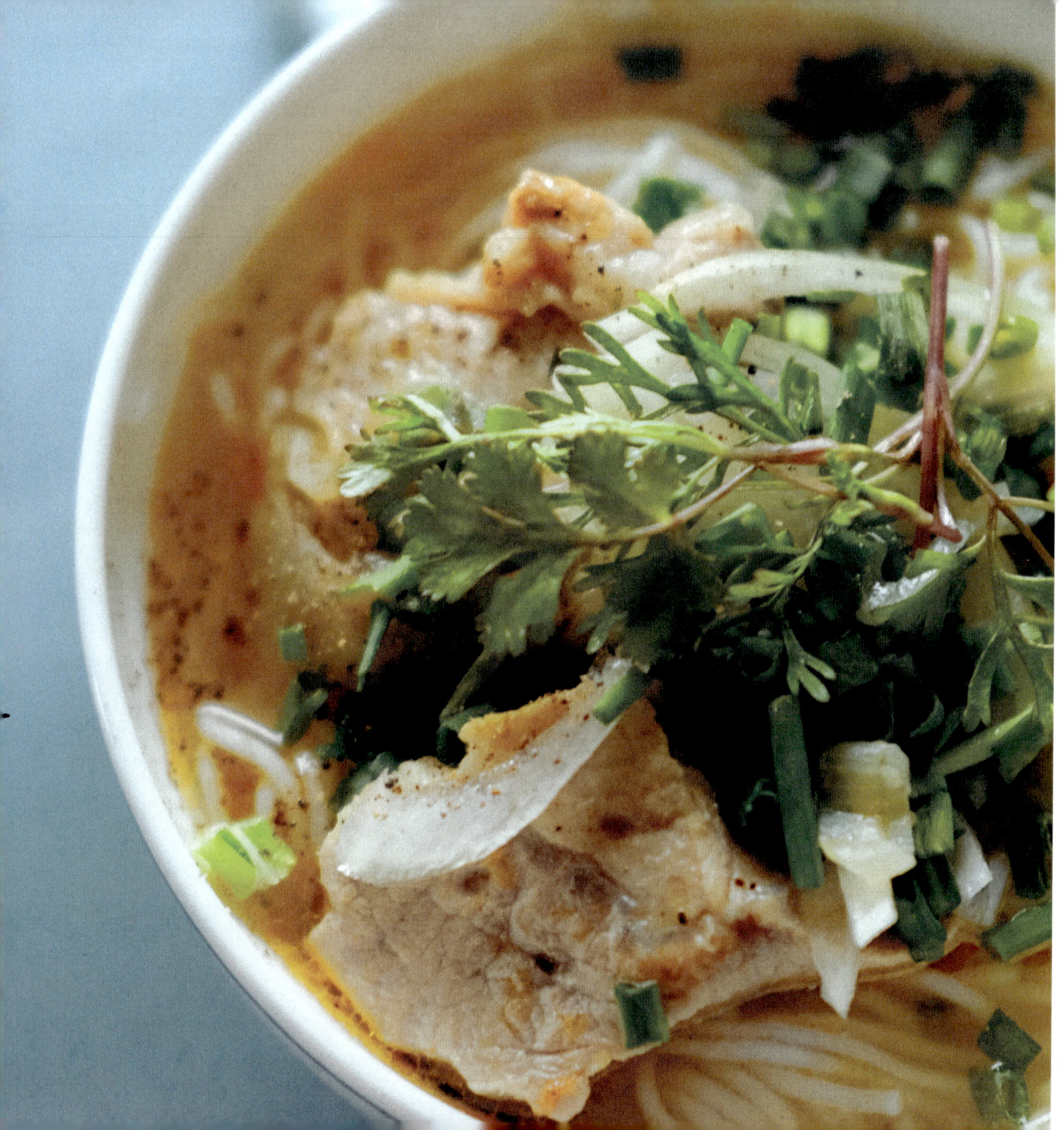

Chef Andrew Johnson

# Mushroom Ramen with Shirataki Noodles

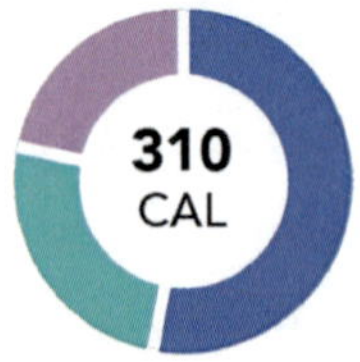


14g Fat
12g Net Carb
30g Protein

**Makes 4 servings:** each 1½ cups, 367 grams

## Ingredients

1 pkg (1 oz) dried shiitake mushrooms

2 cups hot water

1 tbsp olive oil

3 cloves garlic, minced

½ cup shallots (approx. 2 large), minced

1 tbsp freshly grated ginger

6 cups bone broth (chicken or turkey)

1½ tbsp white miso paste

2 tsp soy sauce

3 slices bacon

¾ lb Baby Bella mushrooms, sliced thin

2 pkg (7 oz each) Shirataki noodles (e.g. Miracle Noodle)

1 tbsp rice wine vinegar

Freshly ground black pepper to taste

4 soft-boiled eggs, peeled and halved

2 green onions, thinly sliced

## Directions

**1.** In a large bowl, combine shiitake mushrooms and 2 cups hot water; let stand until softened, about 20–30 minutes. Drain, reserving the mushroom water. Coarsely chop the mushrooms, then set aside.

**2.** Heat olive oil in a large stockpot or Dutch oven over medium heat. Add garlic, shallots, and ginger, and cook, stirring frequently, until fragrant, about 2 minutes. Stir in reserved shiitake mushrooms until golden brown (about 3 minutes).

**3.** Stir in reserved mushroom water, bone broth, white miso paste, soy sauce, and bacon. Bring to a boil, then reduce the heat, cover, and simmer until the flavors have blended (about 15–20 minutes). Remove and discard the bacon.

**4.** Stir in Baby Bella mushrooms and simmer until softened (about 3–5 minutes). Add the Shirataki noodles and cook until they are just tender (about 3 minutes), then stir in the rice wine vinegar and season with additional soy sauce and pepper, to taste.

**5.** Serve immediately, and garnish with soft-boiled eggs and green onions.

**Carb-conscious or ketogenic options:**

Add 2 cups of heavy cream and increase to 8 servings (1 cup each). This provides 360 calories, 28 grams fat, 8 net carbs, 16 grams protein. This recipe is automatically dairy, nut, and wheat free.

## Fierce Foods Facts

This well-balanced ramen has just about every nutrient you need for a satisfying and nutritious meal. Fortified mushrooms provide almost half of the daily requirement for the immune-supporting and bone-building vitamin D needed daily. The dried shiitake mushrooms recipe also provides over 50% of vitamin B5 (Pantothenic Acid), important for the breakdown and utilization of healthy fats and carbohydrates.

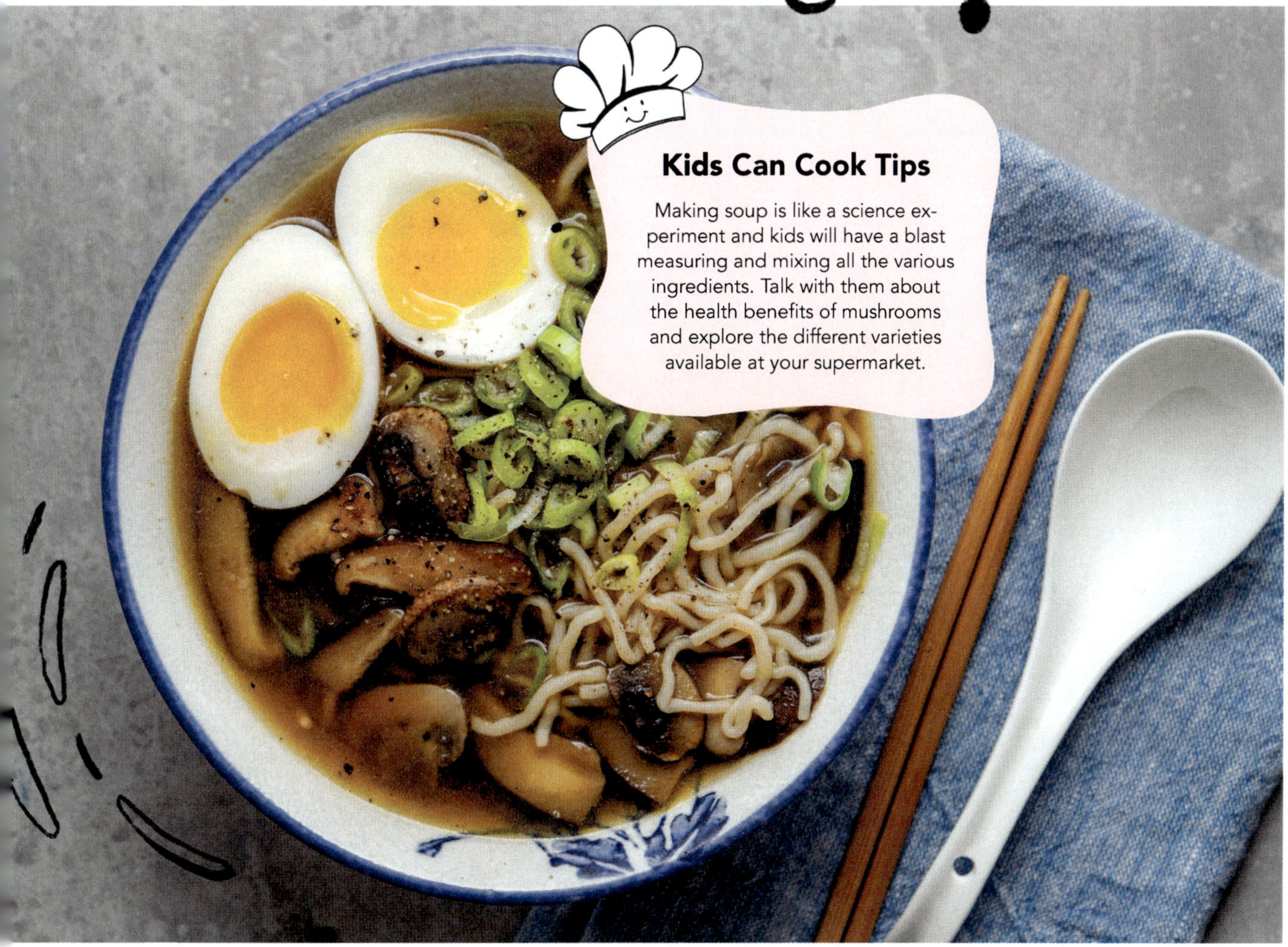

### Kids Can Cook Tips

Making soup is like a science experiment and kids will have a blast measuring and mixing all the various ingredients. Talk with them about the health benefits of mushrooms and explore the different varieties available at your supermarket.

Chef Andrew Johnson

# Thai-Style Curried Pumpkin Soup

**Makes 6 servings:** each ~1 cup, 226 grams

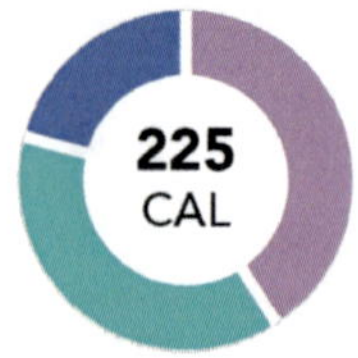


15g **Fat**
16g **Net Carb**
8g **Protein**

## Ingredients

2 tbsp olive oil

½ cup yellow onion, diced

1 tbsp ginger, minced

8 oz crimini mushrooms, sliced thin, stems removed

2 tbsp gluten-free flour

32 oz chicken bone broth

2 cans (15 oz each) pumpkin purée

1 tsp kosher salt

1 tsp black pepper

1 tbsp curry powder

16 oz unsweetened coconut milk

⅛ tsp nutmeg

2 tbsp fresh Thai basil, chiffonade sliced

1 tbsp honey

## Directions

**1.** Heat a stockpot over medium heat. Add olive oil when hot, then add onions, ginger, and mushrooms. Sweat the mixture for 5 minutes or until the onions are translucent. Add flour to the mixture and cook for 5 minutes. Add bone broth, pumpkin purée, curry, salt, and pepper. Bring to a boil and simmer for 20 minutes, then turn the heat to low.

**2.** Temper the coconut milk to avoid curdling it by shaking your can of room-temperature coconut milk and pouring it into a bowl. Slowly add a half cup of the soup mixture to the coconut milk while stirring steadily. Add another half cup and whisk steadily. Return the coconut milk mixture to the stockpot with the remaining soup and continue to stir.

**3.** Finish with honey, nutmeg, and chiffonade Thai basil and serve immediately. Allow to cool before storing for leftovers.

### Fierce Foods Facts

This recipe's superpower is vitamin A, coming in at 125% of the daily recommended value. It is also loaded with selenium and iron, helpful for healthy blood cells, thyroid, and immune systems.

### Instant Pot version:

1. Press Sauté on the Instant Pot and add the olive oil. Once the oil is hot but not smoking, add the onion, ginger, and mushrooms, and sauté until softened, about 5 minutes. Press Cancel and stir in the flour while the pot is still hot. Add the broth, pumpkin purée, curry, salt, and pepper to the pot.
2. Secure the lid and move the steam release valve to Sealing. Select Manual/Pressure Cook to cook on high pressure for 5 minutes. When the cooking cycle is complete, let the pressure naturally release for 10 minutes, then move the steam release valve to Venting. When the floating valve drops, remove the lid. Stir in the coconut milk, and season with a drizzle of honey, a dusting of nutmeg, and a few pieces of Thai Basil.

   **Carb-conscious options:**
   Reduce pumpkin purée to 1 can (15 ounces). This will reduce net carbohydrate grams to 9 grams per serving.

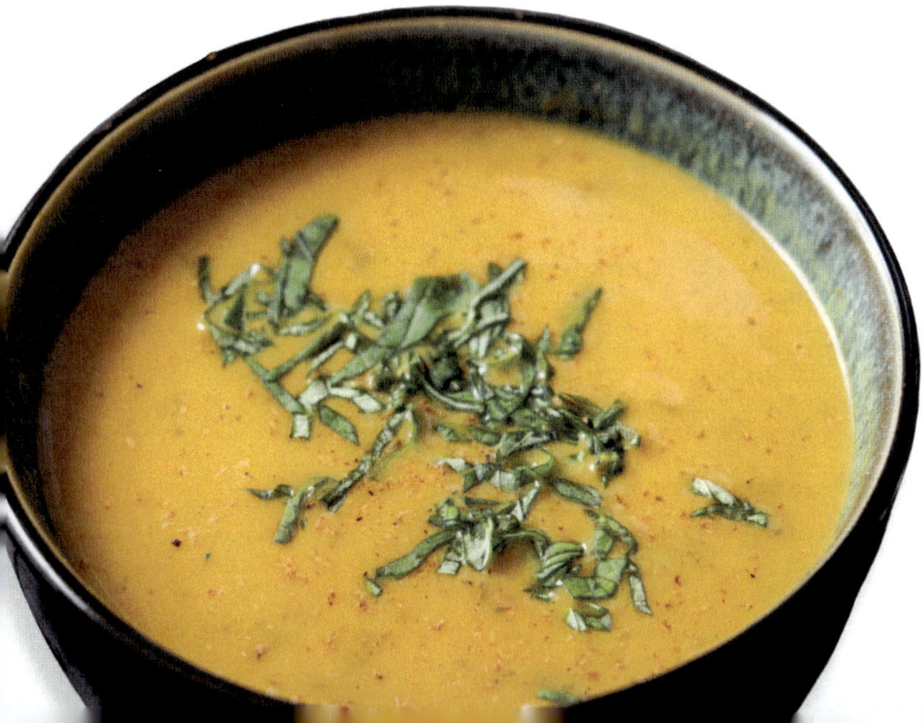

Chef Alexia Hall, RDN

# Mom's Vegetable Minestrone Soup with Cauliflower

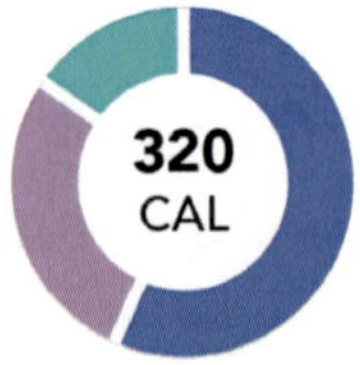


9g Fat
17g Net Carb
35g Protein

**Makes 6 servings:** each ~1.5 cups, 363 grams

## Ingredients

1 lb thin-cut chicken

2 tbsp olive oil

½ cup yellow onion, diced fine

½ cup carrot, cut into ¼" coins

2 cloves garlic, minced

½ tsp dried rosemary leaves, crushed (or 1 tsp fresh)

2 large zucchini (approx. 3 cups), sliced into ½" chunks

½ tsp Italian seasoning or poultry seasoning)

1 tsp dried basil

1 tsp dried oregano

1 tsp dried parsley

¼ tsp rosemary salt

Salt and pepper to taste

4 cups chicken bone broth

1 can (14.5 oz) diced tomatoes (including canning liquid)

1 can (15 oz) cannellini or white northern beans, rinsed and drained

2 cups riced cauliflower

1 cup frozen peas

¼ cup grated parmesan cheese or dairy-free alternative (e.g. VioLife Parmesan)

## Directions

1. Using a sharp knife, slice chicken into 1" strips, then sprinkle the chicken breast with poultry seasoning and rosemary salt. Add olive oil to a sauté pan and heat over medium heat, then add the chicken and sauté until just cooked. Set aside.
2. Using a 6-quart saucepan, heat olive oil over medium-high heat. Add the onion, carrot, garlic, and rosemary, then sauté for 2 minutes. Add the zucchini and Italian seasoning (or poultry seasoning) and cook until the carrot is tender-crisp.
3. Stir the broth and tomatoes in the saucepot and heat to a boil. Reduce the heat to low, then cover and cook for 10 minutes.
4. Increase the heat to medium, then stir in the beans, riced cauliflower, and peas. Cook for an additional 10 minutes or until the cauliflower is tender. Season further to taste, and serve with cheese, if desired.

**Carb-conscious options:**
Removing beans and peas will reduce net carb to 7.5 grams per serving.

### Fierce Foods Facts

This nicely balanced and fiber-filled soup is the perfect comfort food for any day. It's like a hug from mom! Richly flavored and filled with almost every vitamin and mineral, this is the food that nourishes the body and soul!

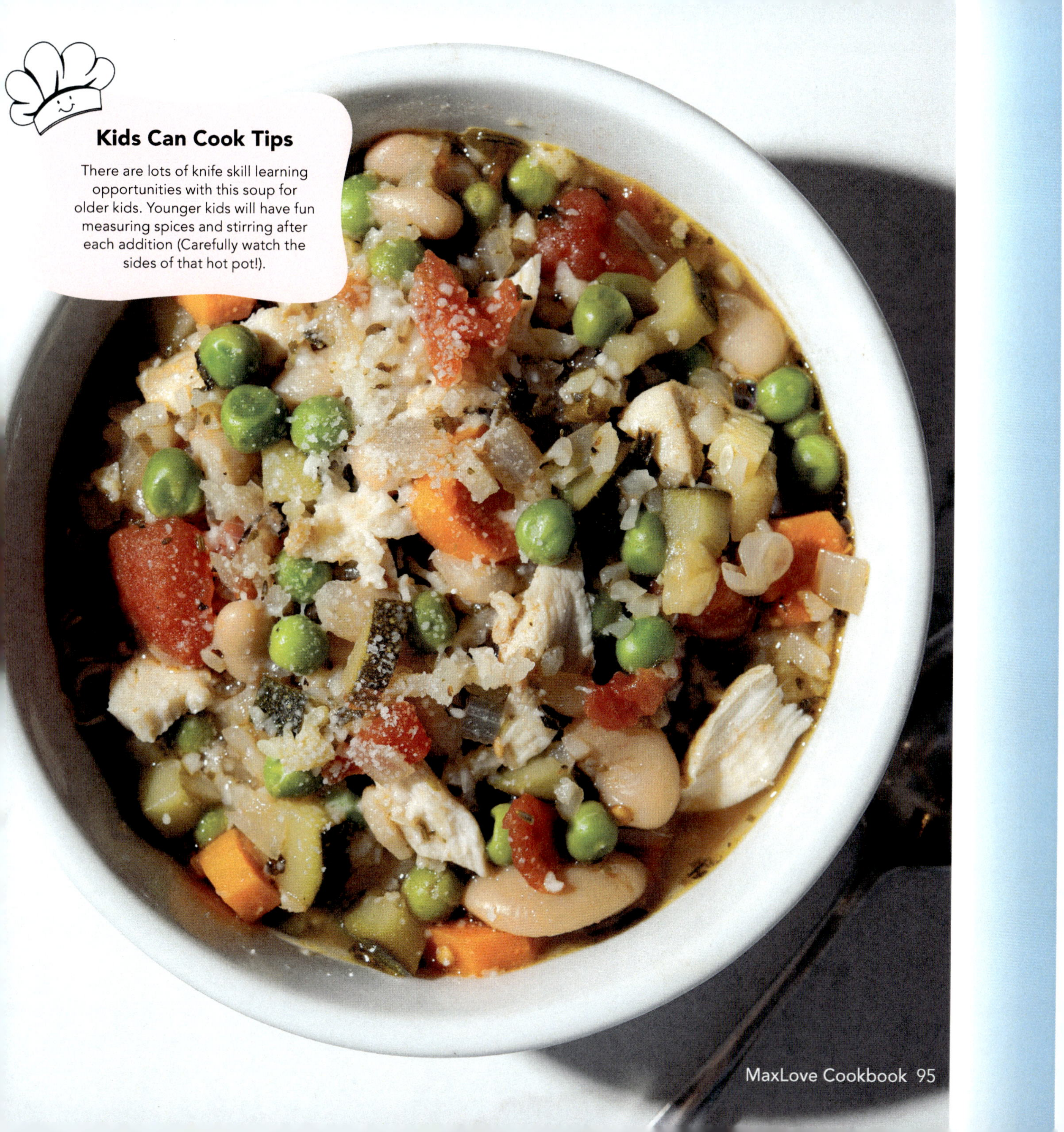

## Kids Can Cook Tips

There are lots of knife skill learning opportunities with this soup for older kids. Younger kids will have fun measuring spices and stirring after each addition (Carefully watch the sides of that hot pot!).

Chef Catherine McKnight

# Vinnie's Pozole with Cauliflower Florets

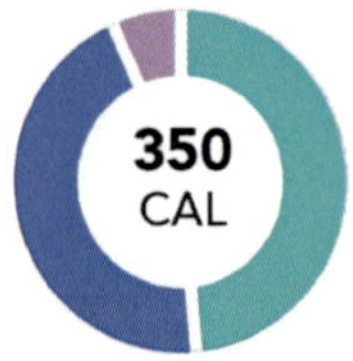


25g Fat
3g Net Carb
23g Protein

**Makes 10 servings:** each ~10 ounces, 300 grams

## Ingredients

**Pork Shoulder Broth**

3 lb bone-in pork shoulder

4 garlic cloves, peeled

1 onion, chopped

1 tbsp cumin

3 qt water

2 tsp salt

**Ancho Chili Sauce**

1 pkg (4 oz) dried ancho chili

1 lime, peeled

1 tsp salt

**Pozole**

3 cups cauliflower florets

3 tbsp extra virgin olive oil or avocado oil

3 garlic cloves, minced

1 onion, diced

1 jalapeño, small dice

2 tbsp chili powder

1 tsp fresh oregano

1 tsp fresh thyme

1 tsp salt and pepper, coarsely ground

2 cups ancho chili sauce

## Directions

1. In a Dutch oven or heavy-duty pot, add 2 tablespoons of oil on medium heat. Pat the pork shoulder dry and sprinkle with salt and pepper. Place fat-side down in the oil and sear for 5 minutes per side. Add the water, cumin, garlic, and onion, bring to a boil, then reduce to simmer for 45 minutes.
2. While the broth simmers, prepare the ancho chili sauce. Place the dried chilis in a sauté pan and cover with water. Simmer for 15 minutes until tender. In a blender, purée the chilis with the cooking liquid, lime, and salt, then chill.
3. After 45 minutes of simmering, carefully remove the pork and broth and reserve both. Using the same pot, sauté the onion, jalapeño, and garlic in the new oil. Stir to coat on medium heat, then cook for 3–5 minutes.
4. Cube the pork into 1" pieces and add into the pot with the oregano, chili powder, thyme, salt, and pepper. Cover with the reserved broth, simmer for 55 minutes, then add the cauliflower florets. Cook until the florets are tender (about 2 minutes).
5. Serve with ancho chili sauce, fresh cilantro leaves, shaved radish, shredded cheese, limes, and corn tortillas.

**Variation:** Consider utilizing the meat pulled from a rotisserie chicken instead of the pork shoulder.

## Fierce Foods Facts

Cauliflower florets have the wonderful mouthfeel of hominy from traditional pozole without the added carbohydrate. Cauliflower also adds a nice amount of fiber and vitamin C. This flavorful soup is also loaded with iron, important for a strong blood supply as well as helping to stave off depression.

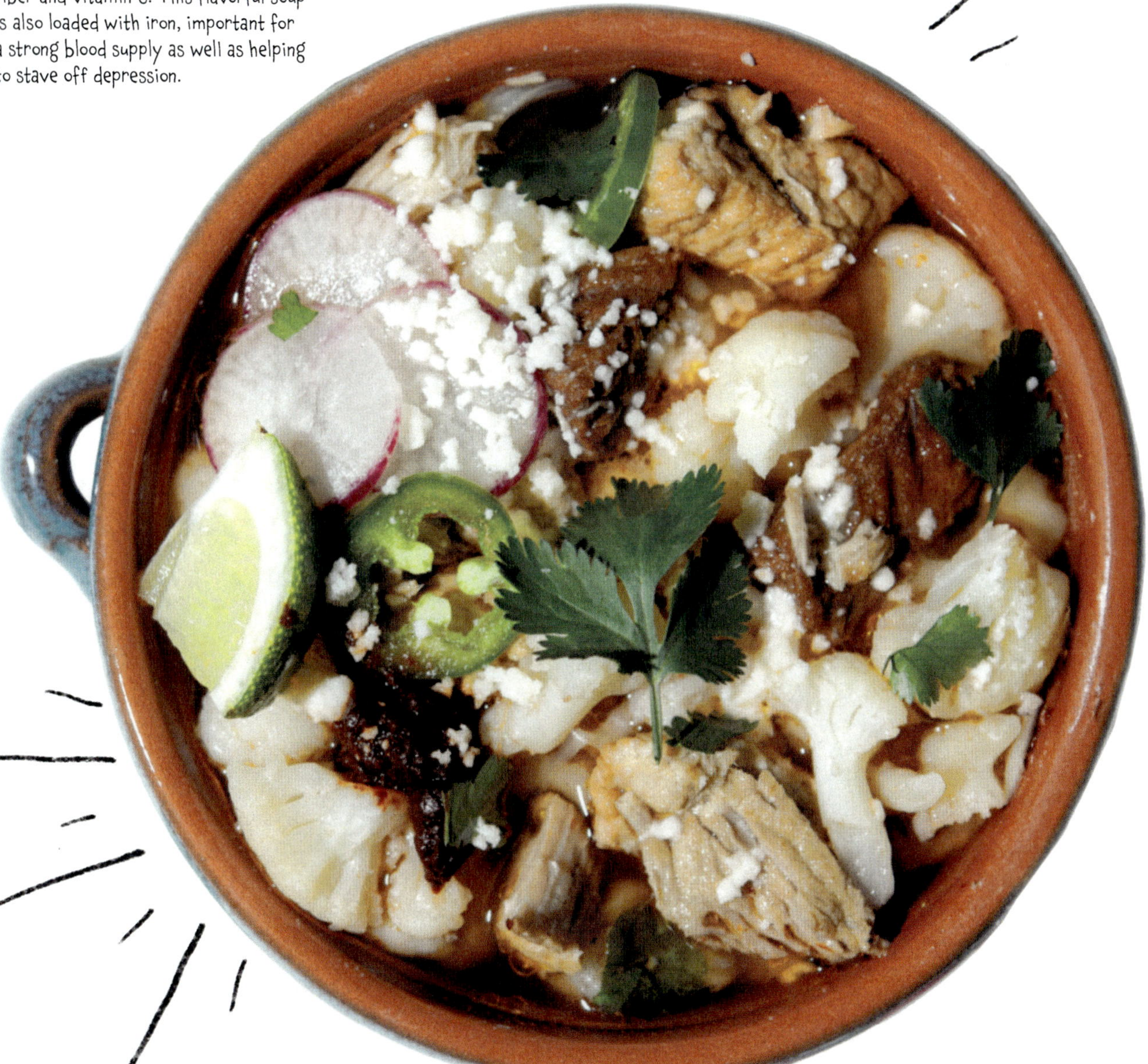

Chef Cathy McKnight

# Hearty Italian-Style Meat Sauce

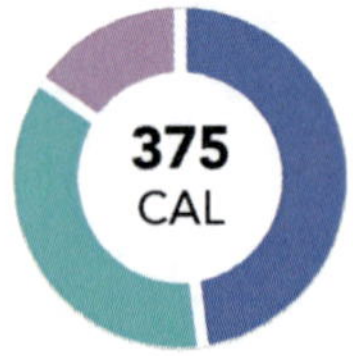


23g **Fat**
10g **Net Carb**
31g **Protein**

**Makes 4 servings:** each ~1 cup, 241 grams

## Ingredients

2 tbsp extra virgin olive oil

1 lb ground beef

1 medium onion, diced

8 oz carrot, diced

4 cloves garlic, minced

2 tsp salt

1 tsp black pepper, ground

8 oz cherry tomatoes

2 tsp fresh oregano, minced (or 1 tsp dried)

1 tsp thyme, minced

2 bay leaves

## Directions

**1.** Add olive oil to a large sauté pan over medium heat, then add ground beef, stirring and breaking up clumps with the back of a spoon. While cooking, add the onion, carrots, and garlic, then stir through and continue to sauté for 4 minutes.

**2.** Sprinkle with salt and pepper, stir well, then mix in the cherry tomatoes. Add oregano, thyme, and bay leaves and cook uncovered, stirring occasionally until the beef is cooked through and the juices have almost evaporated. Remove and discard the bay leaves. Serve over low-carb noodles or vegetable zoodles.

### Fierce Foods Facts

This easily doubled or tripled recipe freezes wonderfully, making it great for batch cooking! Cooked tomatoes are a major source for the powerful antioxidant lycopene as well as potassium, reducing risk of heart disease and cancer. This recipe also provides almost 120% of the daily required vitamin A, supporting not only the immune system but skin, eye, and bone health as well.

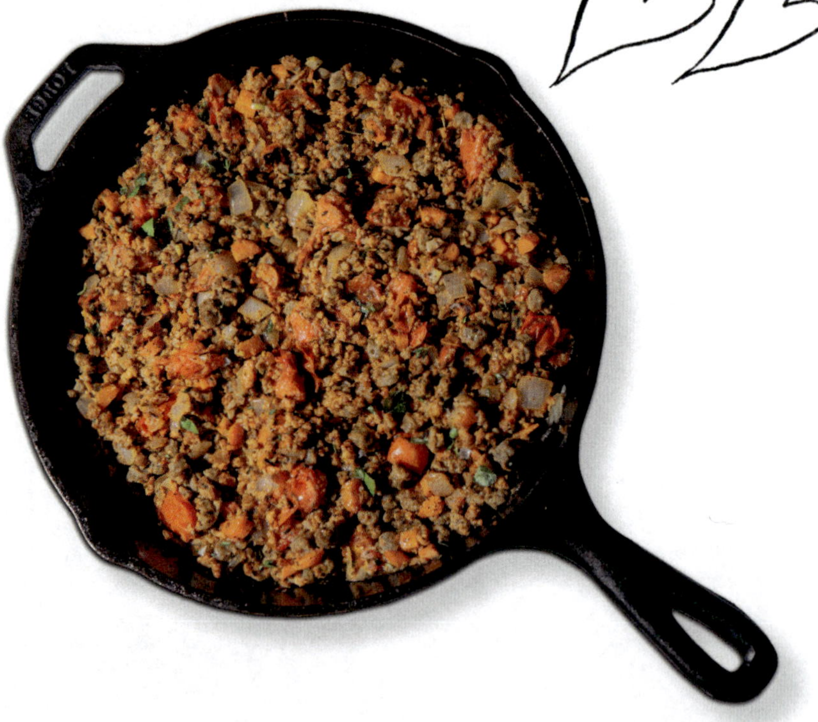

Chef Cathy McKnight

# Keto Beef Stroganoff

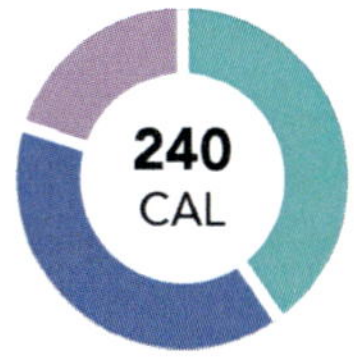


17g Fat
6g Net Carb
15g Protein

**Makes 10 servings:** each ~1 cup, 248 grams

## Ingredients

2 tbsp extra virgin olive oil

1 medium onion, diced

1 lb ground beef

8 oz crimini mushrooms, sliced

2 garlic cloves, crushed

1 cup bone broth, beef or chicken

2 tbsp coconut aminos

4 oz crème fraîche

2 oz heavy cream

2 tsp salt

1 tsp coarse black pepper

3 lb zucchini, spiralized

1 bunch fresh parsley, chopped (approx. ½ cup)

1 bunch fresh thyme, chopped (approx. ½ cup)

## Directions

1. Using a large sauté pan, heat the extra virgin olive oil over medium heat. Add the diced onions and sauté for 3 minutes. Add the beef and stir to break up any lumps. Cook the beef until the juices start to brown, then add the mushrooms and garlic to the pan. Continue cooking until the beef is cooked through and no longer pink.
2. Add the bone broth and coconut aminos, and simmer for about 5–8 minutes until most of the liquid is evaporated. Reduce heat to low, stir in the crème fraîche and the heavy cream. Continue stirring until very smooth.
3. Season with salt and pepper and serve over spiralized zucchini noodles (zoodles). Top with a sprinkle of fresh chopped parsley and thyme. **Serve immediately.**

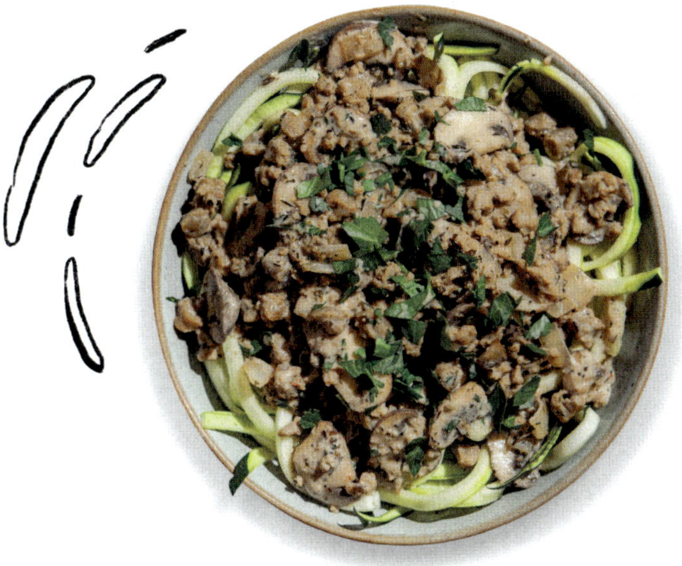

### Kids Can Cook Tips

Kids can help tear the fresh herbs, zest the lemon, and measure the other ingredients. Older kids with knife skills can help mince the garlic and the onion.

Chef Andrew Johnson

# Roasted Spaghetti Squash with Super Simple Marinara

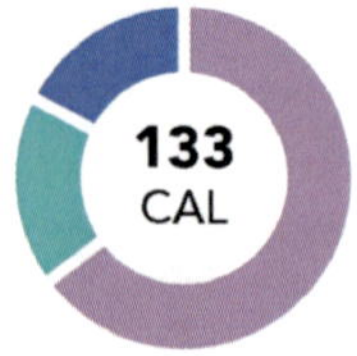


4g **Fat**
14g **Net Carb**
4g **Protein**

**Makes 6 servings:** each ~½ cups sauce and ¾ cup squash, 347 grams

## Ingredients

1 spaghetti squash (approx. 4 lb) halved lengthwise, seeds removed

1 tsp coarse salt

1 tsp freshly ground pepper

½ tsp dried oregano

½ tsp dried garlic granules

½ tsp rosemary powder

½ cup grated parmesan cheese, vegan alternative, or nutritional yeast (approx. 2½ oz)

¼ cup fresh flat-leaf parsley, chopped

1 lb meat (e.g. ground sausage, ground meat, or shredded rotisserie chicken)

**Sauce**

3 tbsp olive oil, divided

½ cup onion ( approx. 1 medium), diced

½ cup carrot (approx. 1 large), diced

3 lb ripe Roma tomatoes, blanched and deseeded

1 cup white wine

2 tsp salt

1 tbsp fresh basil, minced

1 tbsp fresh oregano, minced

1 tbsp fresh thyme, minced

Pinch of chili flakes

¼ tsp ground black pepper

1 tsp salt

*For pre-made sauce, consider Rao's without added sugar*

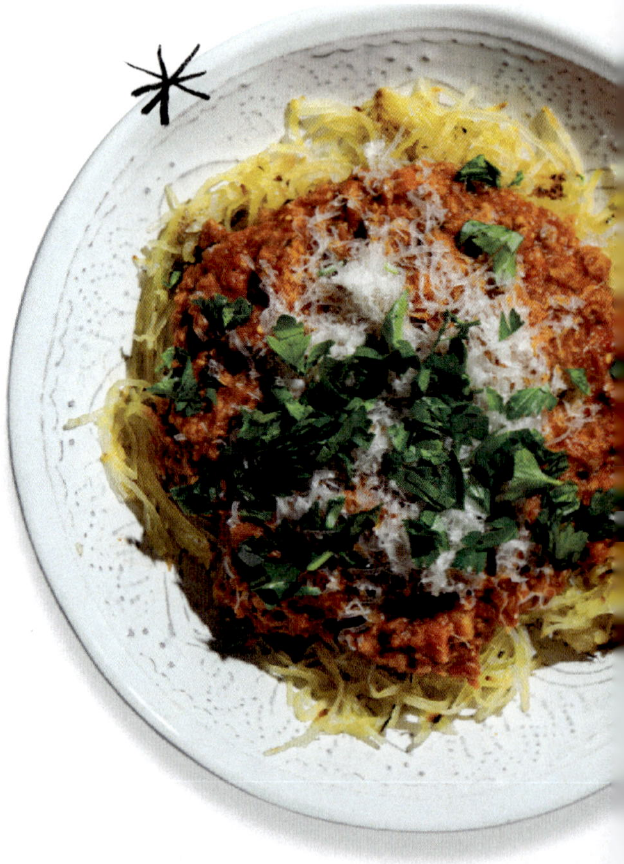

## Directions

1. If using pre-made sauce, skip ahead to the instructions for the squash.
2. To make the sauce, boil a pot of water and prepare an ice bath. Core out the stems from each tomato and slice a shallow "x" on the bottom of each fruit. Blanch the tomatoes in the boiling water for about 45 seconds or until you see the skin start to pucker and split. Immediately lift out the tomato and place in the ice bath to stop cooking. Repeat with all the tomatoes.
3. When finished blanching, peel tomatoes with a knife or your hands. To deseed, cut through the center of the tomato and then into quarters. Use a teaspoon to scoop the seeds out.
4. In a large stockpot, heat 2 tablespoons of olive oil over medium heat. Add the onion and carrots, cooking and stirring until translucent (about 2–3 minutes). Add the tomatoes, fresh herbs, wine, and salt and pepper to taste. Simmer for 30–90 minutes, then blend with an immersion blender.
5. Meanwhile, preheat the oven to 400°F. Brush the cut sides of squash with the remaining 1 tablespoon of oil, and sprinkle with salt, pepper, oregano, garlic powder, and dried rosemary to taste.
6. Place the squash cut sides down on a rimmed baking sheet. Roast until tender (about 45 minutes). Let cool slightly on the sheet or on a wire rack for about 10 minutes, then scrape the inside of the squash with a fork to remove the flesh in long strands.
7. Place the strands in a large bowl, then add marinara sauce and cooked meat. Top with parmesan, fresh parsley, and salt and pepper to taste.

### Fierce Foods Facts

Dietary fiber and lycopene are stars in this recipe. Lycopene, a key nutrient of cooked tomatoes, functions as a key antioxidant. It may even be more bioavailable when consumed with fat (thank you, olive oil). Using spaghetti squash in this recipe increases the fiber content while decreasing the carbohydrate content when compared to pasta. This duo will keep you satisfied longer and your blood sugar more stable.

Chef Alexia Hall, RDN

# Pumpkin Lentil Chili

**Makes 10 servings:** each ~1 cup, 216 grams

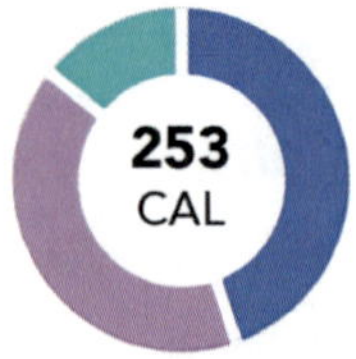


7g **Fat**
21g **Net Carb**
23g **Protein**

## Ingredients

1 can (15 oz) kidney beans, drained

2 cups vegetable or chicken broth

2 cans (15 oz each) fire-roasted diced tomatoes

1 cup dry split red lentils

1 cup pumpkin purée

1 cup chopped yellow onion (approx. ½ medium onion)

1 medium jalapeño pepper, minced

1 tbsp cocoa powder

1 tbsp chili powder

2 tsp ground cumin

½ tsp ground cinnamon

⅛ tsp ground cloves

1 tsp kosher salt

1 lb ground turkey or ground beef

### Recommended Toppings

Diced tomatoes

Diced or sliced scallions

Sour cream or dairy-free alternative (e.g. Forager sour cream)

Shredded cheddar or gruyere or dairy-free alternative (e.g. VioLife shredded cheddar)

Toasted pumpkin seeds/pepitas

## Directions

1. Add all the ingredients (excluding the toppings) to a 3-quart (or larger) slow cooker and stir.
2. Cook on high for 4–5 hours or on low for 8–10 hours, until the lentils are tender and the chili is thick and hearty.
3. An hour before the end of your chosen cook time, use a large sauté pan and brown the ground beef or ground turkey over medium heat. Drain the fat (or use if following a ketogenic diet), then season with salt and pepper. Add browned meat to chili during the remaining cooking time. Serve with assorted toppings as desired.

## For carbohydrate-conscious options:

1. Reduce pumpkin purée to ½ cup. Omit kidney beans and lentils. Add 15 ounces unsweetened full-fat coconut milk.
2. Serve with 2 tablespoons each shredded cheese, sour cream, and scallions.

**Carb-conscious options:**
This will reduce net carbohydrates to 5 grams per serving, 357 calories, 26 grams of fat, and 22 grams of protein.

### Kids Can Cook Tips

This recipe is simple for such a busy day, though it has lots of opportunities for the kids to measure ingredients and toss them into the slow cooker. Have the kids help taste and decide when more seasoning is necessary.

## Fierce Foods Facts

Perfect for a pre-Halloween dinner, this recipe is a sure bet to fix those "too-much-sugar blues." The abundant protein and fiber can help kids feel full, lessening the desire to overeat sweets later. It also helps to slow the rush of sugar into the bloodstream, preventing the blood sugar crash that ultimately follows. The abundant B vitamins also help to ensure a sustained energy release, specifically B6 which is important in every energy transaction in the body. This recipe is also loaded with vitamin A, thanks to the pumpkin, which helps to support excellent eyesight!

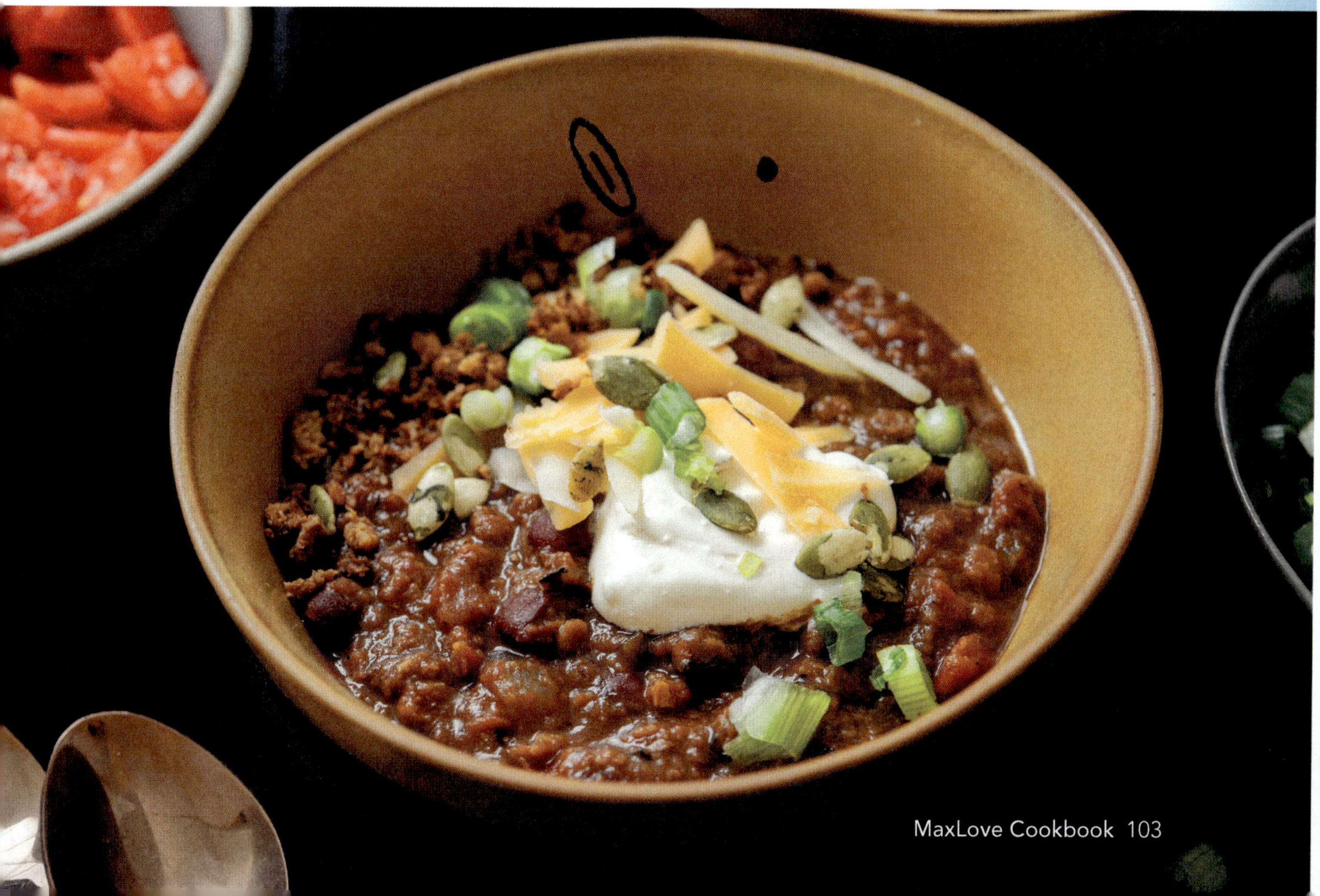

Chef Cathy McKnight

# Thai-Style Lettuce Cups

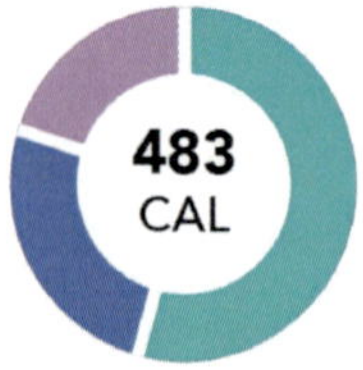


40g Fat
15g Net Carb
19g Protein

**Makes 8 servings:** each ~1 cup, 256 grams

## Ingredients

2 tsp sesame oil

1 lb ground beef

3 cloves garlic, minced

½ inch ginger, minced

1 medium shallot, minced

1 tsp fish sauce

16 Bibb Lettuce leaves, cleaned and dried

2 tsp sugar-free garlic chili sauce

1 pkg mung beans

8 oz carrot, julienne

6 oz daikon radish, julienne

2 oz scallion, minced

2 medium cucumbers, half moons

2 avocados, sliced

1 bunch cilantro, chopped

8 oz cashew or macadamia nut, crushed

### Dipping Sauce

¼ cup sesame oil

¼ cup rice vinegar

2 dashes garlic chili sauce

## Directions

1. In a large sauté pan on medium heat, add the sesame oil and the beef. Stir in the garlic, ginger, shallot, and fish sauce. Sauté until the beef is done and no longer pink, then stir in the chili sauce and adjust the seasoning.
2. On a large platter, set the cleaned lettuce leaves on the back of the platter. Pile the seasoned beef in the middle of the platter, then arrange the mung beans, carrot, daikon, cucumber, scallions, and sliced avocados in rows around the beef. Sprinkle the cilantro and crushed nuts over the beef before you serve.
3. To make the dipping sauce, add the remaining sesame oil and rice vinegar to a small bowl and whisk in a dash of garlic chili to taste. Serve immediately.

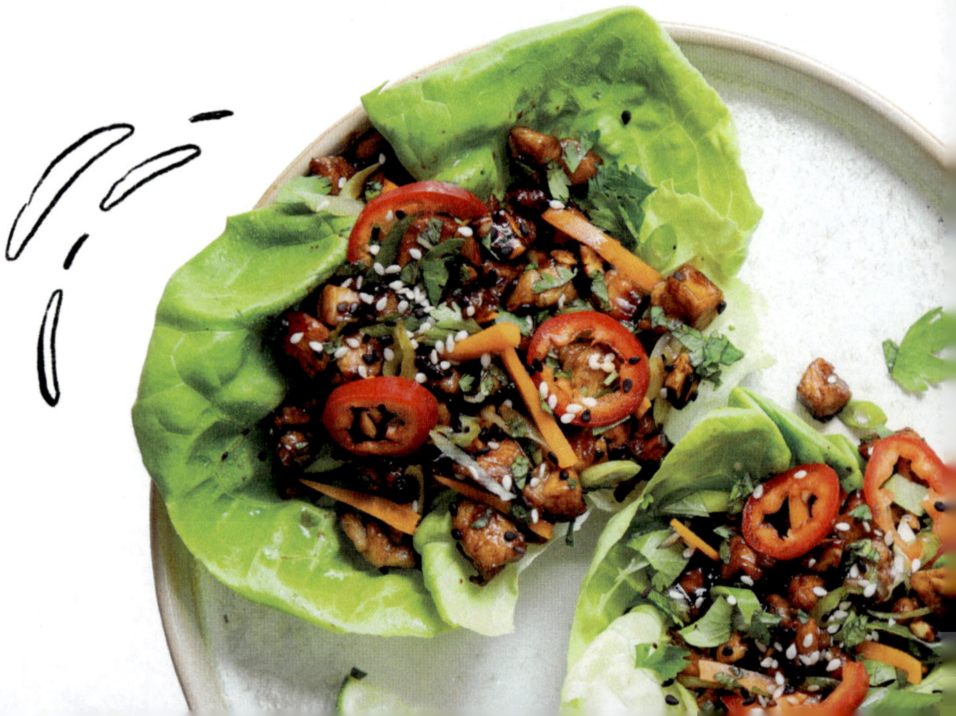

Chef Andrew Johnson

# Taco Stuffed Avocados

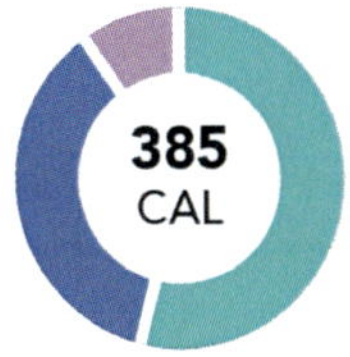


30g Fat
5g Net Carb
20g Protein

**Makes 8 servings:** each ~¾ cup filling in ½ avocado shell, 193 grams

## Ingredients

1 tbsp olive oil

½ cup yellow onion (approx. 1 medium), minced

4 cloves garlic, minced

1 lb ground beef (70% lean)

½ tsp chipotle chili powder

½ tsp salt

1 tsp cumin

1 tsp coriander

1 tsp dried oregano

4 oz tomato sauce

3 avocados, halved

1 cup cheddar cheese, shredded

¼ cup cherry tomatoes, sliced

¼ cup lettuce, shredded

1 cup fresh cilantro (approx. 3 oz), sliced

1 cup sour cream, full-fat

## Directions

1. Using a medium size sauté pan, add the olive oil and heat over a medium flame. Once the oil is hot, add the diced yellow onion and garlic and sauté for 2 minutes or until they are translucent.
2. Add the ground beef, breaking it up with the back of a spoon, cooking until browned. Add the chili powder, salt, cumin, dried oregano, and tomato sauce, then stir to combine. Cook for another 3–4 minutes, then remove from flame and set aside.
3. Meanwhile, halve and remove the pits from the avocados Using a spoon, carefully remove the majority of the flesh from the avocados, while retaining the shell of the avocado. Using a small bowl and a fork, mash the fruit from the avocados.
4. Combine the mashed avocados with the cheddar cheese, tomatoes, lettuce, cilantro, and sour cream. Spoon the avocado mixture evenly among the 6 avocado shells. Divide the meat mixture and spoon this evenly over the filled avocado shells. Sprinkle with additional fresh cilantro, if desired. Serve and consume immediately.

### Fierce Foods Facts

This nutrient-packed dinner has everything—it's balanced with plenty of muscle-building protein and heart-healthy fat. It is also super flavorful and is a rich source in just about every mineral category (calcium, copper, iron, magnesium, phosphorus, potassium, and selenium).

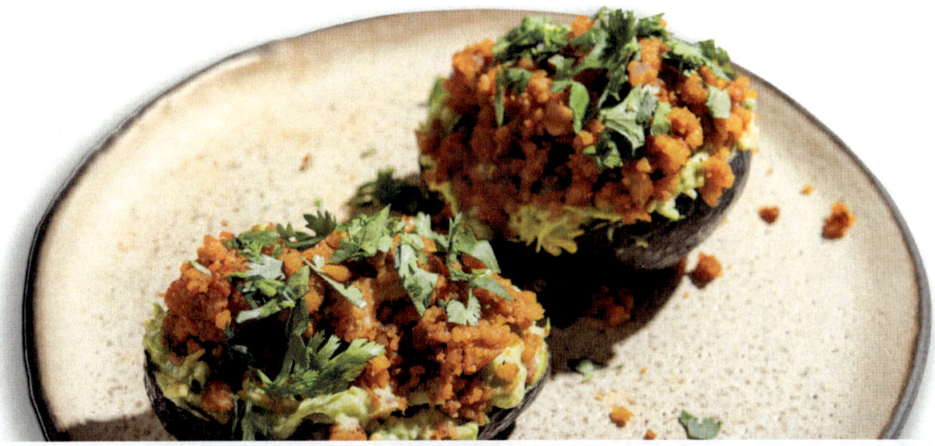

Chef Andrew Johnson

# Southern Oven-Fried Chicken

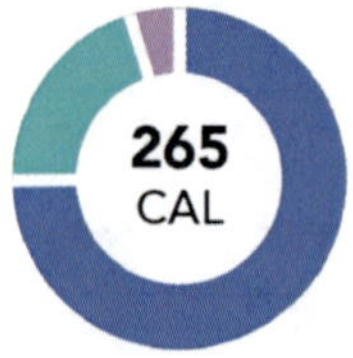


10g Fat
2g Net Carb
38g Protein

**Makes 20 servings:** each 4 ounces, 127 grams

## Ingredients

5 lb chicken, any variety (use bone-in/skin-on for the most classic fried chicken results)

1½ cups ground flaxseed

½ cup parmesan cheese, grated

3 tbsp paprika

2 tbsp black pepper

1 tbsp ground ginger

1 tbsp sea salt

1 tbsp mustard powder

1 tbsp smoked paprika

1 tbsp coriander

2 tsp dried thyme

2 tsp garlic powder

1 tsp dried oregano

1 tsp dried basil

1 tbsp mayonnaise

1 tbsp Dijon mustard

Oil spray

## Directions

1. Preheat the oven to 400°F. In a large mixing bowl add the ground flaxseed, parmesan, and all of the herbs and spices, and mix until fully incorporated to create your spice mixture. Remove the chicken from the refrigerator for 12–20 minutes prior to coating and cooking the chicken (this helps to maintain a better crust in the chicken).
2. In another large mixing bowl, add the chicken parts, mayonnaise, and Dijon mustard and mix to completely cover the chicken. The secret is to coat the chicken in a thin layer of the mayo-Dijon mixture, which will act as a glue to adhere the spices. Then, pour enough of the spice mixture onto the chicken and toss until coated evenly, adding more spice mixture until every piece of chicken is thoroughly coated.
3. Place the chicken on a baking sheet with a wire rack, making sure that the pieces are not touching. Spray the chicken liberally with oil spray before baking.
4. Bake bone-in/skin-on chicken for approximately 40–45 minutes until golden brown.
5. For chicken tenders, slice large boneless breasts into approximately 6 or 7 pieces on an angle (about ¾-inch thick), then follow the same steps to coat the chicken. Bake chicken tenders for 10–15 minutes, then serve with your favorite dipping sauce.

### Fierce Foods Facts

This healthified fried chicken provides loads of healthy fat with Omega 3s for growing brains. It is also loaded with protein for strong muscles and a great supply of B vitamins for sustaining energy and focus levels for those long school days!

## Kids Can Cook Tips

There are so many opportunities to measure all of the flavorful spices in this dish. Kids will also have fun tossing the chicken with the mayonnaise and Dijon and making sure to coat all the pieces of chicken in the spice mixture. Who doesn't love cold fried chicken in a lunchbox? Be sure to pack with an ice pack to maintain safety throughout the day.

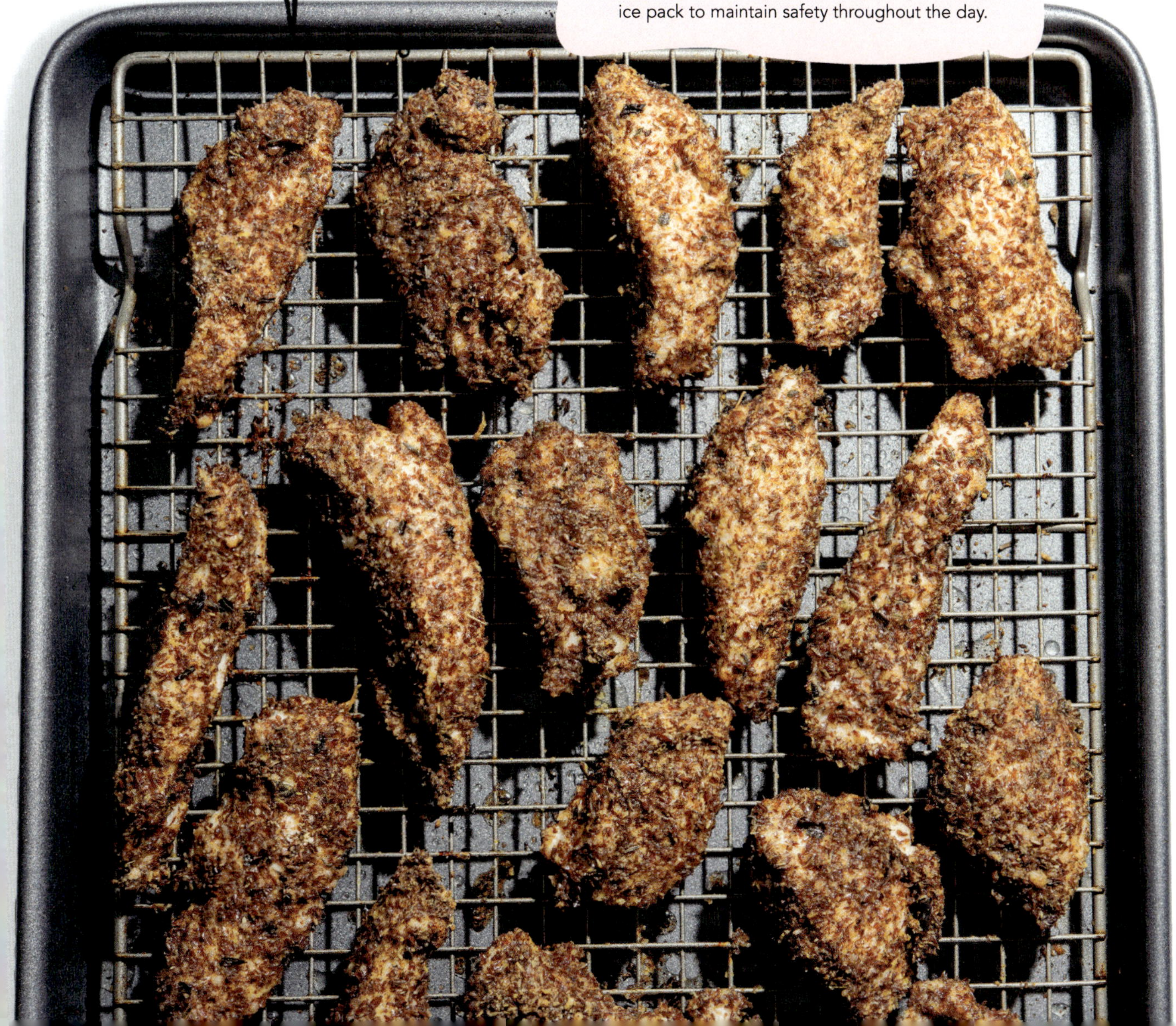

Chef Andrew Johnson

# Grilled Chicken Panzanella Salad

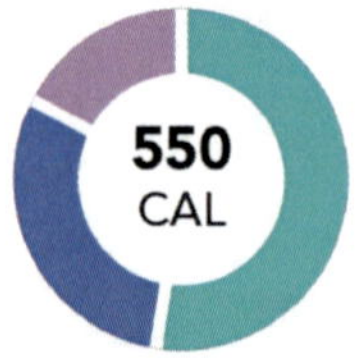


44g Fat
14g Net Carb
25g Protein

**Makes 8 servings:** each 1 cup salad, 3 ounces chicken, 260 grams

## Ingredients

1 lb chicken breasts, sliced in half lengthwise

### Marinade

4 tbsp olive oil

2 lemons, zested and juiced

4 garlic cloves, peeled and minced

4 tbsp fresh oregano, chopped

1 tbsp vinegar (e.g. apple cider, red, white wine, champagne, or rice)

1 tsp smoked paprika

Sea or kosher salt and black pepper to taste

### Salad

4 cups heirloom tomatoes, sliced into wedges

1 cup cherry tomatoes, halved

1 English cucumber halved, cut into ½" half-moon shapes

¼ cup red onion thinly shaved

½ cup pitted olives

Fresh basil leaves to garnish

### Croutons

6 slices keto bread, cut into ¾-inch cubes or torn

8 tbsp olive oil

½ tsp paprika

½ tsp dried oregano

½ tsp dried thyme

4 cloves garlic, peeled and minced

### Dressing

1 tsp Dijon mustard

1 shallot, finely minced

1 clove garlic, peeled and minced

1 lemon, zested and juiced

4 tsp vinegar (e.g. apple cider, red, white wine, champagne, or rice)

⅓ cup olive oil

Sea or kosher salt to taste

## Directions

1. In a large mixing bowl combine the marinade ingredients, mix well, then add chicken and refrigerate and marinate for 2 hours.
2. Preheat grill to medium/high, remove chicken from the marinade, and grill both sides until just cooked through–approximately 10 minutes. Transfer to a large clean mixing bowl, cover with plastic wrap or foil and let rest 10 minutes. Slice chicken into strips, toss it back into the bowl, and pour off the excess juices.

3. Into the chicken bowl add: tomatoes, cucumber, olives and red onion.

4. To make the croutons: Preheat oven to 400°F. In a large clean mixing bowl add: 8 tablespoons of olive oil, 4 cloves minced garlic, paprika, oregano, thyme, salt and pepper–then mix well. Add keto bread cubes or torn bits and toss until evenly coated.

5. On a parchment lined sheet pan add croutons in a single layer. Bake in the oven for 5–10 minutes until golden brown. Remove and let cool.

6. In a mason jar add the dressing ingredients in order listed. Place a lid on the jar and shake vigorously to emulsify.

7. Lightly drizzle veggies and chicken with dressing and gently toss to evenly coat. Then throw in the croutons and toss again. This step will allow the croutons to capture some of the dressing, but not get overly soggy. Then transfer the salad to your favorite serving dish. Garnish liberally with fresh basil leaves. Enjoy!

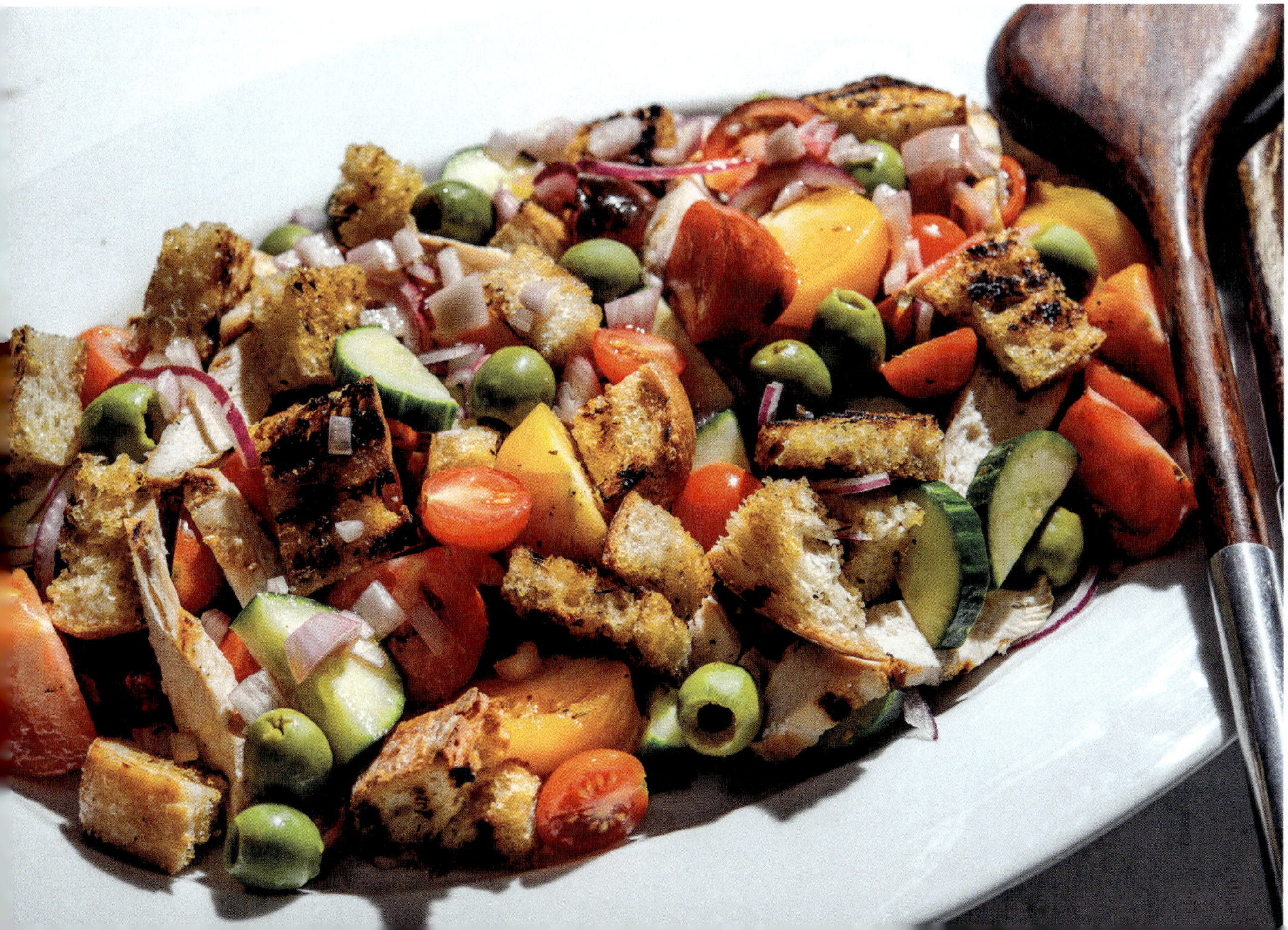

Chef Cathy McKnight

# Cold Thai Zoodle and Shrimp Salad

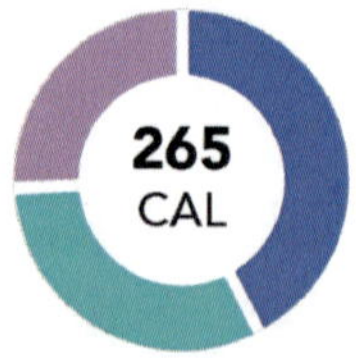


15g **Fat**
12g **Net Carb**
20g **Protein**

**Makes 8 servings:** each ~1½ cups, 302 grams

## Ingredients

### Salad

6 cups raw zucchini noodles or cooked and chilled Thai rice noodles (or 50/50 mix)

1 lb (16–20 count) shrimp, peeled and deveined (consider pre-cooked)

1 small head Napa cabbage, chopped

1 cup red, yellow, or orange bell peppers, diced

Chopped cilantro

1 red jalapeño, thinly sliced (optional)

Fresh Thai basil leaves (optional)

### Vinaigrette

¼ cup toasted sesame oil

2 tsp ginger root, freshly grated

1 clove garlic, minced

½ tsp Red Boat Fish Sauce (optional)

1 large lime, juiced

1 tbsp unsweetened rice vinegar

2 tbsp toasted sesame seeds

1 tsp Sambal chili paste

### Marinade

1 lime, juiced

1 clove garlic, crushed

½ tsp ginger, grated

Dash of salt and pepper

### Garnish recommendations

½ cup toasted cashews, macadamia, or almonds, chopped

## Directions

1. Using a small bowl, whisk the ingredients for the marinade together. Add the shrimp and marinate for at least 5 minutes and up to 20 minutes.
2. Grill the shrimp (if uncooked) until no longer pink and cooked through. If using cooked shrimp, marinate for at least 5 minutes and use immediately on the salad.
3. To assemble the salad, combine the raw zoodles or cooked and chilled rice noodles with the cabbage and lightly toss to mix. Add the shrimp, bell peppers, and jalapeño, then toss with the vinaigrette and garnish with nuts, cilantro, and Thai basil leaves. Best served chilled and immediately.

## Fierce Foods Facts

What to do when it's too hot to cook? Make a cold zoodle salad, of course! This flavorful salad provides almost 100% of the daily vitamins C and K. And thanks to the shrimp, we also get over 45% of the day's selenium, 25% of the day's magnesium, and some zinc and calcium: a winning combination to support the immune system and strong bones!

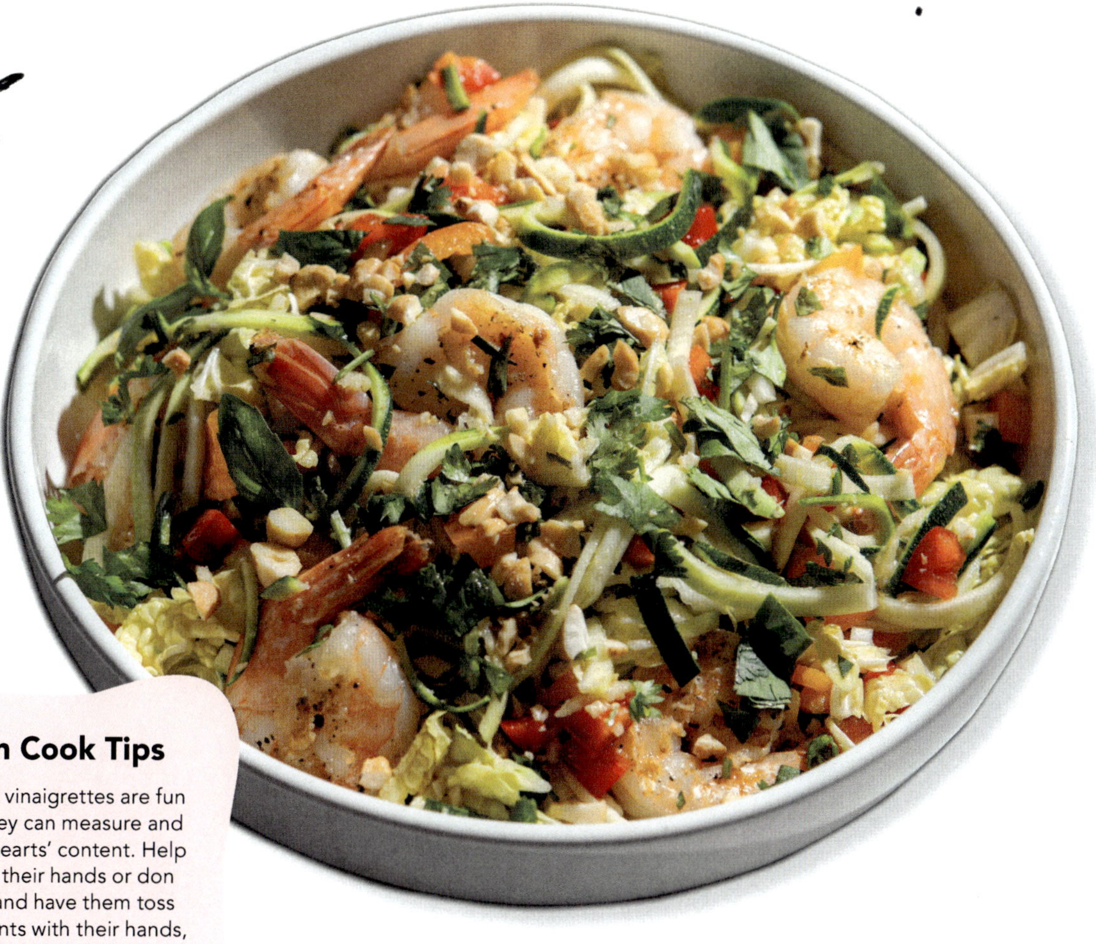

## Kids Can Cook Tips

Marinades and vinaigrettes are fun for kids and they can measure and whisk to their hearts' content. Help the kids wash their hands or don some gloves and have them toss all the ingredients with their hands, one of the best tools they have! Pro tip: Use a larger bowl with a rubber bottom to help contain spills.

Chef Andrew Johnson

# Slow Cooker Turkey Breast with Grain-Free Gravy

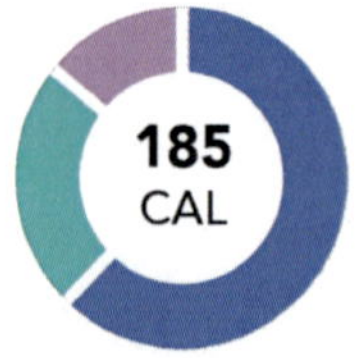


13g Fat
7g Net Carb
35g Protein

**Makes 8 servings:** each ~4 ounces and ¼ cup gravy, 149 grams

## Ingredients

2 lb boneless turkey breast, skin on

¾ tsp paprika

¾ tsp dried thyme

1¼ tsp kosher salt, plus more for seasoning

½ tsp black pepper

1¼ tsp garlic powder

4 tsp extra virgin olive oil

6 cloves garlic, roughly chopped

1 cup yellow onion, 1" dice

3 sprigs rosemary

3 tbsp ghee or coconut oil, drippings, or lard

4 tbsp tapioca flour or arrowroot powder

2½ cups chicken broth or bone broth

½ tbsp soy sauce or coconut aminos

¼ tsp poultry seasoning

## Directions

1. Rinse the turkey breast and dry thoroughly with a towel or paper towel. Place turkey breast on a sheet pan or baking stone.
2. In a small bowl combine paprika, thyme, salt, pepper, garlic powder, and olive oil. Using hands, rub the spice mixture evenly over both sides of the turkey breast. Sprinkle the garlic cloves, onions, and rosemary evenly over the bottom of a 6-quart slow cooker. Place the turkey breast inside, cover, and cook on low for 3 hours.
3. Cook until the turkey reaches an internal temperature of 165°F. Check at 2½ hours and continue to cook as needed. Remove the turkey from the slow cooker and place on a sheet pan lined with foil. Set oven to broil. Place the turkey inside about 12" away from the top. Broil until the skin is golden brown and crispy, about 5–7 minutes. Keep a close eye that the skin does not burn.
4. Allow to rest for 10 minutes before slicing. Strain the contents of the slow cooker into a bowl, reserving only the juices. It should yield about a ½ cup of liquid.
5. For the gravy, use a small saucepan over low heat to keep turkey stock from the slow cooker hot (the mixture should not be boiling). Add additional turkey (or chicken bone) broth until there are about 2½ cups of stock total.

6. Using another medium saucepan over medium-low heat, heat the ghee or other fat. Using a whisk, add tapioca starch and stir vigorously until smooth. Continue cooking for 1 minute, whisking constantly. The mixture should be golden and bubbling. Slowly pour in the warm stock while continuing to whisk until the mixture is smooth.
7. Cook the gravy for a couple of minutes or until thickened, whisking regularly. Gravy will be a very light tan. For a darker, richer gravy, add the soy sauce or coconut aminos to taste. Add the poultry seasoning. If necessary, season the gravy with more salt and pepper to taste.

## Fierce Foods Facts

This super-star of the Thanksgiving table is a piece of cake to prepare thanks to the Crockpot! It also supplies an excellent dose of tryptophan filled protein which can be a wonderful mood booster. The iron and Vitamin A are also a nice bonus, thanks to the dark meat on the turkey.

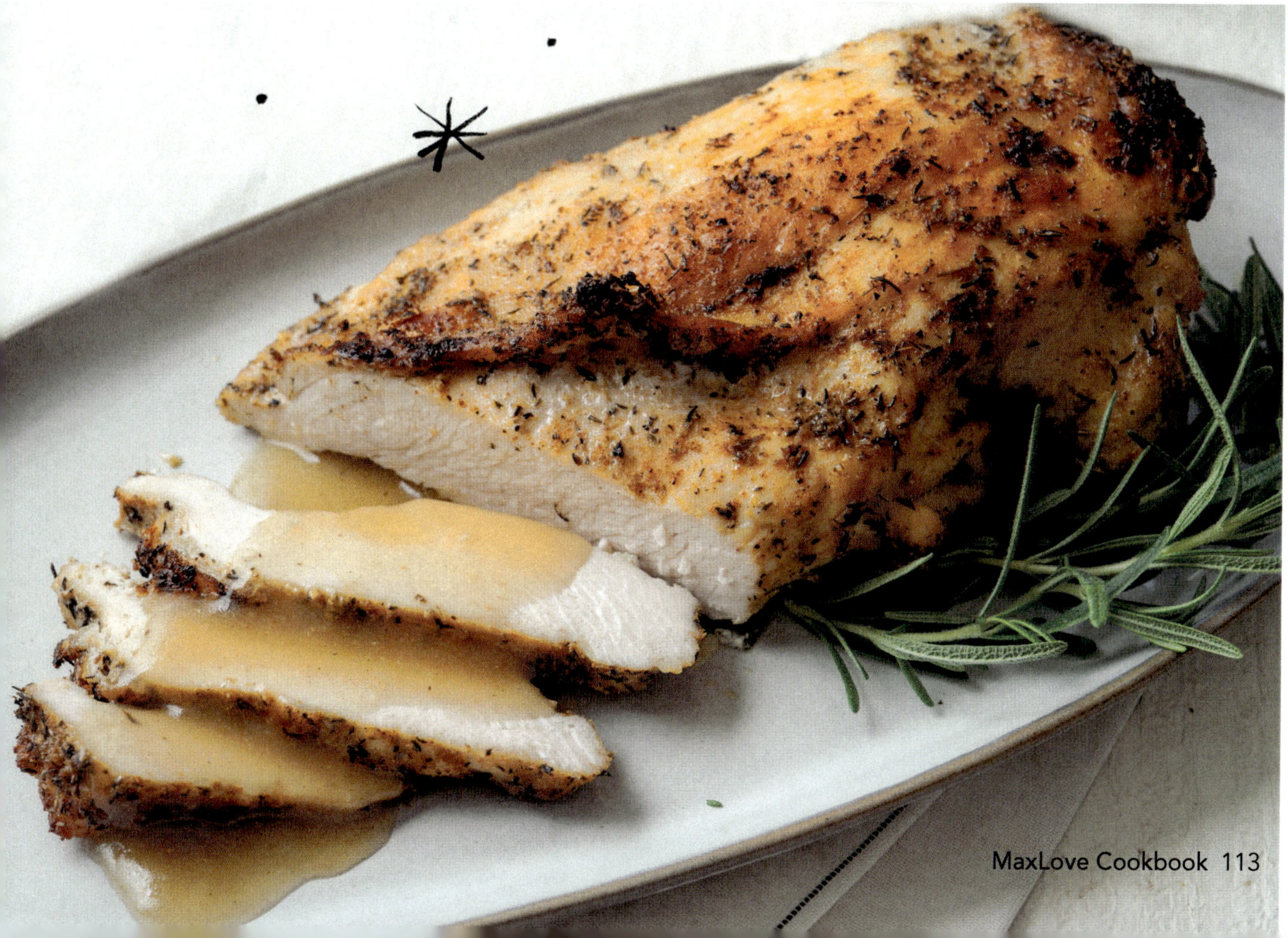

Chef Andrew Johnson

# Chilled Summer Garden Soup

**Makes 8 servings:** each ~1 cup, 254 grams

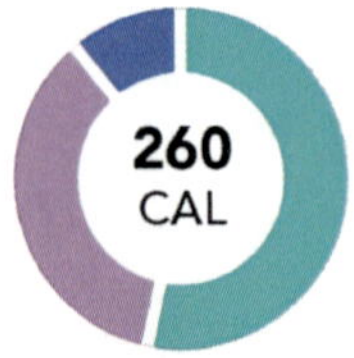


21g **Fat**
14g **Net Carb**
4g **Protein**

## Ingredients

4 ears corn, cut off the cob

2 cups yellow heirloom tomatoes, chopped

2 yellow bell peppers, seeded and chopped

2 cups cucumber, peeled and chopped

½ cup extra virgin olive oil

¼ cup seasoned rice vinegar or apple cider vinegar

1 tbsp kosher or sea salt

Freshly ground black pepper to taste

1 tsp Sambal chili paste (optional)

### Garnish recommendations

1 cup cherry tomatoes, sliced

2 avocados, sliced

1–2 tbsp tender herbs, chopped (basil, oregano, marjoram, lemon verbena, etc.)

1–2 tbsp pepitas, roasted

## Directions

1. In a blender or food processor, add the corn, tomato, bell peppers, cucumber, vinegar, salt, and pepper and blend until smooth. Drizzle in the olive oil until you achieve the desired consistency.
2. Serve immediately or refrigerate before serving. Garnish with cherry tomatoes, sliced avocado, herbs, seeds, a drizzle of olive oil, and coarse salt.

### Fierce Foods Facts

This recipe is a great, wonderfully easy way to stay out of a hot kitchen with its no-cook instructions. And, by using a lot of farm-fresh veggies, it comes loaded with nutrients including everything from B and C vitamins to lots of minerals too! Try pairing it with grilled meat for a balanced meal.

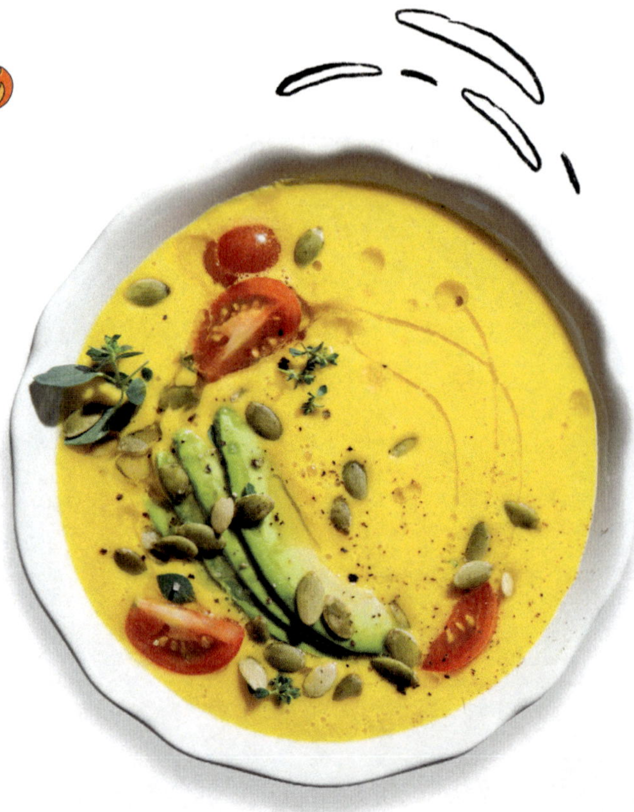

Chef Andrew Johnson

# Easy Pan Southwest Bake

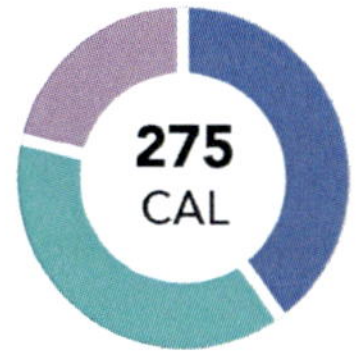


24g Fat
13g Net Carb
25g Protein

**Makes 10 servings:** each ~1¼ cups, 264 grams

## Ingredients

5 cups chicken, peppers, and onions (leftovers from Easy Pan Chicken Fajitas)

1 cup sour cream

10 low-carb tortillas (6"– 8"), cut into chip-sized wedges

8 oz baby spinach

4 cups shredded Monterey Jack or cheddar cheese

1 can (28 oz) green or red enchilada sauce

**Garnish recommendations**

Sliced scallions or chopped cilantro

## Directions

1. Preheat the oven to 400°F. In a greased 9"x13" baking dish, pour in half of the enchilada sauce and layer in half of the tortilla wedges.
2. In a large mixing bowl, toss together the chicken fajita mixture, sour cream, 2 cups of shredded cheese, and spinach, then add that to the baking dish. Layer in the rest of the tortilla wedges and cover with the remaining enchilada sauce.
3. Cover with foil and bake for 30–40 minutes. Uncover and add the rest of the shredded cheese and bake for 10 minutes or until the cheese is melted and golden. Garnish with scallions or cilantro.
4. To save for later, cool completely and wrap tightly to store in the freezer for up to 6 months.

### Fierce Foods Facts

This recipe is a great way to easily turn one healthy dinner into another. This recipe is loaded with vitamins A and E, both of which are important in fighting off free radical damage, especially damaging in a growing brain. Eat these recipes twice this week to double the antioxidant delivery!

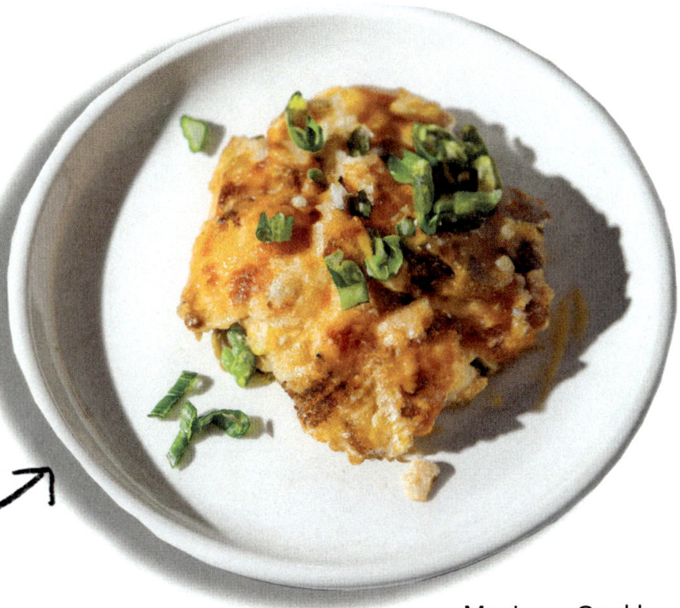

Chef Cathy McKnight

# Cauliflower Mac 'n' Cheese

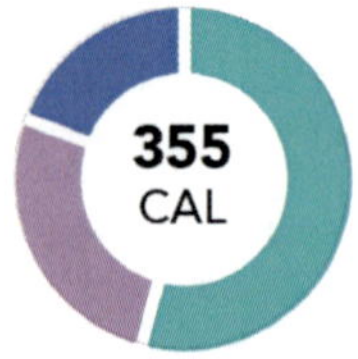


29g Fat
14g Net Carb
10g Protein

**Makes 8 servings:** each ~¾ cup, 175 grams

## Ingredients

4 cups cauliflower florets

2 tsp salt

1 cup heavy cream

1 cup half and half

1 white onion, cubed

4 garlic cloves, minced

1 lb cheddar cheese, shredded

1 cup panko bread crumbs

4 tbsp butter or ghee, melted

**Notes:** This recipe creates double the amount of cheese sauce needed. Freeze the remaining half for future use.

## Directions

1. Break the cauliflower florets into small pieces, about the size of penne pasta. Lay the cauliflower on a cookie sheet, sprinkle with salt, and bake at 400°F for 25 minutes, adding time until the cauliflower is soft and slightly browned.
2. While the cauliflower is cooking, add the heavy cream and half and half to a 2-quart saucepan. Bring to a simmer and add the onion and garlic. Simmer for 25 minutes, stirring a few times and making sure not to let the cream boil or curdle.
3. Strain the cream into a large saucepan on low heat. Stir in the shredded cheese a cup at a time, reserving 1 cup of the cheese. Once the cheese is melted, turn off the heat and let it rest while you get the cauliflower.
4. Drain off any water from the cauliflower before placing in a 10"x10" casserole dish. Stir in the cheese sauce and mix gently until distributed evenly. Sprinkle the remaining cheese on top.
5. Mix the panko and melted butter or ghee and sprinkle it over the top of the casserole and bake at 400°F for 25 minutes or until bubbling and crisp. For a crunchy topping, broil on high for 3 minutes before taking it out of the oven.
6. Once out of the oven, let it rest for 10 minutes before serving.
7. For a 50-50 variation, consider using 2 cups of cooked high-protein pasta (such as bean or lentil) in place of 2 cups of the cauliflower.

**Pro Tip:** Like most casseroles and baked pasta dishes—especially cheesy ones—it's important to let the dish rest for 10 minutes before serving. Digging in too quickly will result in a liquid, soupy scoop, plus, letting it sit will allow the dish to cool to an edible temperature.

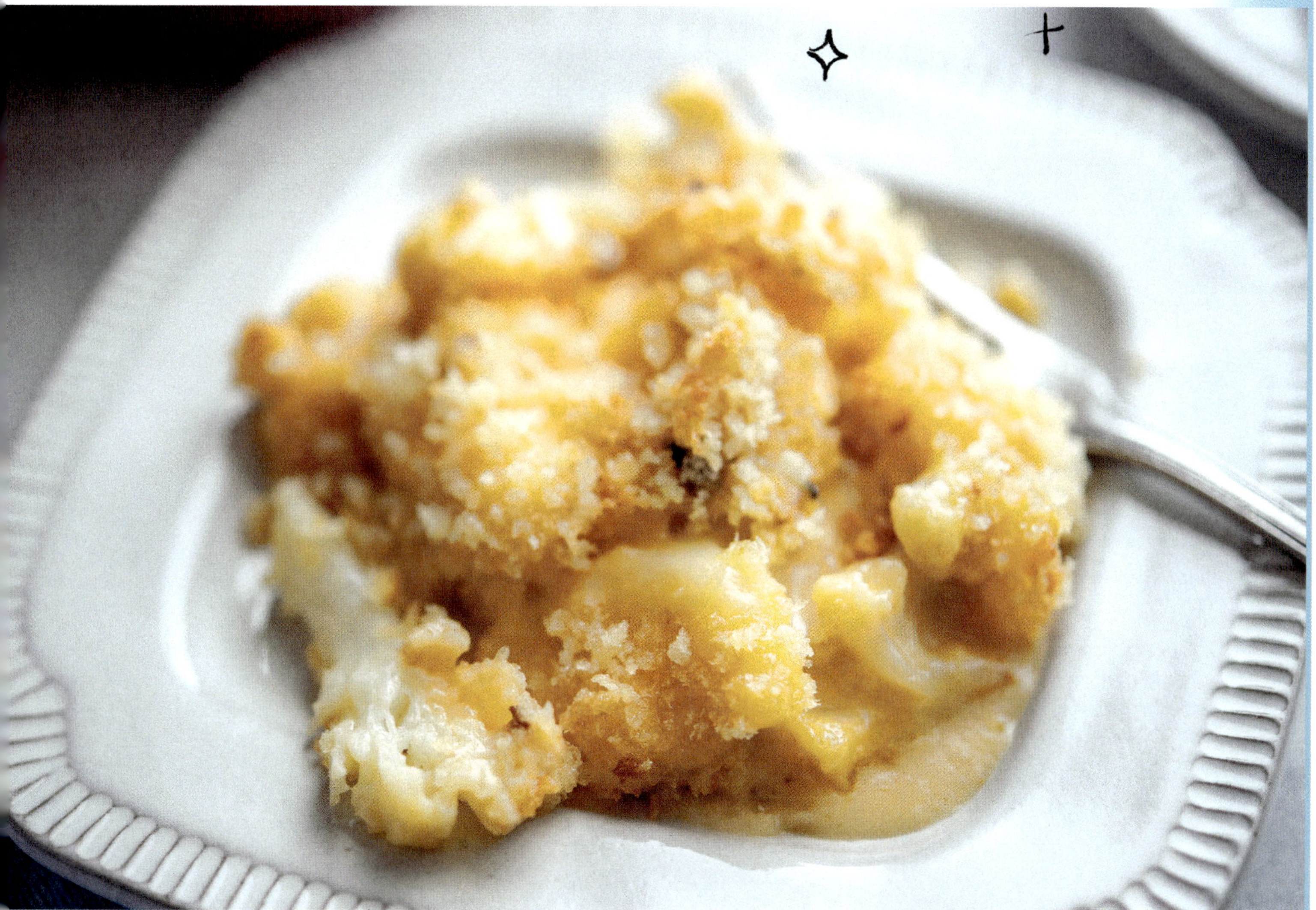

Chef Alexia Hall, RDN

# Salad Shakers

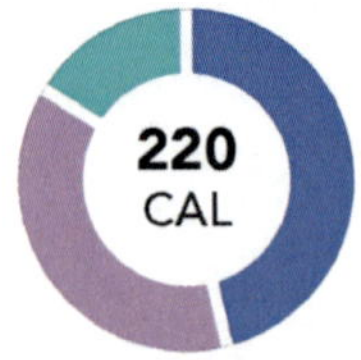


7g **Fat**
17g **Net Carb**
21g **Protein**

**Makes 4 servings:** 1 salad each, ~235 grams

## Ingredients

½ cup uncooked quinoa

1½ cups water

1 rotisserie chicken, de-boned and shredded

½ cup carrot, shredded

½ cup cherry or grape tomatoes, sliced

¼ cup currants

¼ cup pumpkin seeds

5 oz spring mix

### Dressing

½ cup plain Greek yogurt

1 tsp honey or alternative (e.g. Pyure Hunny)

2 tbsp apple cider vinegar

¼ tsp sea salt

1 bunch cilantro

1 lemon, juiced

2 cloves garlic crushed

*Will also need:*
4 wide-mouth mason jars, quart size

## Directions

1. Using a medium-sized saucepan, add quinoa and 1½ cups of water. Cover and bring to a boil over high heat. Once boiling, reduce the temperature to low. Cook 10–15 minutes until able to fluff with a fork and all water has been absorbed. Cool completely.
2. Using a blender or food processor, combine the Greek yogurt, honey, apple cider vinegar, sea salt, fresh cilantro, lemon juice, and garlic cloves. Whir or blend on high until well combined, set aside.
3. Add 2 tablespoons of dressing to the bottom of each jar. Layer the remaining salad ingredients in each mason jar in the following order, from the most sturdy vegetables to the most tender vegetables at the top. This order will ensure that what comes in contact with the acidic dressing will not wilt before the week is up.
4. On top of the dressing layer 2 tablespoons carrot, 2 ounces chicken, 2 tablespoons tomatoes, 1 tablespoon dried currants, 2 tablespoons quinoa, 1 tablespoon pumpkin seeds, and finally the most tender, about 1 cup spring mix lettuce.
5. When ready to serve, shake the salad to incorporate dressing through ingredients. You may eat directly from the jar. Will stay fresh in the refrigerator for up to 5 days.

**Mix it up with these variations:**

*Poppy Seed:* poppy seed dressing, jicama shreds, carrot shreds, pomegranate seeds, sliced almonds, feta cheese, baby spinach

*Asian:* Asian ginger dressing, snap peas, carrot shreds, cabbage shreds, water chestnuts, quinoa, toasted sesame seeds, shredded lettuce

*Italian:* balsamic dressing, shredded carrots, sliced bell peppers, chopped cauliflower, mini mozzarella balls, cherry tomatoes

*Chicken Caesar:* Caesar dressing, carrot shreds, diced grilled chicken, olives, lettuce, shredded parmesan

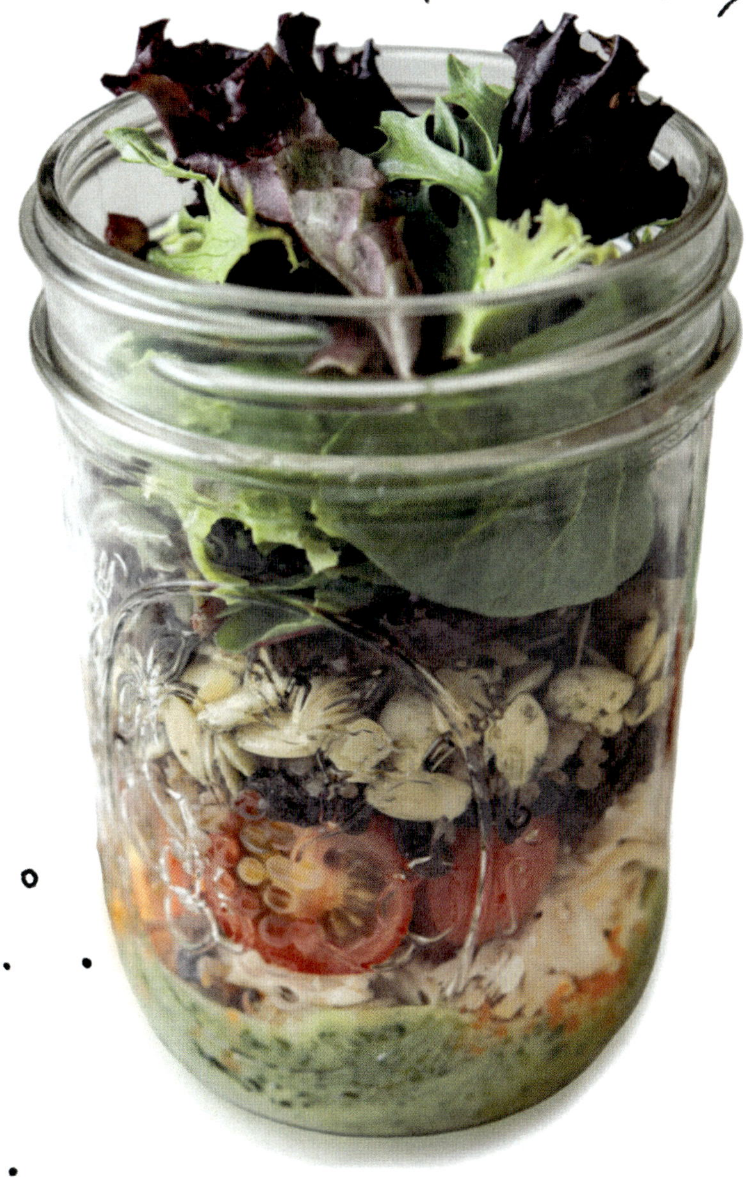

## Fierce Foods Facts

This salad is loaded with fiber for a happy set of gut bugs. It also has almost 90% of the day's vitamin A, helpful for a strong immune system. It provides a nice amount of zinc, magnesium, phosphorus, and calcium, which is great for strong bones, hair, skin, and nails.

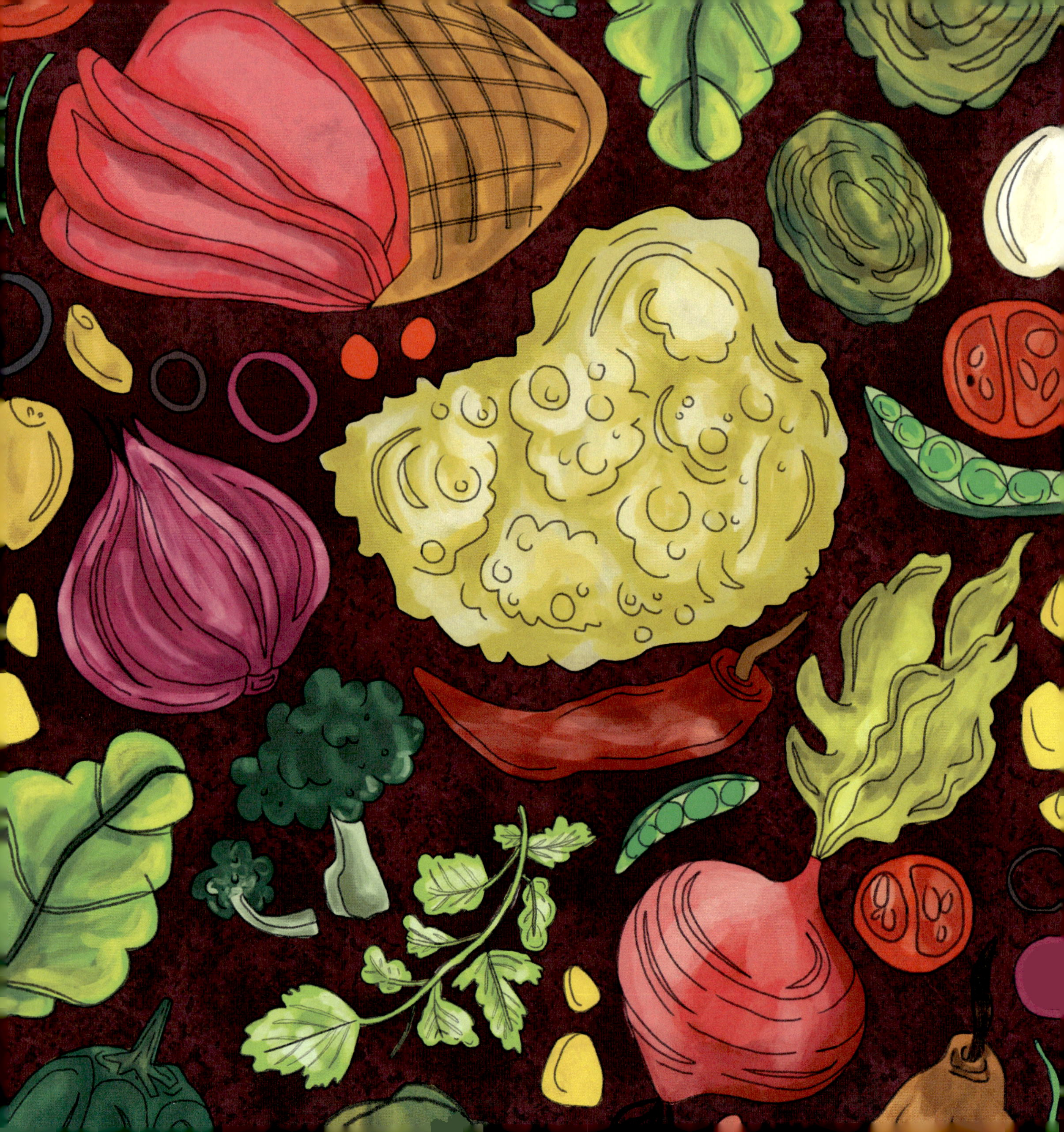

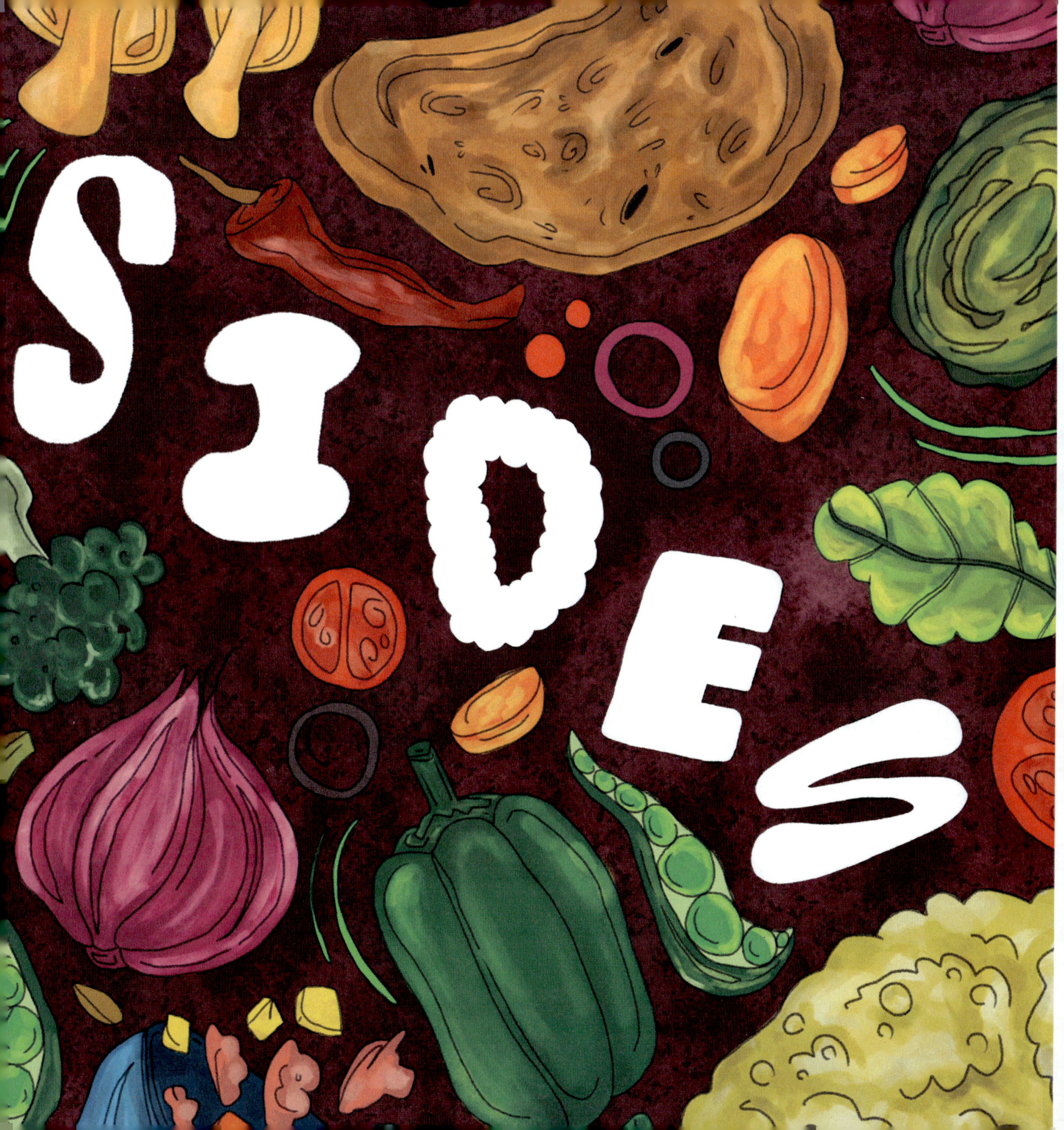
SIDES

# Sides



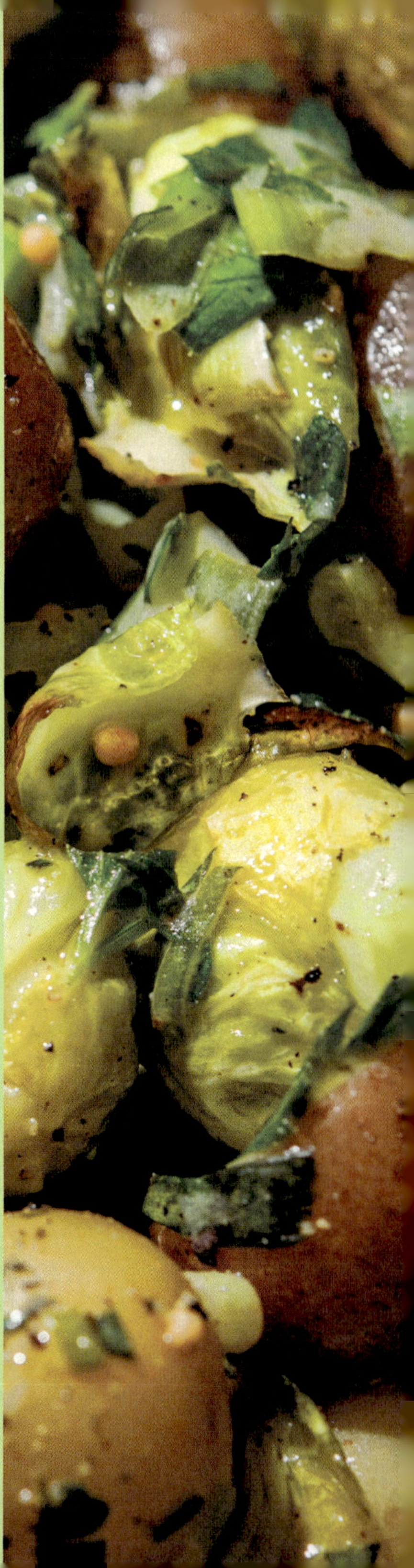

If proteins are the star of the main dish, then vegetables are the star of the sides. However, as important as they are to nutrition, vegetables are likely going to get more refusals than anything else on the table. Increased fruit and vegetable consumption is associated with lower health risks including the development of cancer, and are now shown to be inversely proportional to severe symptoms of ADHD.

So why do we refuse vegetables and what can we do about it? One of the best ways to encourage children to eat vegetables is for their parents to model enjoyment of them at a young age. Sadly though, less than 7% of the adults in this country eat the recommended 2½ cups of vegetables in a day. Not liking the flavor or texture is one of the biggest stated reasons and experts think this may be because of food scientists who work hard to make ultra-processed food palatable. If the stronger-tasting vegetable is competing with high sugar and added chemical flavors, they often come out on the losing side.

To fight this battle, we must gradually make the change by intentionally serving vegetables each day. Using other foods (or dips or dressings) as a bridge to take in more vegetables is one way to do it. Folding them into favored foods (like eggs or tacos) is another. Changing taste buds take time. Start with a goal of one vegetable a day and ease your way into it. Making use of the 50-50 rule is also a great way to gradually introduce vegetables by replacing half of pasta or rice with a chopped veggie.

The good news is that flavor preferences can be changed and using some of the kid-tested recipes in this chapter should help!

While any vegetables are better than no vegetables at all, some vegetables contain more nutrition than others. Non-starchy vegetables include dark green leafy vegetables like broccoli, spinach, bok choy, and kale. Cauliflower is included in that category, and so are onions and garlic. These vegetables tend to have a much lower impact on blood sugar and a lot more vitamins and minerals than the starchier varieties like potatoes, corn, and peas.

However, one saving grace of the potato is the idea of resistant starch. Once potatoes are cooked and cooled, they form "resistant" starch meaning that they resist breaking down in the first portion of the gut (small intestine) and travel to the second portion (large intestine) to be used as food for good gut bacteria. They can be considered almost like fiber in this instance. The key point is that they are not absorbed and turned into glucose as much as digestible starches and have less of an impact on blood sugar. To make this type of resistant starch, simply cook and then cool the potatoes overnight in the fridge. Re-heating will not make them more digestible and will not reduce their resistant starch content.

Keep reading for some of our favorite healthy, easy sides that are sure to be a highlight of the meal!

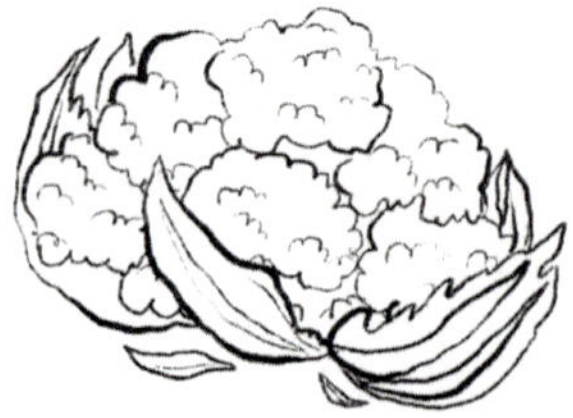

## Cauliflower Rice

Cauliflower is a cruciferous vegetable that is well known for its health benefits. It is rich in glucosinolates, a super-food property that helps to prevent disease (especially heart and stroke), as well as infection and cancer. In fact, a large review found that more than 70% of studies found a link between cruciferous vegetables and protection against cancer.

One unique aspect of cauliflower is the fact that it is mild in flavor and can take on the flavors of just about any dish. The texture of cauliflower is also similar to rice, making it easy to use in place of or in combination with many rice dishes. By using cauliflower, you increase nutrient density while also lowering the carbohydrate load of the rice due to the extra fiber it contains.

Cauliflower contains vitamins that dissolve in water as well as phytonutrients and antioxidants to support health. Consider incorporating raw or steamed cauliflower into many dishes. With only 27 calories, 2 net grams of carbohydrate, and 3 grams of fiber per one cup raw serving, as well as half a day's need for vitamins C and a healthy dose of vitamin K, it is a great addition to any meal. Cauliflower can be wholly substituted for or used in a 50-50 addition, to not just rice dishes but in potato, pasta, and pizza crusts too.

Cauliflower comes in several colors though most grocery stores carry just the white variety. Look for densely packed florets, creamy white in color without blemishes or wet spots. There should not be a strong odor, as this would indicate an aged product. Keep it whole until the day of use, and remove any cellophane to avoid trapped moisture prior to placing it in the refrigerator. Once ready to use, discard outer leaves, remove the center core, chop or rice and then rinse well before adding to recipes.

Read on for a beautiful variety of recipes that are guaranteed to gain acceptance and put more vegetables on the table!

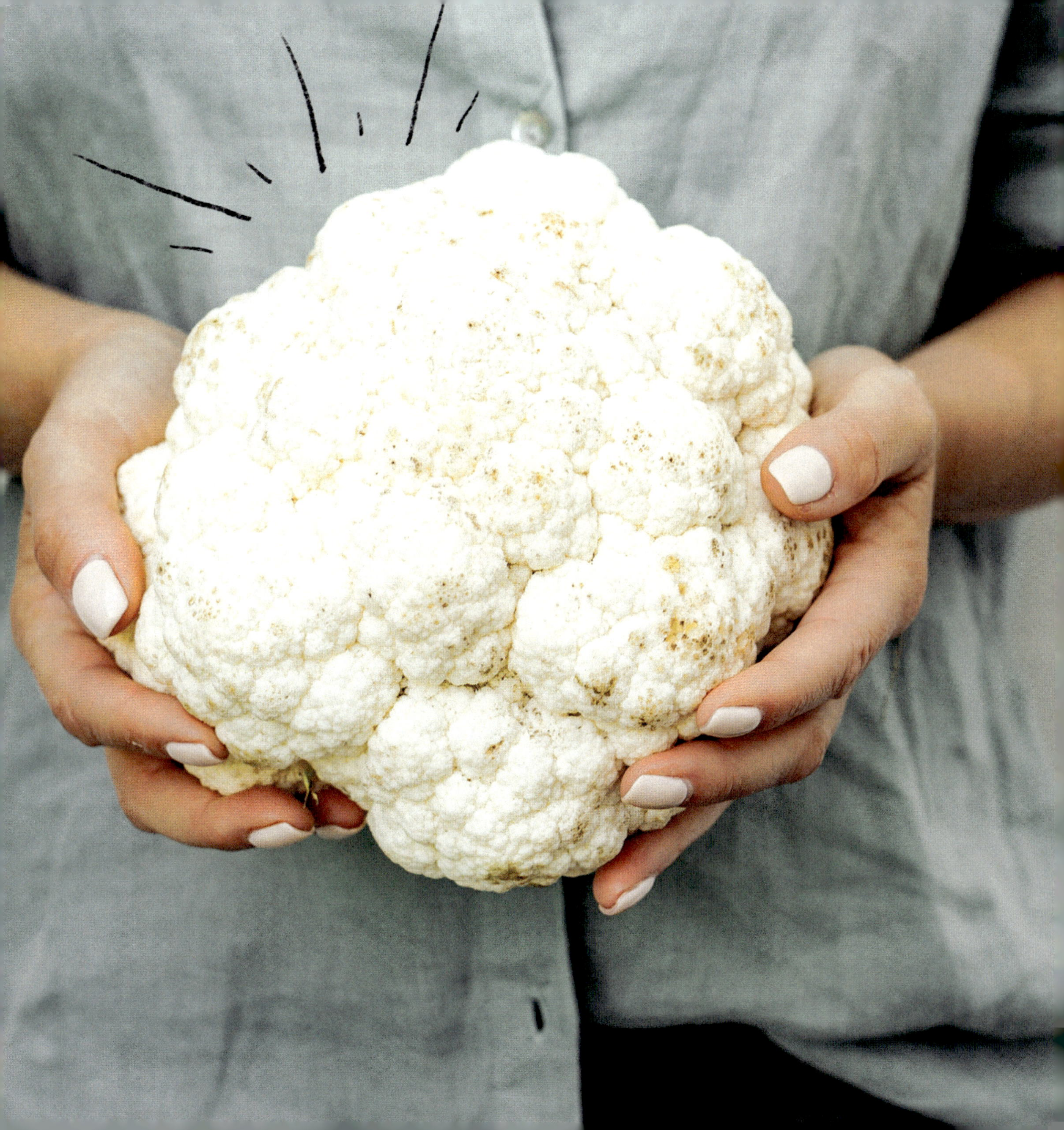

Chef Andrew Johnson

# 50-50 Cauliflower Fried Rice

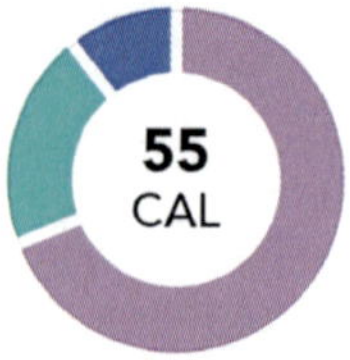


2g **Fat**
7g **Net Carb**
1g **Protein**

**Makes 6 servings:** each ~¾ cup, 156 grams

## Ingredients

3 cups cauliflower, riced

2 cups long-grain rice, cooked

1½ cups frozen mixed vegetables: corn, carrots, peas, green beans, broccoli (e.g. Birds Eye with water chestnuts)

2–3 whole garlic cloves, grated or finely minced

1 tsp ginger, grated or finely minced

½ cup scallions, thinly sliced

1 oz soy sauce or coconut aminos

1 oz coconut oil

½ tsp sesame oil

Salt and pepper to taste

## Directions

1. Heat a large sauté pan on medium/high heat. Once hot, add the coconut oil and cauliflower, then cook for 5–7 minutes. Add the garlic, ginger, and frozen vegetables, then sauté for 5–7 minutes or until fragrant.
2. Then add the cooked rice, soy sauce, and sesame oil and cook for another 1–2 minutes. Season with salt and pepper to taste and garnish with scallions.
3. **For a complete leftover makeover dinner:** Preheat the oven to 400° F. On a parchment-lined sheet pan, arrange portions of **Easy Baked Salmon,** then brush on **Sugar-Free Teriyaki Sauce** and bake for 6–8 minutes. Garnish with sesame seeds and serve on top of a bowl of the **50-50 Cauliflower Fried Rice**.

### Kids Can Cook Tips

Older kids will have fun ricing the cauliflower and grating the ginger. Have the younger ones help with measuring all of the ingredients.

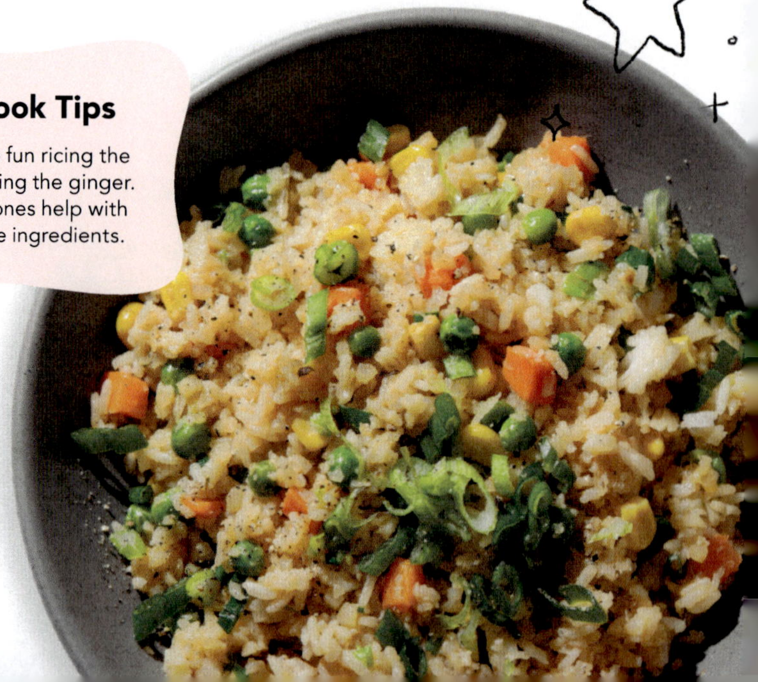

### Fierce Foods Facts

This recipe is a great way to include tasty vegetables in a kid-friendly favorite, and it will be finished and on the table in no time, making it a parent favorite too! Add a scrambled egg for protein or include salmon for a balanced dish.

Chef Andrew Johnson

# Curried Cauliflower Rice

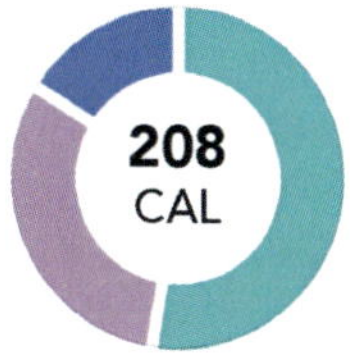


17g Fat
10g Net Carb
5g Protein

**Makes 6 servings:** each ~1 cup, 221 grams

## Ingredients

2 pkg (16 oz each) frozen cauliflower rice

1 medium leek, thinly sliced, green tops removed

3 garlic cloves, minced

1 tbsp avocado or coconut oil

1 cup heavy cream or full-fat coconut milk

2 tbsp red or green Thai curry paste

1 tsp Red Boat fish sauce

2 tbsp Lakanto golden monk fruit sweetener

2 tsp salt

½ tsp ground pepper

### Garnish recommendations

Lime wedges

## Directions

1. In a large skillet over medium, heat the oil. Sauté the leeks and garlic until the leeks start to brown and the garlic is aromatic.
2. Turn the heat to high and add 1 bag of frozen cauliflower rice. Spread cauliflower out across the skillet to see if you have room in the pan for the second bag. If not, cook in batches.
3. Once all of the rice is cooked, add it back to the sauté pan and add heavy cream or full-fat coconut milk. Stir in the curry paste, fish sauce, and sweetener. Add salt and pepper, reduce heat to low, and simmer until liquid is reduced. Serve immediately.

### Kids Can Cook Tips

Kids can help mince garlic with a garlic press and measure all of the ingredients. Older kids with knife skills can help to slice the leeks and sauté the cauliflower.

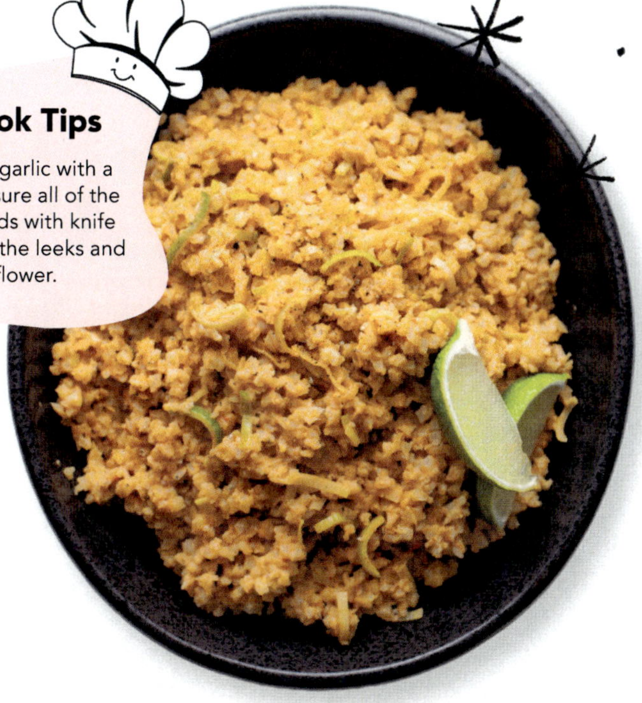

### Fierce Foods Facts

This flavorful low-carb side dish is quick to put together and loaded with plenty of fiber. It also has over 100% of the daily needed vitamin C, which the body uses to help fight off infections, as well as keep skin and connective tissue in tip-top shape.

Chef Audra DiPadova Wilford

# Italian-Style Cauliflower Rice

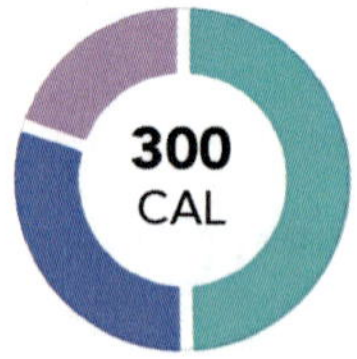


23g **Fat**
9g **Net Carb**
14g **Protein**

**Makes 6 servings:** each ~1 cup, 250 grams

## Ingredients

2 pkg (16 oz each) frozen cauliflower rice

1 medium leek (green tops removed), thinly sliced

3 garlic cloves, minced

1 tbsp avocado or extra virgin olive oil

1 cup of heavy cream

½ cup grated parmesan cheese

1 cup grated asiago cheese

¼ cup fresh basil, chiffonade sliced

1 lemon, juice only

¼ cup rinsed capers (optional)

2 tsp salt

½ tsp ground pepper

## Directions

1. In a large skillet over medium, heat the oil. Sauté the leeks and garlic until the leeks start to brown and the garlic is aromatic.
2. Turn the heat to high and add 1 bag of frozen cauliflower rice. Spread cauliflower out across the skillet to see if you have room in the pan for the second bag. If not, cook in batches.
3. Once all of the rice is cooked, add it back to the sauté pan and add heavy cream, salt, pepper, and cheese. Reduce heat to low and simmer until liquid is reduced. Just before serving, add the basil, lemon juice, and capers. Serve immediately.

### Kids Can Cook Tips

Have the younger kids help measure the oils and cream and grate the cheeses and juice the lemons. Older kids with knife skills can help chiffonade the basil and slice the leeks.

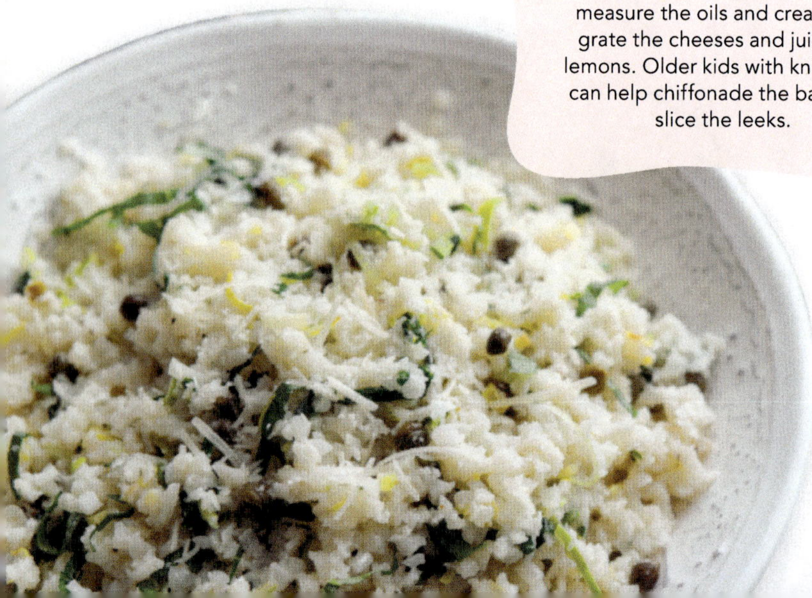

### Fierce Foods Facts

This easy-to-put-together, low-carbohydrate side dish has a nice punch of vitamins A, C, and K along with 20% of the daily needs for calcium. The fresh herbs also provide wonderful flavor along with anti-oxidants and polyphenols to help support your immune system.

Chef Andrew Johnson

# Mexican-Style Cauliflower Rice

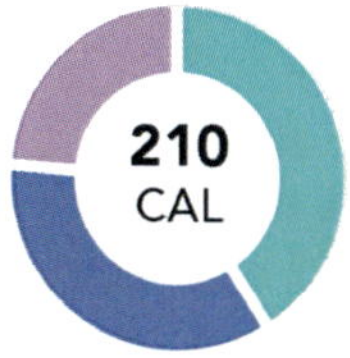


14g Fat
8g Net Carb
12g Protein

**Makes 6 servings:** each ~¾ cup, 156 grams

## Ingredients

2 pkg (16 oz each) frozen cauliflower rice

16 oz sugar-free uncased chorizo

1 white onion, diced

1 red bell pepper, diced

½ green bell pepper, diced

2 garlic cloves, crushed

1 tbsp fresh lime juice

2 tsp salt

1 tsp coarse ground pepper

1 tbsp chipotle purée (optional)

2 tsp Mexican seasoning blend

½ cup chopped fresh cilantro leaves

1 cup grated Mexican cheese blend

## Directions

1. Heat a large sauté skillet over medium. Sauté the chorizo until cooked thoroughly. Remove chorizo with a slotted spoon and set it aside in a bowl.
2. Cook the onion in the same skillet with pan drippings for 5 minutes or until translucent. Add the bell peppers and sauté for 3–4 minutes. Remove the peppers and onions from the pan and add them to the same bowl as the chorizo.
3. If needed, add more fat to coat the bottom of the skillet. Turn the heat to high and add 1 bag of frozen cauliflower rice. Spread the cauliflower out across the skillet to see if you have room in the pan for the second bag. If not, cook in batches.
4. Once all of the rice is cooked, add the chorizo, peppers, and onions back to the pan. Mix in the lime juice, cilantro, and chipotle, then sprinkle with cheese and gently mix. Serve immediately.

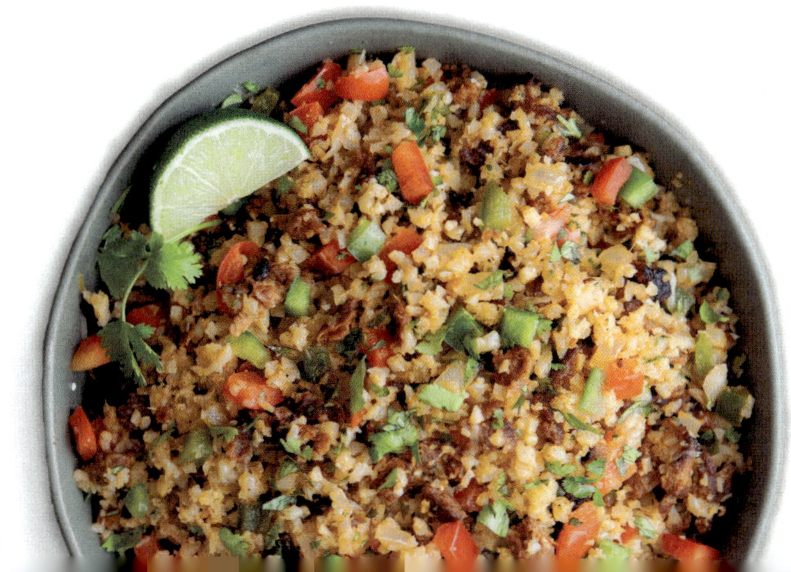

### Fierce Foods Facts

These versatile cauliflower rice dishes can be made in just about any flavor, this Mexican-inspired variety adds a nice punch of vitamin A with the addition of the peppers. It is also complete with a nice dose of satiating muscle-building protein and the cheese provides almost one-third of the day's calcium.

Chef Andrew Johnson

# Cauliflower Risotto

**Makes 8 servings:** each ~¾ cup, 156 grams

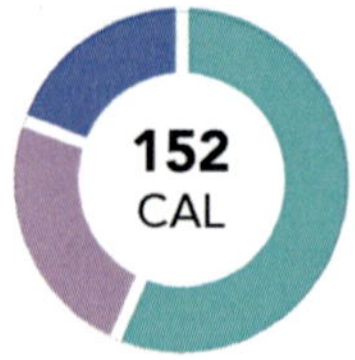


12g **Fat**
5g **Net Carb**
4g **Protein**

## Ingredients

2 pkg (16 oz each) frozen cauliflower rice

1 medium leek (green tops removed), thinly sliced

3 garlic cloves, minced

1 tbsp coconut or extra virgin olive oil

1 cup heavy cream or full-fat coconut milk

2 tsp salt

½ tsp ground pepper

## Directions

1. In a large skillet over medium, heat the oil. Sauté the leeks and garlic until the leeks start to brown and the garlic is aromatic.
2. Turn the heat to high and add 1 bag of frozen cauliflower rice. Spread cauliflower out across the skillet to see if you have room in the pan for the second bag. If not, cook in batches.
3. Once all of the rice is cooked, add it back to the sauté pan and add the heavy cream or full-fat coconut milk. Add salt and pepper, reduce heat to low, and simmer until the liquid is reduced. Serve immediately.

### Kids Can Cook Tips

Have the younger children help measure the oil, cream, salt, and pepper. Older kids with knife skills can help slice the leek and mince the garlic.

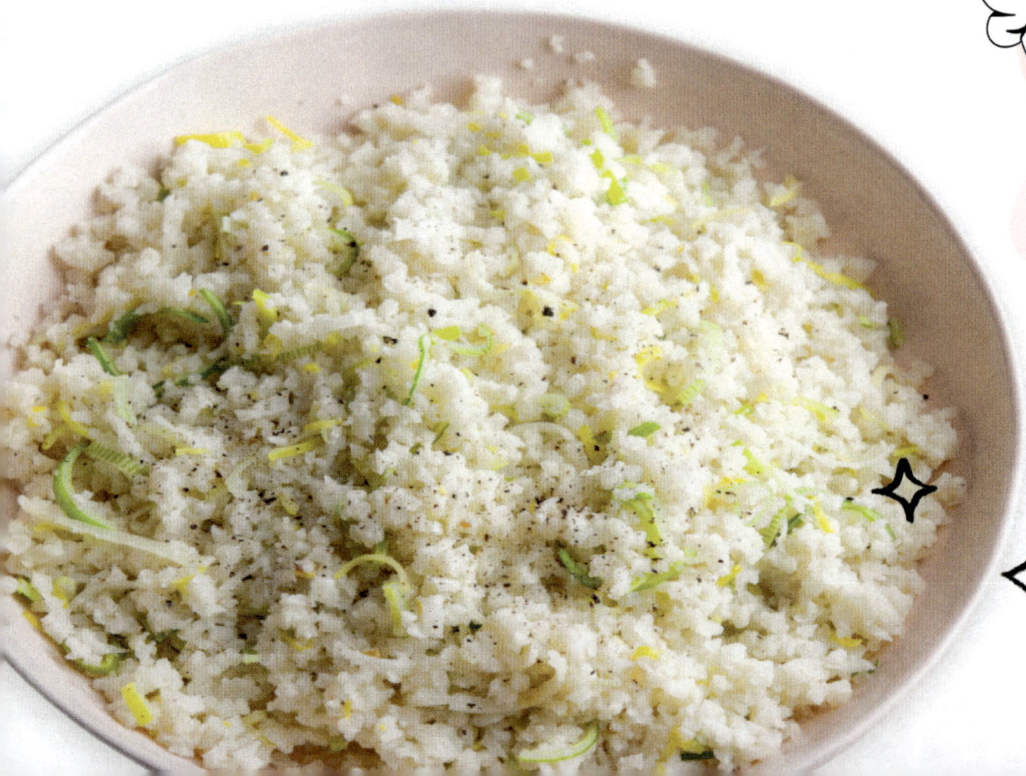

Chef Cathy McKnight

# Creamy Cauliflower Mash with Brown Butter and Sage

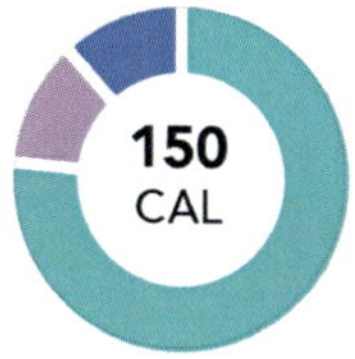


14g Fat
2g Net Carb
2g Protein

**Makes 8 servings:** each ~½ cup, 94 grams

## Ingredients

2 heads cauliflower, whole

¼ cup heavy cream or whole milk

1 stick unsalted butter

10 fresh sage leaves

Flaked sea salt

### Fierce Foods Facts

The fried sage adds both beauty and flavor to this gorgeous dish. The cauliflower adds vitamins C and K along with the superstar phytonutrients that are known for fighting cancer and lowering inflammation.

## Directions

1. Clean and core the cauliflower heads. In a large glass bowl, break into uniform florets, then cover with plastic wrap and microwave for 5 minutes until very soft. Set aside without uncovering the bowl (watch out for the steam when you uncover it later).
2. In a large sauté pan, melt the butter over medium heat. Once it is fully melted, add the sage leaves, vein-side down. Swirl the butter slightly to coat the leaves. Do not burn the butter—it will slowly brown as you swirl it over the sage leaves. Turn off the heat once the leaves are crispy. Remove the crispy leaves with a slotted spoon and drain on a paper towel. Try to leave as much butter in the pan as possible.
3. Drain any water off of the cooked cauliflower. Using a potato masher or a food processor with the S blade, mash into smooth consistency, using 2 tablespoons of the sage-infused butter and ¼ cup of heavy cream or whole milk. It should have the consistency of mashed potatoes.
4. Place into your serving bowl, then pour the reserved butter over the mash and sprinkle the crispy sage leaves over the top. Give it a soft swirl, and sprinkle it with the flaked salt.

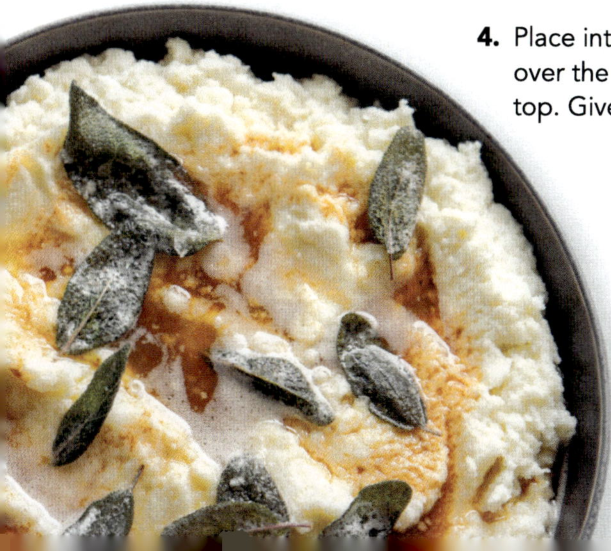

Chef Andrew Johnson

# Devilish Green Eggs and Ham

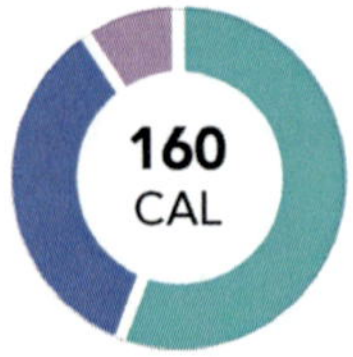


13g Fat
2g Net Carb
8g Protein

**Makes 6 servings:** 2 halves each, 91 grams

## Ingredients

6 large eggs

1 medium or large avocado

3 slices prosciutto

½ lemon, zested and juiced

1–3 tsp mayonnaise

1 tsp celery seed

Salt and black pepper to taste

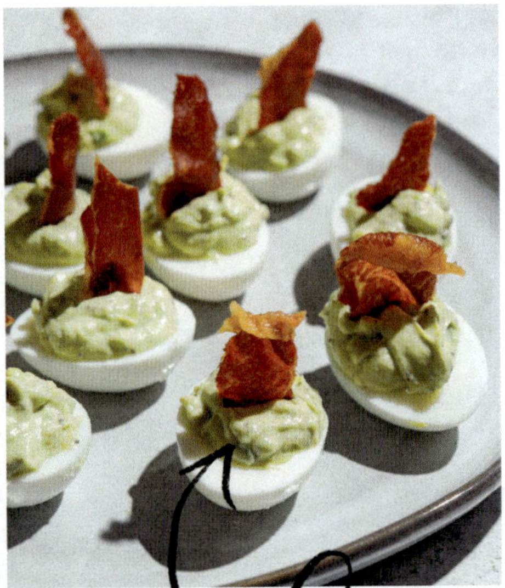

## Directions

1. Preheat the oven to 350°F. Lay out the prosciutto on a parchment-lined baking pan and bake for 10–12 minutes until golden brown and crispy.
2. In a medium saucepan add the fresh, uncooked eggs and cover with cold water (at least ½" deep). Bring the pot to a boil, then once it reaches a rolling boil, cook for 10 minutes. Carefully pour off the boiling water and add ice to cover the eggs.
3. Once the eggs are cool, peel and slice the eggs in half, top to bottom with a sharp knife. Scoop out the egg yolks and arrange the hard-boiled egg whites on a nice tray or plate.
4. In a large mixing bowl, add egg yolks, avocado, lemon zest and juice, mayonnaise, celery seed, salt, and pepper. With a potato masher or the back of a large fork, mash and thoroughly incorporate the ingredients until you reach your desired consistency.
5. With a small ice cream scoop (or spoon) add a dollop of the deviled egg mixture to each egg white. Break the crispy prosciutto into shards and top each deviled egg with prosciutto. It looks great if the prosciutto is standing up tall on top of the yolk mixture. Serve cold.

### Fierce Foods Facts

Eggs are such an awesome appetizer or snack, with a great balance of protein and fat to help satiate hunger. This flavorful twist on the deviled egg favorite comes loaded with monounsaturated fat, choline, zinc, and iodine—perfect for fueling those energy factories called mitochondria in the body. In fact, choline has been studied extensively for its effectiveness in warding off anxiety and depression!

Chef Andrew Johnson

# French Picnic Potato Salad

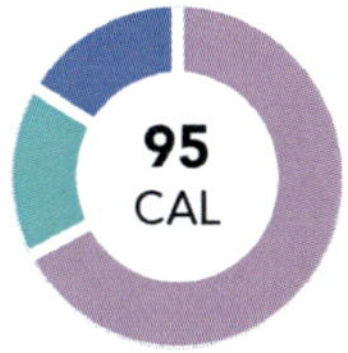


3g **Fat**
13g **Net Carb**
3g **Protein**

**Makes 8 servings:** each ~½ cup, 133 grams

## Ingredients

1 lb baby potatoes, ¾" in diameter

1 lb Brussels sprouts, small to medium size

¼ cup scallion, chopped

¼ cup parsley, chopped

2 tbsp Dijon mustard

1 tbsp olive oil (plus more to drizzle)

½ lemon, juiced

1 tbsp mustard seeds

1 tsp tarragon

Salt and black pepper to taste

## Directions

1. Preheat the oven to 350°F. Trim the stems and any less-than-pretty leaves from the Brussels sprouts, and cut larger sprouts in half. In a large mixing bowl, toss the Brussels sprouts, olive oil, salt, and pepper. Lay out the Brussels sprouts on a parchment-lined baking pan and bake for 15–20 minutes.
2. Fill ⅔ of a large stock pot with water and bring to a boil. Once boiling, add salt until it tastes like the ocean. To the boiling stock pot, carefully add the baby potatoes. Boil the potatoes for 10–15 minutes until they are fork-tender. Remove potatoes from the pot and strain.
3. Allow the potatoes and sprouts to cool before adding them to a large mixing bowl. Then add the scallions, parsley, wet and dry mustards, lemon, and seasonings. Gently toss or fold the salad to completely incorporate the ingredients. Serve at room temperature or cold.

**Pro Tip:** If you want to eliminate the Brussels sprouts and if minimizing carb consumption is not a requirement, simply double the potatoes and continue with the rest of the recipe.

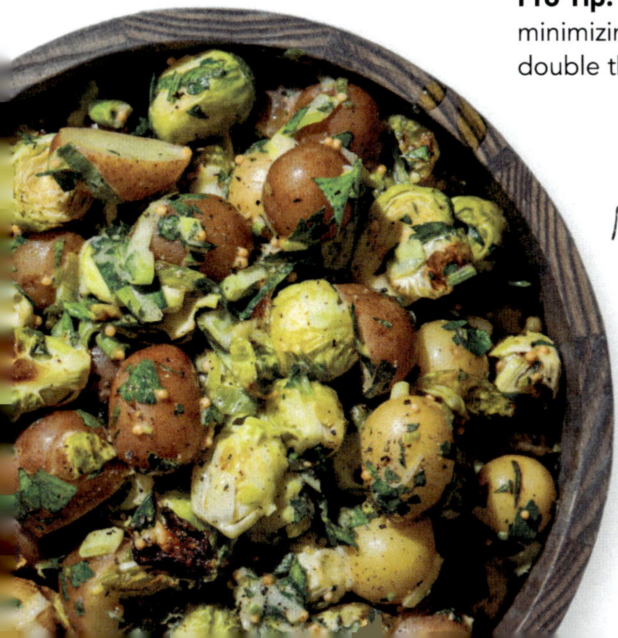

### Fierce Foods Facts

Brussels sprouts provide this favorite barbecue side dish with a huge nutrient infusion, adding vitamins A, C, and K, which are excellent for eyesight, skin, and blood. Known as the "sunshine vitamin," optimal levels of vitamin C have been correlated with improved mood and cognitive function!

Chef Andrew Johnson

# Hasselback Sweet Potatoes with Romesco Sauce

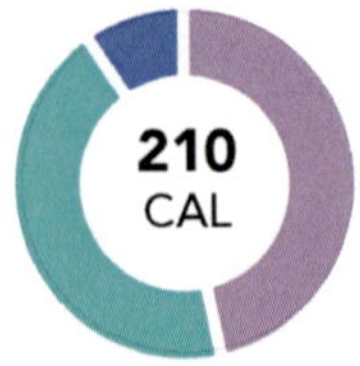


15g Fat
16g Net Carb
3g Protein

**Makes 12 servings:** each ~½ cup,144 grams

## Ingredients

3 large red bell peppers, roasted or 12–15 oz jarred

2–3 scallions, green and white

1 tbsp fresh thyme

½ cup pepitas, toasted

¼ cup tomato purée

2 tbsp apple cider vinegar

2 tsp smoked paprika

½ cup extra virgin olive oil

½ tsp sea salt, finely ground

¼ tsp black pepper, freshly ground

3½ lb (~6 medium) garnet sweet potato

2 tbsp butter or vegan alternative (e.g. Miyoko Creamery vegan butter)

2 cloves garlic, minced

## Topping

2 tbsp butter or vegan alternative (e.g. Miyoko Creamery vegan butter)

2 tbsp brown sugar or Lakanto brown monk fruit sweetener

2 tbsp pepitas, roasted and salted

Fresh thyme, chopped

## Directions

1. Preheat the oven to 425°F. Cut and remove the stems of peppers, then slice peppers into wide strips. Over a fast grill or stove flame, use tongs to roast the peppers directly in the flame, turning until the skins are black. Seal in a bowl with plastic wrap over the top. Allow to cool, then remove the skin and seeds. Alternatively, consider using roasted peppers pre purchased in the jar to allow for a time-saving tip.

2. In a food processor, pulse the bell peppers, scallions, thyme, pepitas, tomato purée, apple cider vinegar, and paprika until they are incorporated, but still somewhat chunky and intact. Turn the food processor on and drizzle in olive oil until incorporated. Add salt and pepper to taste, then set the mixture aside.

3. Wash and peel sweet potatoes. Using a mandolin slicer or food processor slicer attachment, slice all sweet potatoes to ¼" thick slices. In a large bowl, combine sweet potatoes with prepared sauce and toss to coat. May refrigerate any unused sauce and store it in a glass jar in the refrigerator for up to 5 days or freeze it for future use.

4. In a round oven-safe baking dish, arrange sweet potatoes in a circular pattern. Place in oven covered and bake for 1 hour and 15 minutes.

5. Combine melted butter and brown sugar in a small bowl. Using a basting brush, baste sweet potatoes with this mixture and bake uncovered for another 15 minutes. Remove from oven and top with fresh thyme and toasted pepitas. Serve immediately.

6. Additional time-saving options: Consider purchasing a prepared romesco sauce, and if you don't have time for the pictured presentation, simply chop the sweet potatoes into a medium dice, toss with the prepared sauce, and follow the remaining baking instructions.

## Kids Can Cook Tips

This is where the kids get creative! Have them help measure all of the ingredients for the romesco sauce. Have them stack the sweet potato coins and stand on end to help create the circle in the pan. Come up with a new pattern for even more adventure in the kitchen! Have the kids pull fresh herbs to help decorate after the dish is out of the oven.

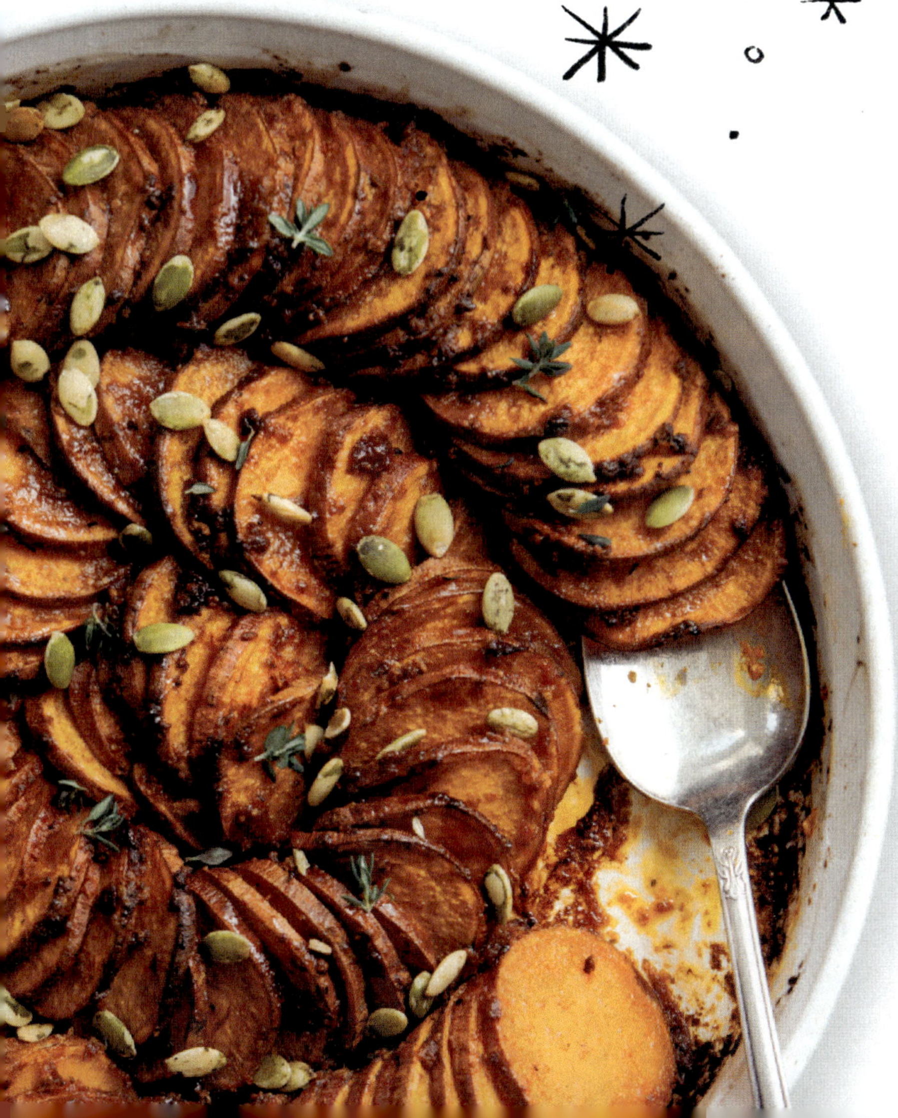

## Fierce Foods Facts

This delicious side is full of quality carbohydrates, packing over 200% of the daily vitamin A, with almost 100% of the vitamin C. It's a great side dish and supports eyesight and the immune system! It also sports a lot of magnesium and potassium, helpful for every energy transaction in the body as well as strong bones.

Chef Andrew Johnson

# Oven-Baked Garlicky Mushrooms

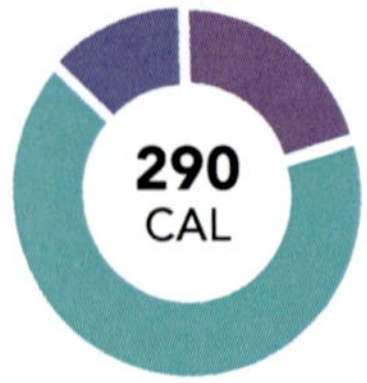


26g **Fat**
5g **Net Carb**
8g **Protein**

**Makes 6 servings:** each ~3 mushrooms, 96 grams

## Ingredients

8–10 oz Baby Bella or crimini mushrooms, medium size

½ cup ground flaxseed

⅓ cup almond flour or lupin flour

½ tsp sea salt

1 tsp garlic powder

½ tsp paprika

½ tsp dried parsley

4 tbsp parmesan cheese or dairy-free alternative (e.g VioLife vegan parmesan)

½ cup mayonnaise or egg-free alternative (e.g. Primal Kitchen avocado mayonnaise)

## Directions

1. Preheat the oven to 400°F degrees. Prepare a baking sheet with parchment paper or use a baking stone. Prepare mushrooms by using a dry cloth or paper towel to remove any debris.
2. In a shallow bowl combine ground flaxseed, almond flour, sea salt, garlic powder, paprika, parsley, and parmesan cheese. Coat each mushroom in mayonnaise, then fully coat with flour mixture and place on the prepared baking sheet. Repeat with the remaining mushrooms.
3. Bake for 7–8 minutes, carefully turn mushrooms then bake for another 7–8 minutes or until crispy and golden brown.

### Kids Can Cook Tips

Have kids help to clean mushrooms and measure all ingredients for the flour mixture. Kids will also enjoy dipping the mushrooms in the mayonnaise and again in the flour mixture.

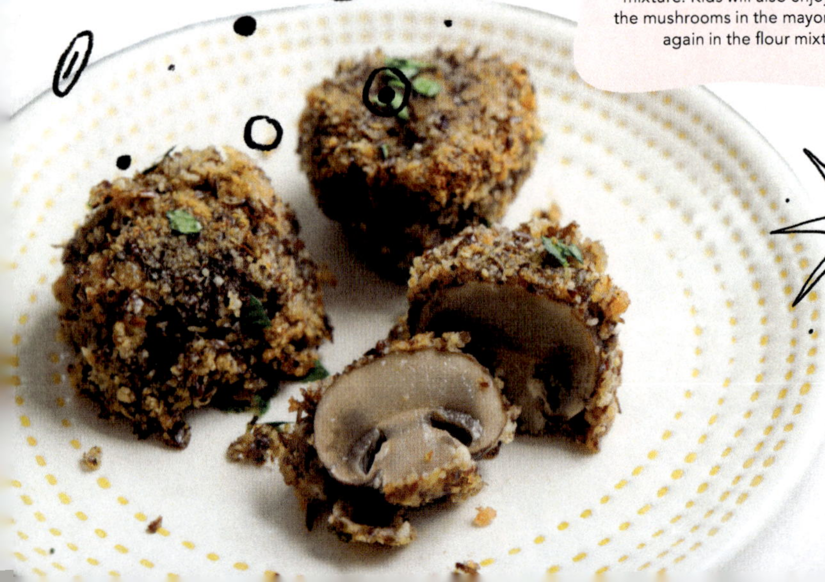

### Fierce Foods Facts

Mushrooms are loaded with B vitamins and the mushrooms in this recipe are no exception. Riboflavin, niacin, and pantothenic acid all combine to provide sustained energy. The addition of the flax and almond flours provide plenty of fiber (Almost 7 grams per serving!) and has an almost 3:1 ratio of Omega-3 to Omega-6 fats.

Chef Alexia Hall, RDN

# Rainbow Vegetable Fritters

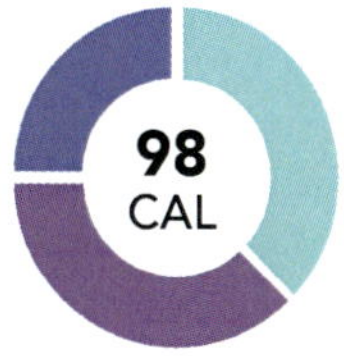


6g Fat
6g Net Carb
4g Protein

**Makes 8 servings:** 1 fritter each, 67 grams

## Ingredients

- ½ cup almond flour, finely ground
- 2 tbsp flaxseed, finely ground
- 2 large eggs, whisked
- ½ tsp sea salt
- 2 cloves garlic, minced
- ½ cup onion, finely diced
- 2 tbsp fresh parsley, finely chopped
- ¼ cup parmesan cheese, grated
- ½ cup zucchini, grated
- ½ cup sweet potato, peeled and grated
- ½ cup red bell pepper, finely chopped
- 2 tsp olive oil

## Directions

1. Preheat the oven to 425°F. Using a large bowl, add almond flour, ground flaxseed, egg, sea salt, garlic cloves, onion, parsley, and parmesan cheese, then stir to combine.
2. Peel and shred the sweet potato, and shred the zucchini with skin on. Remove the seeds and white pith of the bell pepper and mince. Wrap all the prepared vegetables in a kitchen towel and squeeze tightly, wringing out excess liquid into a bowl. Discard the liquid.
3. Add all the shredded and chopped vegetables to the bowl with the egg and flour mixture, and combine well. Use a large scoop or mold and form fritters by hand. This mixture should make about 8 evenly-sized fritters.
4. Add fritters to a cookie sheet lined with parchment paper or place on a lightly oiled baking stone. Brush the top of each fritter with olive oil. Bake at 425°F for 20–22 minutes. When done, they should be firm, light brown, and slightly crispy. Consider serving with our **Avocado Pepita Dip.**

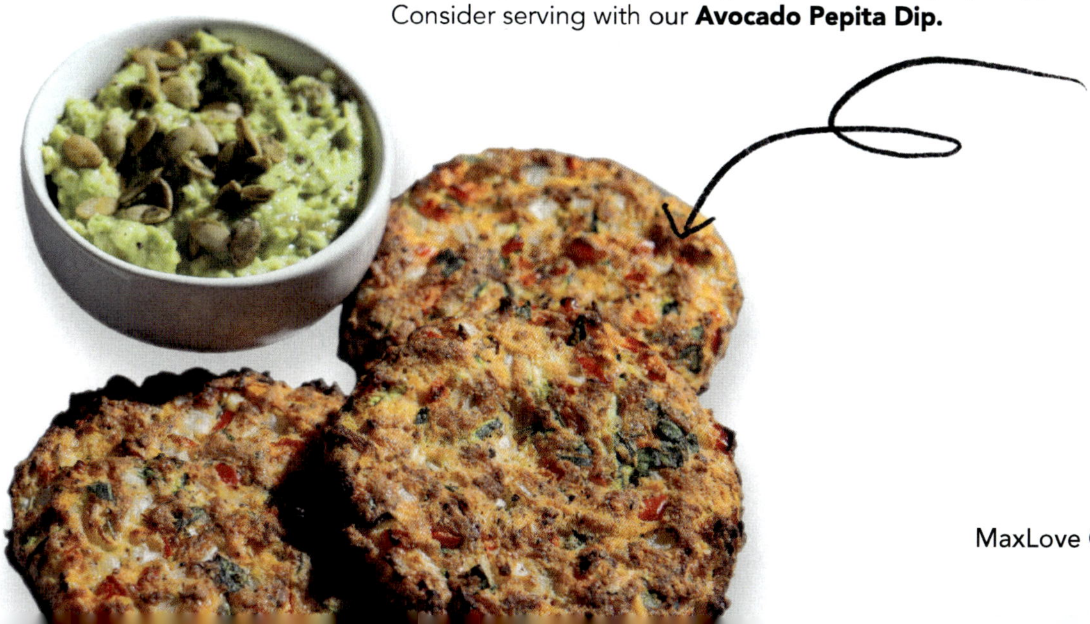

Chef Andrew Johnson

# Braised Collard Greens

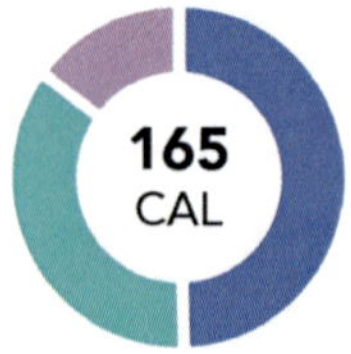


10g Fat
4g Net Carb
14g Protein

**Makes 8 servings:** each ~½ cup, 122 grams

## Ingredients

2 large bunches collard greens (approx. 4 oz), stems removed and chopped

2 cups chicken stock

½ lb uncured bacon, diced

4–5 garlic cloves, peeled and thinly sliced

1 bunch fresh oregano, tied with twine

2 shallots, thinly sliced

1 lemon, thinly sliced into rounds

1 tbsp unfiltered apple cider vinegar, rice vinegar, or red wine vinegar

1 tsp Sambal Oelek chili paste (optional)

1 tsp smoked paprika

Sea or kosher salt and pepper to taste

## Directions

1. Add bacon to a large Dutch oven or stock pot over medium heat and cook for 5–6 minutes, stirring frequently. Add garlic and shallots, then continue to cook until the bacon is crispy and the shallots and garlic are beginning to caramelize and soften. Remove with a slotted spoon and set aside in a mixing bowl.
2. Deglaze the pot with the vinegar, scraping the bacon bits from the bottom of the pot. Add the greens, chicken stock, lemon, chili paste, smoked paprika, salt, pepper, and oregano. Mix to combine; the greens won't be fully submerged.
3. Cover and let cook on medium to low/medium for 30–40 minutes. The greens release their own water, creating a braising liquid called potlikker. Remove the lid and let cook for another 5–10 minutes to reduce the potlikker. Then return the cooked bacon, garlic, and shallots to the pot and season to taste before serving.

### Fierce Foods Facts

Collard greens hit the top of the scale in terms of nutrient density, in fact, they contain every B Vitamin, as well as vitamins A, C, & E. They also come stocked with a wide array of minerals, making this dish a superstar. The savory bacon provides a wonderful mouth-watering taste that is sure to entice any kid (and adult). Bacon also has a superstar quality that most are unaware of: about 50% of bacon fat is a type of fat called oleic—the same kind that olive oil contains! Oleic acids have been shown to support healthy cholesterol and downplay inflammation. Try to buy your bacon nitrate free to avoid problematic substances in your food.

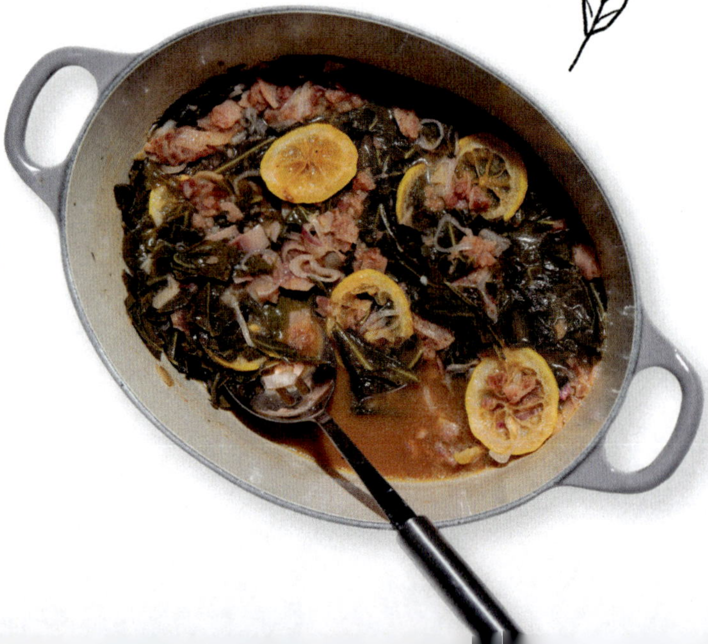

Chef Andrew Johnson

# Cauliflower Tabbouleh

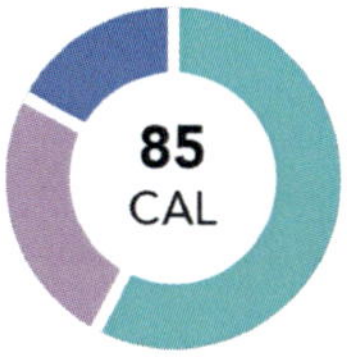


**Makes 8 servings:** each ~½ cup, 111 grams

7g Fat
3g Net Carb
2g Protein

## Ingredients

2 cups cauliflower, grated

⅓ cup scallions, green and onion parts, chopped

1 cup flat or curly parsley leaves, chopped

¼ cup fresh mint leaves, oregano, or marjoram, chopped

1 clove garlic, peeled and minced

1 cup cherry tomatoes, halved

1 cup cucumber, medium diced

1 lemon, juiced

4 tbsp olive oil

1 tsp sumac

Salt and pepper to taste

## Directions

1. Using a box grater or a food processor with a grater blade, grate the cauliflower into rice-size bits.
2. In a large mixing bowl add cauliflower, scallions, fresh herbs, garlic, tomatoes, cucumber, and sumac. Toss to fully incorporate the ingredients, then drizzle in the olive oil and the juice of a lemon. Season with salt and pepper and toss again to fully incorporate. Taste and reseason if necessary.
3. Enjoy right away or place in a sealed container in a refrigerator for up to a week.

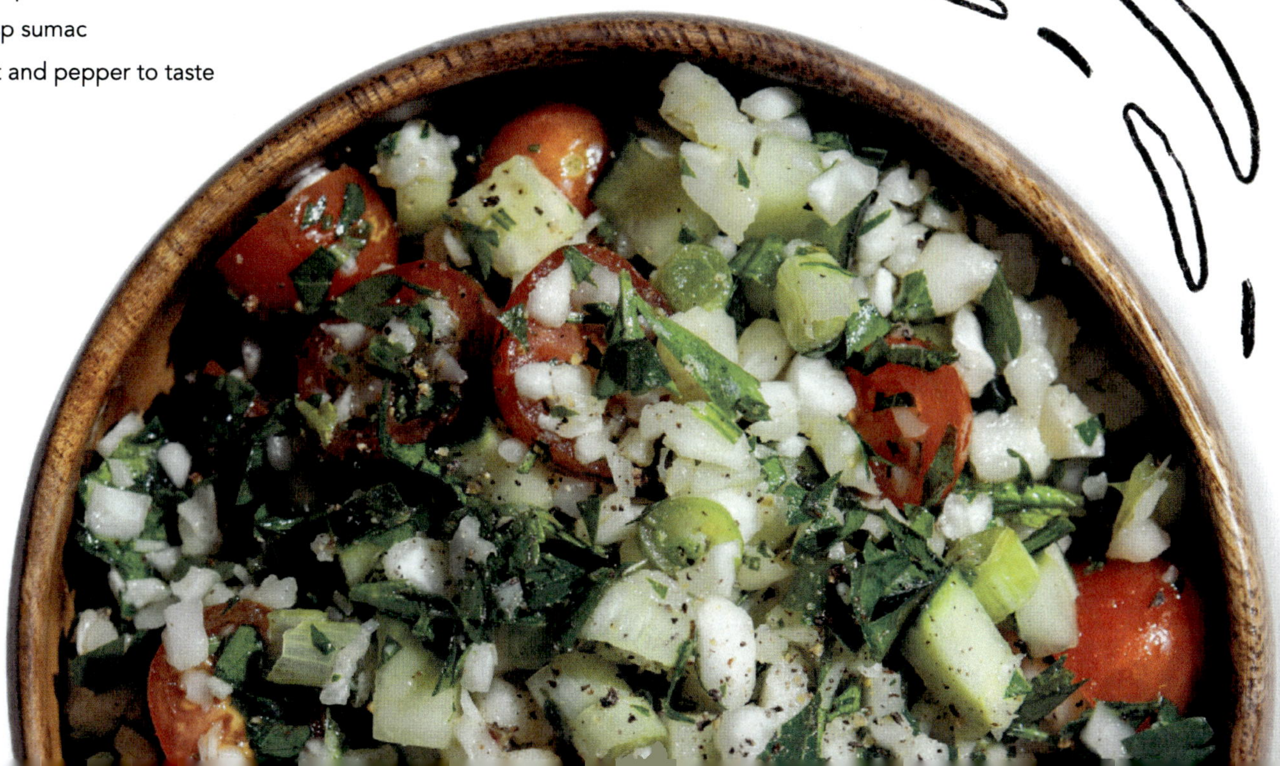

Chef Cathy McKnight

# Roasted Beet Poke

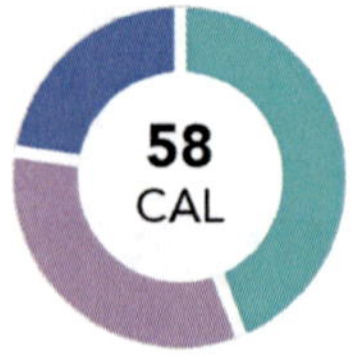


4g Fat
3g Net Carb
2g Protein

**Makes 16 servings:** each ~¼ cup, 45 grams

## Ingredients

4 fresh beets, any color

2 tbsp extra virgin olive oil

2 tbsp coarse salt, divided

2 tbsp sesame oil

3 tbsp yuzu or any citrus juice

1 tsp white sesame seeds

1 tsp black sesame seeds

2 tsp dulse flakes

1 pinch Korean chili flakes

1 tbsp chives, minced

## Directions

1. Remove the beet tops and set them aside for another use. Scrub any dirt off of the beets. Then place the beets on a large sheet of foil, pour the olive oil and 1 tablespoon of coarse salt over them, and coat to cover the whole beet. Wrap in a foil packet and place on a cookie sheet and roast for 55 minutes at 400°F.
2. Remove the skin from the roasted beets by rubbing them gently with a coarse kitchen towel. The skins will come off very easily.
3. Cut the beets into ½" cubes and place them in a glass bowl. Put the remaining ingredients in the bowl and stir gently to coat all the pieces. Refrigerate for 3–4 hours or overnight. Taste and adjust the seasoning as needed, and serve with watermelon radish coins or Mary's seaweed crackers.

### Fierce Foods Facts

Beets promote the production of nitric oxide, a potent superfood that helps support cardiovascular health, optimize blood pressure, and maintain oxygen status. Packed with fiber, folate, potassium, and vitamin C, this is a great low-carb choice for a snack.

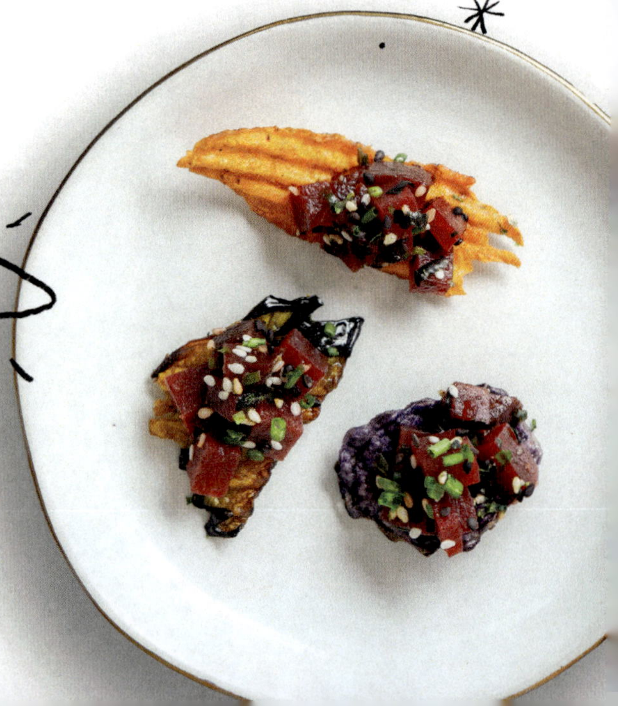

Chef Andrew Johnson

# Roasted Cauliflower

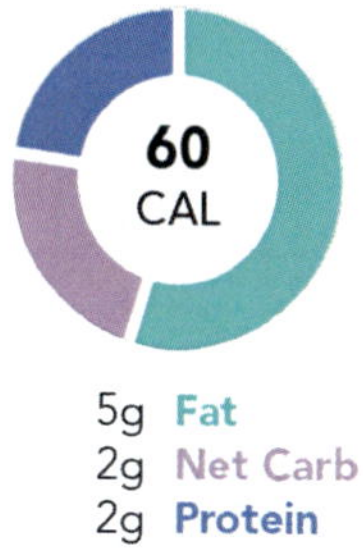


**Makes 6 servings:** each 3 ounces, 85 grams

## Ingredients

1 lb cauliflower, florets (approx. 1 large head)

2 tbsp olive oil

Salt and pepper to taste

## Directions

1. Preheat the oven to 400°F. In a large mixing bowl add cauliflower florets, olive oil, salt, and pepper. Toss to fully coat the florets.
2. On a parchment-lined sheet pan spread out cauliflower evenly in a single layer. Bake for 30–35 minutes until the edges are golden brown. If you are batch cooking it is easy enough to double or triple this recipe and have cauliflower for the rest of the week.

## Fierce Foods Facts

Cauliflower is a low carbohydrate side dish option that is packed with fiber and vitamin C. Easy to prepare, it is also a mild flavor that will take on the flavor of whatever dish that might be cooked with it.

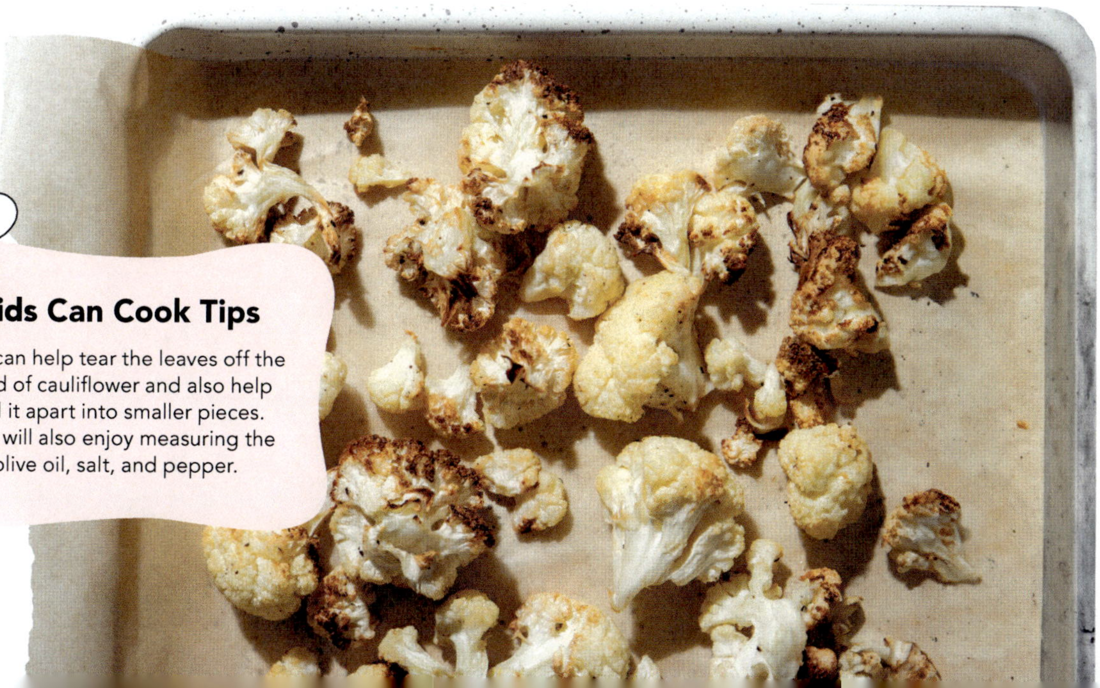

### Kids Can Cook Tips

Kids can help tear the leaves off the head of cauliflower and also help pull it apart into smaller pieces. Kids will also enjoy measuring the olive oil, salt, and pepper.

Chef Cathy McKnight

# Roasted Radish Home Fries

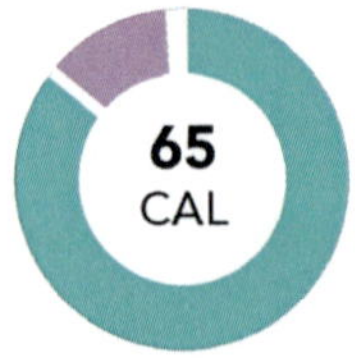


7g **Fat**
1g **Net Carb**
0g **Protein**

**Makes 6 servings:** each ~16 pieces, 26 grams

## Ingredients

3 tbsp olive oil

2 bunches radishes (approx. 24 radishes), cut into quarters

¼ cup yellow or white onion, large diced

¼ cup bell pepper (any color except green), large diced

2 cloves garlic, peeled and minced

½ tsp smoked paprika

½ tsp dried thyme or 1 tsp fresh thyme

Sea or kosher salt and pepper to taste

## Directions

1. Preheat the oven to 450°F. In a large mixing bowl add radish quarters, chopped onion and peppers, olive oil, smoked paprika, thyme, salt, and pepper. Toss until evenly coated.
2. On a parchment-lined sheet pan, pour out the mixture in a single layer. Roast for 15–20 minutes or until they reach your desired doneness.

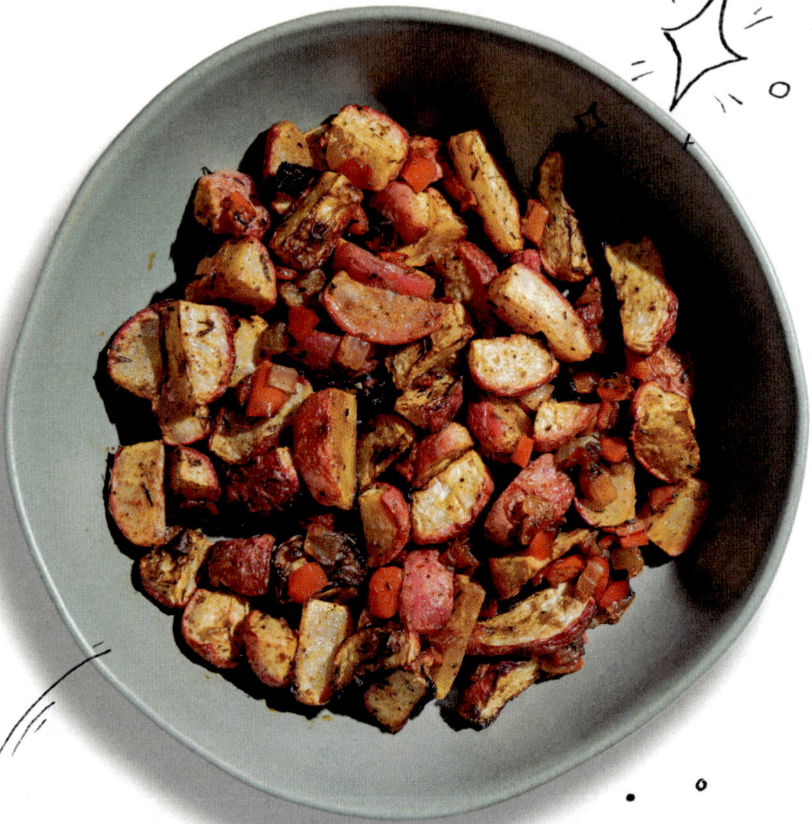

### Fierce Foods Facts

Radishes are crunchy, spicy, and low-carb—a winning combination for a snack. Dark red fruits and vegetables, like radishes, beets, pomegranate, and tart cherries, are good sources of natural nitrates that help reduce inflammation and support healthy blood flow.

Chef Cathy McKnight

# Zesty Cabbage Slaw

Makes 10 servings: each ~1 cup, 251 grams

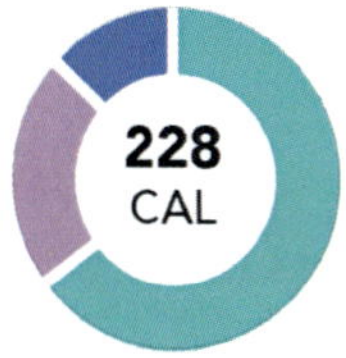


21g Fat
7g Net Carb
4g Protein

## Ingredients

**Slaw**

1 green cabbage, core removed

1 Napa cabbage

¼ cup green onion, green part only

½ cup cilantro

2 watermelon radishes

¼ cup pepitas, toasted

1 tbsp red serrano pepper, minced (optional)

1 tbsp celery seeds (optional)

**Dressing**

1 cup Primal Kitchen mayo

¼ cup unseasoned rice vinegar

2 tbsp yuzu juice or 1 tbsp each lemon juice and lime juice

## Directions

1. In a glass bowl, mix mayo, rice vinegar, and yuzu juice. Add a pinch of salt and set aside.
2. Using a sharp knife, finely shred both cabbages and put in a large glass bowl. Dice the green onion, julienne the radish and add both to the bowl. Chop the cilantro, stems and all, and add to the mix.
3. Toss the slaw mix with the dressing, coating all of the ingredients, and add in the toasted pepitas. You can add celery seed for added crunch and red serrano pepper for a little kick.
4. Chill for 30 minutes. Garnish with fresh cilantro leaves before serving.

### Kids Can Cook Tips

Younger kids can help measure the ingredients and toss the salad. Older kids with knife skills can help shred the cabbages and chop the green onions, cilantro, and peppers

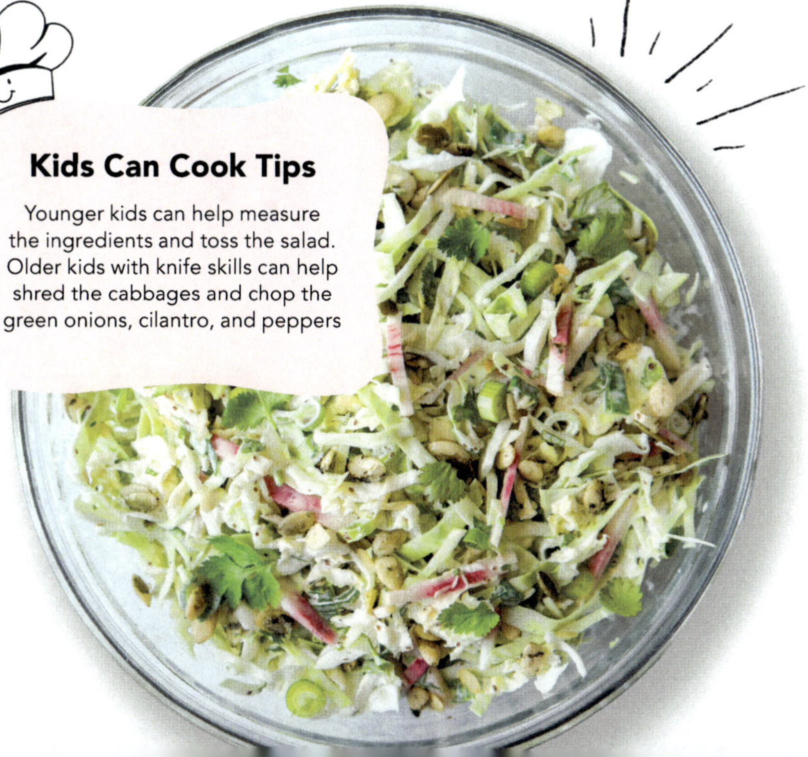

### Fierce Foods Facts

This colorful and zesty side dish is packed with important nutrients like folate and vitamin K which are needed for a healthy blood supply and are involved in the production of DNA and RNA. This dish also comes with a nice dose of vitamins A, C, and K as well as several minerals, helping to support a strong immune system.

Chef Anne Watson

# Anne's Guacamole

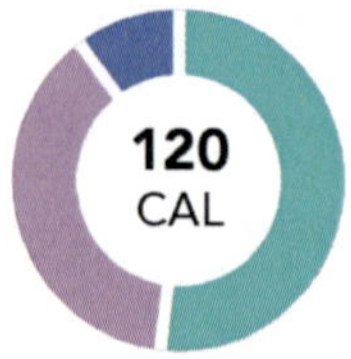


11g **Fat**
8g **Net Carb**
2g **Protein**

**Makes 6 servings:** each ~ ⅓ cup, 100 grams

## Ingredients

2 large or 3 medium Hass avocados, very ripe and soft

3 tbsp red onion, minced

¼–1 whole jalapeño (to taste), seeded and minced

1 small tomato, seeded and chopped

4 tbsp cilantro, chopped

1 lime, juiced

Coarse sea salt to taste

## Directions

1. Place minced onion and pinch of salt in a molcajete and crush to release the onion's juices, then place half of the minced jalapeño in the molcajete and crush a bit more.
2. Add the avocado and mash with a fork, leaving some chunks.
3. Stir in chopped tomato, cilantro, remaining minced jalapeño, lime juice, and salt to taste. Enjoy immediately.

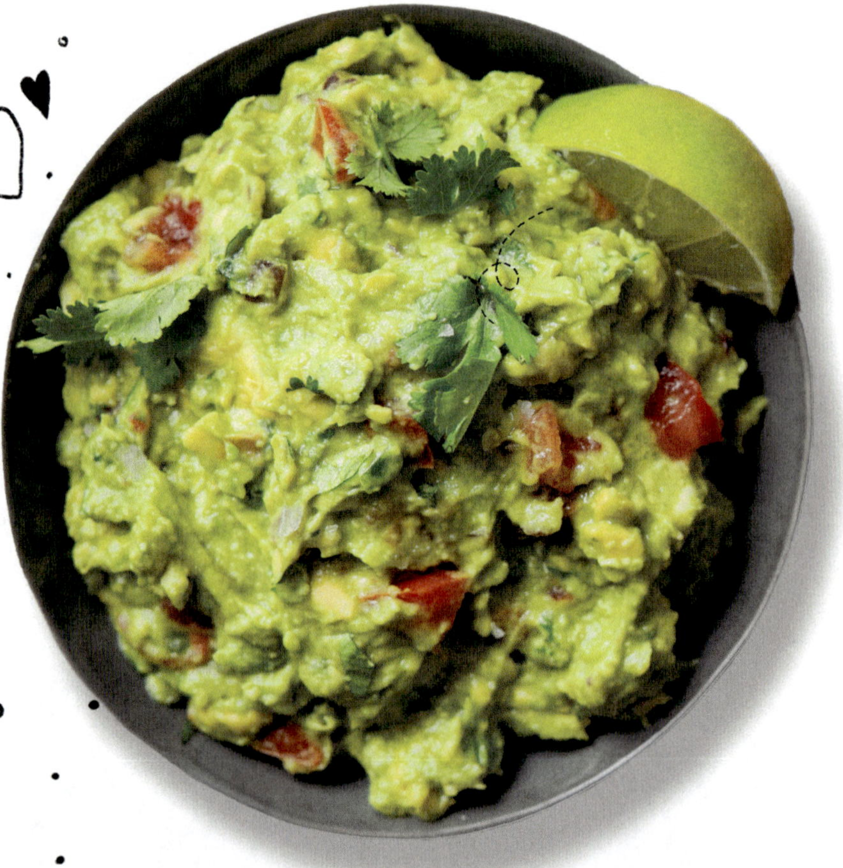

### Fierce Foods Facts

Avocados are filled with monounsaturated heart healthy fats and they make the perfect satiating snack when paired with other fresh vegetables. They are also high in the B Vitamins Folate and B5 (also called pantothenic acid), which is often called the "anti-stress vitamin". So get your yummy snack along with a nice dose of stress reliever!

Chef Alexia Hall, RDN

# Italian Green Beans with Lemon and Garlic

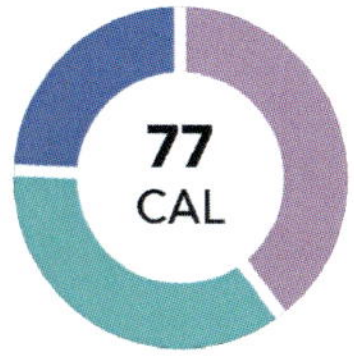


5g **Fat**
5g **Net Carb**
3g **Protein**

**Makes 6 servings:** each ~½ cup, 127 grams

## Ingredients

1½ lb green beans (French or haricot), cleaned and trimmed

1 lemon, zested and juiced

4 cloves garlic, pressed

2 tbsp extra virgin olive oil

¼ tsp salt

¼ tsp pepper

## Directions

1. Trim ends from the green beans. Using a saucepan and steamer basket, add water just to the base of the basket. Bring the water to a boil, then add the green beans and simmer until crisp-tender (about 3 minutes). Remove from heat and drain.
2. Using a zester and juicer, zest and juice the lemon. Heat olive oil over medium-low heat in a sauté pan and add garlic, sautéing for 3 minutes until translucent and lightly browned.
3. Add drained green beans, season with salt and ground black pepper, then add the lemon juice and zest. Enjoy immediately.

### Kids Can Cook Tips

Younger kids can help trim the beans by snapping off the ends or slicing them. They can also help press the garlic and juice and zest the lemon.

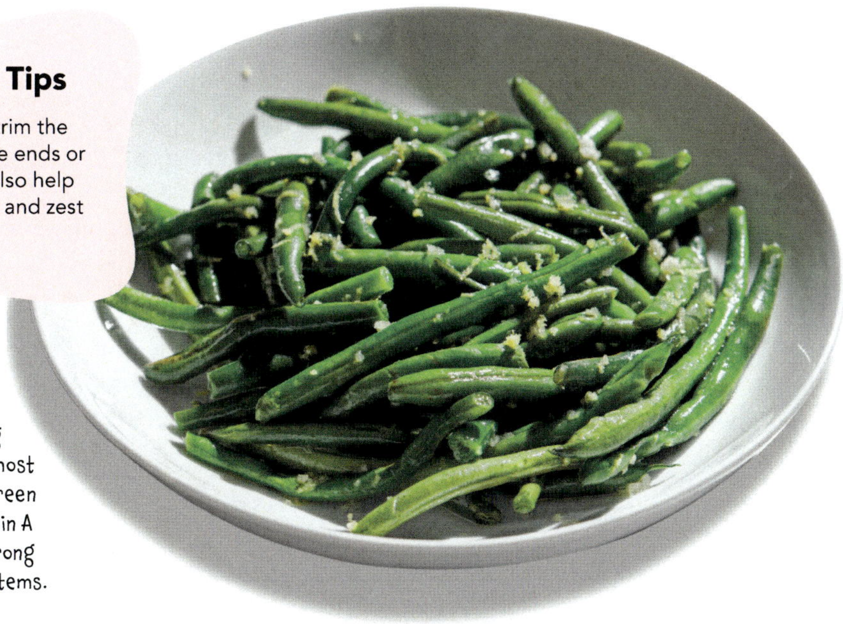

### Fierce Foods Facts

This flavorful side dish provides a wonderful zing from the fresh lemon juice and zest and packs almost 3 grams of fiber per serving. A serving size of green beans also provides almost 20% of the daily vitamin A requirements, helping to support the growth of strong bones, as well as healthy eyesight and immune systems.

Chef Andrew Johnson

# Sunshine Salad

**Makes 4 servings:** each ¼ cup, 67 grams

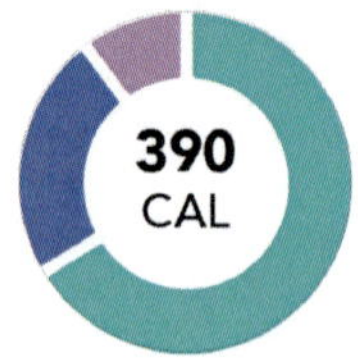


35g Fat
5g Net Carb
12g Protein

## Ingredients

¼ cup extra virgin olive oil

1 clove garlic, thinly sliced

1 tsp ginger, peeled and grated

½ tsp turmeric, ground

¼ tsp chili flakes

1 avocado, peeled, pit removed and sliced

1 lemon, juiced

¼ cup baby spinach

¼ cup baby arugula

¼ cup feta, crumbled

1 oz pepitas, roasted salted

1 tbsp flat leaf parsley

kosher or sea salt, and pepper to taste

## Directions

1. Place the avocado on a cutting board and with a chef knife, cut the avocado in half with the knife parallel to the cutting board by rotating the avocado in a circle. Give the avocado a gently twist to split in half. Place the avocado back on the cutting board and with careful swinging motion, jam the middle of the knife blade into the pit.
2. Give the knife a careful twist and the pit should come out attached to the blade. Then with your thumb from the back of the knife push the pit into the trash can. With a large spoon scoop the avocado flesh from the skin.
3. Slice each avocado half into 4 slices, add them into a medium mixing bowl, and squeeze the lemon juice over the top to keep it from browning. In your favorite family-size serving bowl or plate, arrange the greens on the bottom and top with the sliced avocados.
4. Bring a small/medium sauté pan to medium heat, then add olive oil, garlic, ginger, turmeric, salt, and pepper. Cook, giving it the occasional stir until the garlic starts to sizzle and turns golden and toasty. Cook and stir frequently to fully incorporate the ingredients. Cook until the garlic is starting to caramelize, approximately 3–5 minutes.
5. Let the dressing cool. Lightly drizzle the dressing over top the salad. Top the salad with crumbled feta and pepitas, season with salt and fresh cracked black pepper, and finish with parsley.

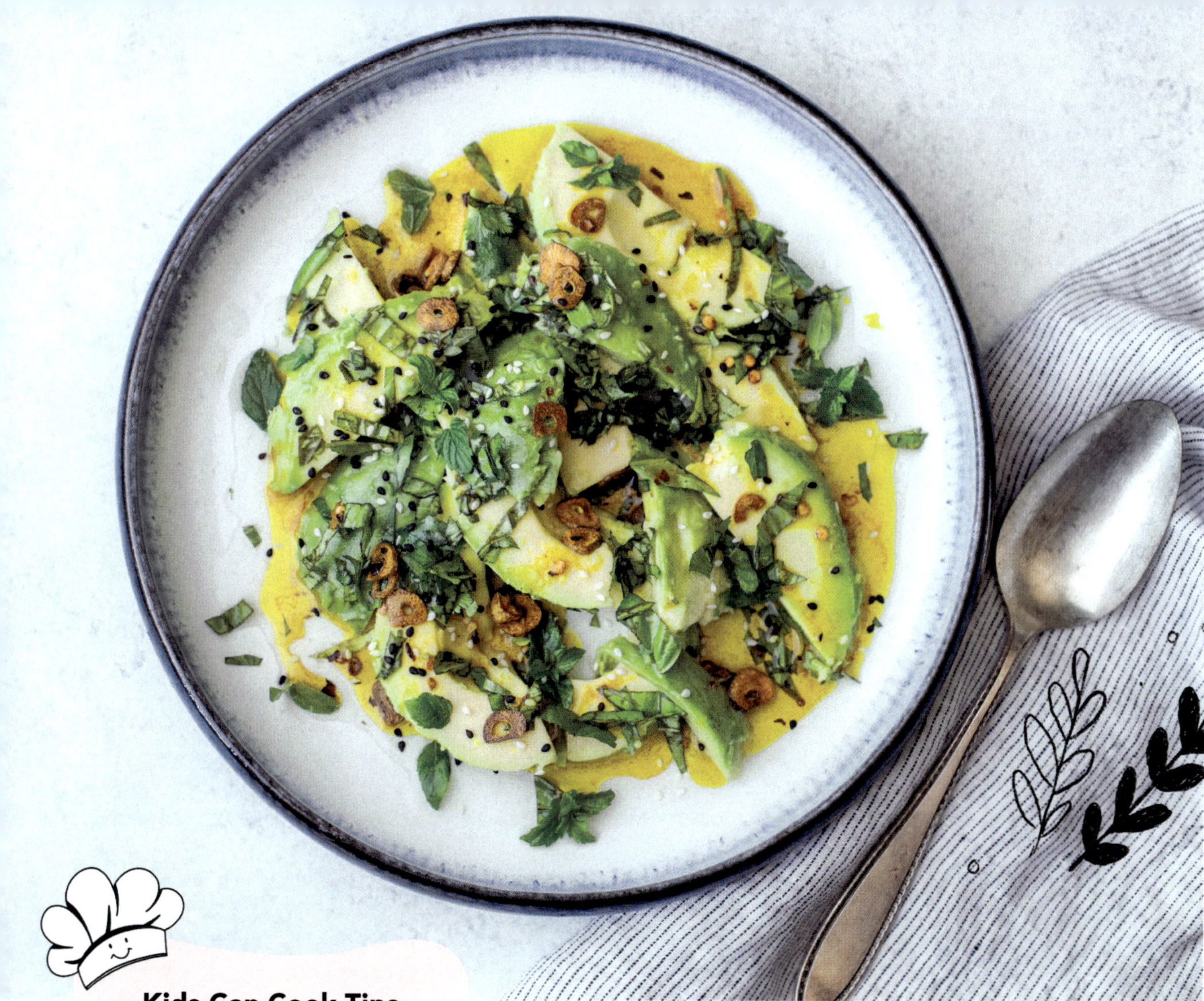

### Kids Can Cook Tips

Younger kids can help prepare the herbs by washing and tearing them into bite size pieces and measuring the oil and juice. Older kids with knife skills can slice the avocado, the lemon, and the garlic.

### Fierce Foods Facts

This fresh and golden summer salad is anti-inflammatory in just about every way. The heart healthy fat from the avocado provides a nice amount of vitamin E, and it makes a winning combination when combined with the anti-inflammatory properties of the dark green leafy vegetables and herbs!

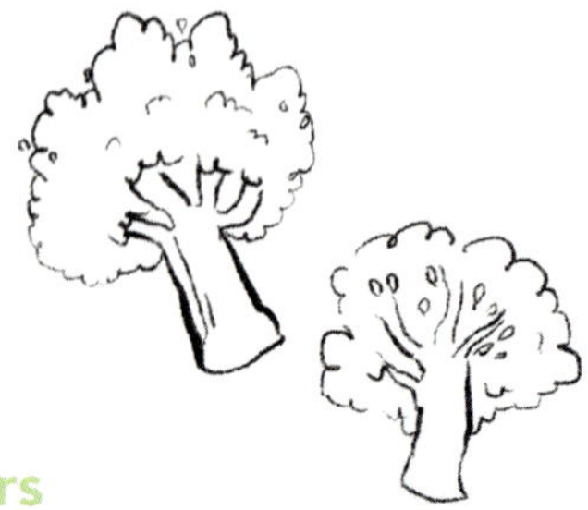

## Roasted Crucifers

Cruciferous vegetables (also known as brassicas) have superstar status in the world of vegetables—and for good reason. Included in this group are broccoli, Brussels sprouts, cabbage, cauliflower, collard greens, kale, and mustard greens. They are loaded with nutrients that support the immune system, lower inflammation, and fight cancer. They also have a very low glycemic impact on blood sugar due to their low net carbohydrate and high fiber contents.

Most dark green cruciferous veggies are high in folate (a B vitamin that is involved in energy production as well as new cell division) and vitamin K which is important in blood clotting. The dark green varieties also contain phytonutrients, which are invaluable for fighting inflammation. A serving of these delicious veggies also keeps gut bugs happy by providing their favorite fuel: fiber. The term for the nutrient in cruciferous veggies that helps to fight cancer is called glucosinolates and is a sulfur-based compound important in ridding the body of unwanted and other toxic compounds.

The cooking method chosen can change the way these nutrients are used in the body. Benefits of eating raw cruciferous vegetables include retaining intact enzymes that will help digest the food, as well as more glucosinolates which can be sensitive to heat. There are also benefits to cooked cruciferous which include decreasing the chance of food-borne illnesses and possibly improving digestion for those that are having trouble tolerating raw.

Some nutrient levels improve when these vegetables are cooked, such as the enzyme released "indole" which is one of the phytochemicals that fight cancer. However, long and high heat cooking can decrease nutrients, especially vitamin C, and can also lower the level of certain flavonoids like beta carotene which are important in their role as antioxidants. Light steaming is generally preferred over higher and longer cooking methods in order to maximize nutrition.

If greens are often high on the refusal list, start with mild-tasting greens and work up to stronger flavors. Milder-tasting spinach or swiss chard might be accepted baked into a frittata before the kale is. Also, consider making a 50-50 or 25-75 substitution by chopping small pieces of darker greens and swapping for portions of lettuce in a salad loaded with other accepted flavors like cheeses and nuts.

Using other accepted foods as a bridge such as blending greens into a spaghetti sauce, or using some in the dip recipes contained in the next section, can help gain acceptance by slowly acclimating taste buds to the new food. Having a novel event such as "pick a green vegetable day" can make the trial of new foods sound like a fun adventure that might pique a child's interest.

Have patience—studies show it could take up to 15 attempts before a child (or an adult!) will accept new foods. Use positive reinforcement and encourage exposure to the new food allowing for safe experimentation. Have kids use their words to explain how they are feeling when trying new foods.

Read on for some vegetable side dishes that are kid-friendly, kid-tested, and kid-approved!

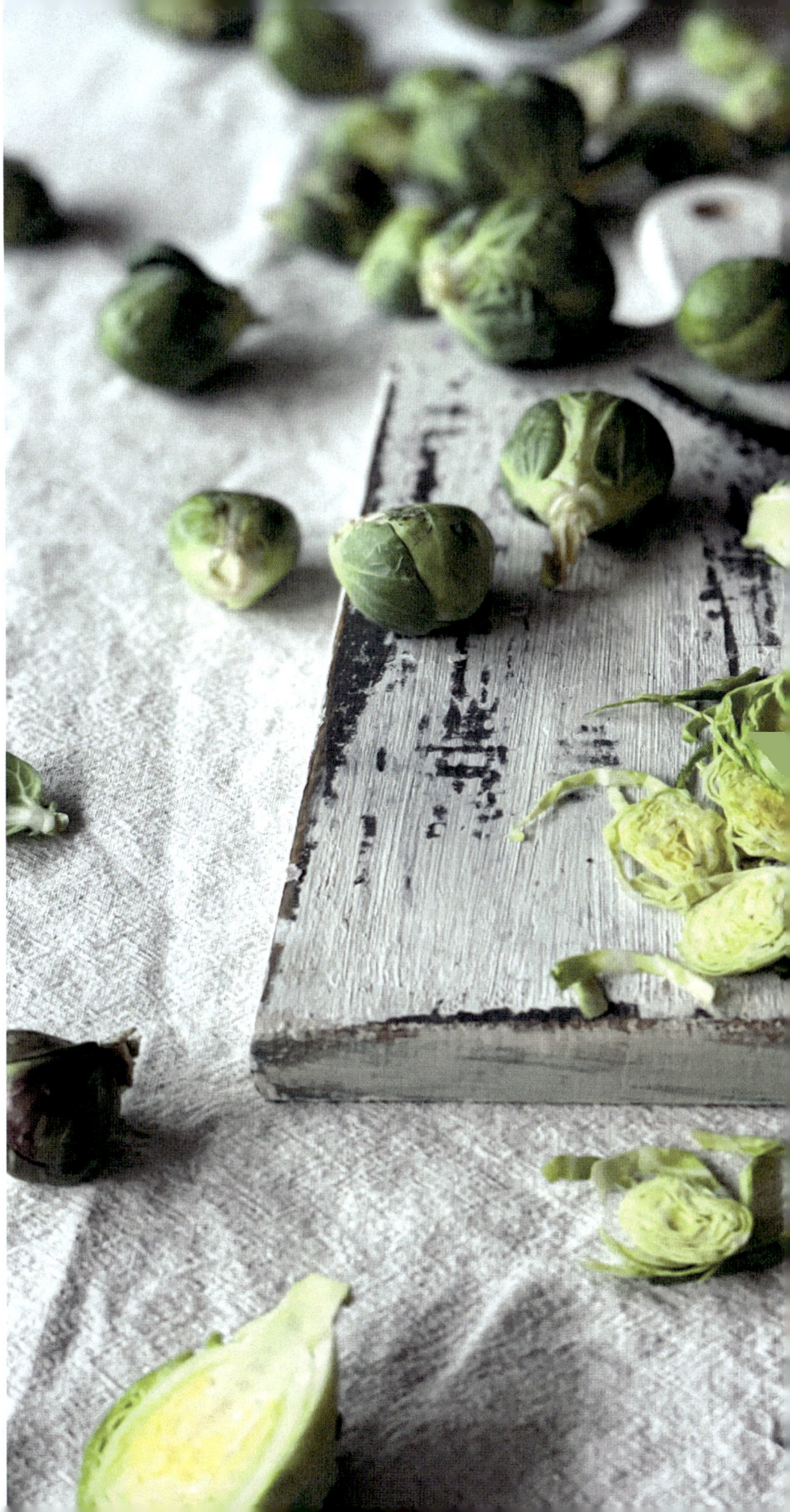

Chef Andrew Johnson

# Sautéed Brussels Sprouts with Bacon

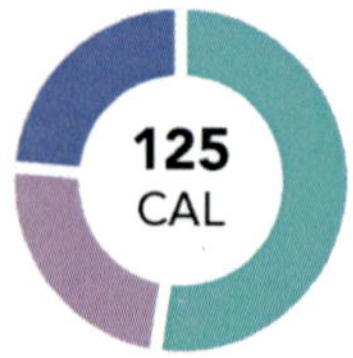


9g Fat
4g Net Carb
4g Protein

**Makes 6 servings:** each ~½ cup, 96 grams

## Ingredients

1 lb fresh Brussels sprouts, halved and sliced thin

5 slices bacon, chopped

2 tbsp fresh chives, chopped

1 tbsp fresh tarragon, chopped

2 tbsp apple cider vinegar

¼ tsp black pepper

⅛ tsp salt

## Directions

1. Cut Brussels sprouts in half and slice them into ⅛" slices. Heat a large cast iron skillet to medium-high, then add chopped bacon. Cook until golden brown, stirring frequently. Remove the bacon from the pan and drain on a plate with a paper towel.
2. Leaving the bacon fat in the skillet and the heat on, add shaved sprouts, then cook and stir for 3–4 minutes. Add salt, pepper, and apple cider vinegar to the pan, and stir to deglaze. Turn off the heat and toss in the bacon and herbs. Enjoy immediately.

### Fierce Foods Facts

This flavorful low carbohydrate side dish packs a wonderful punch of vitamins K and C supporting the heart and the immune system. Cruciferous vegetables are powerful allies in the cancer-fighting world!

### Kids Can Cook Tips

Younger kids can help wash and tear the herbs and help with seasoning. Older kids can practice their knife skills with both the bacon and the Brussels.

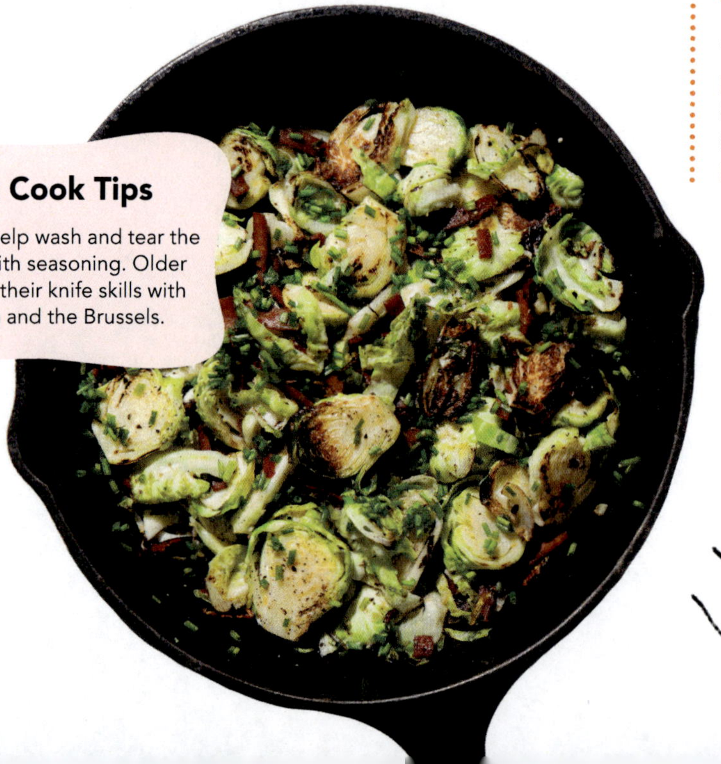

Chef Andrew Johnson

# Tri-Color Pepper Salad

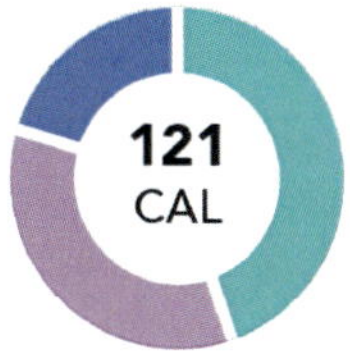


**Makes 6 servings:** each ~4 ounces or ½ cup, 114 grams

## Ingredients

1 clove garlic, minced

3 tbsp champagne vinegar

3 whole mild peppers (e.g. Hungarian wax, hatch, poblano, tri-color bells, or Habanada)

½ cup fresh flat-leaf parsley, oregano, lemon verbena, or basil (approx. 3 oz), minced

2 tbsp extra virgin olive oil

½ tsp salt

¼ tsp black pepper, freshly ground

2 tbsp red onion, peeled and sliced very thin crosswise

½ cup crumbled feta cheese

## Directions

1. Using a large bowl, combine the garlic and vinegar and let sit for 15 minutes. Prepare the peppers by removing the seeds and white membranes, then slice the peppers into thin strips.
2. Separate the parsley leaves (if using) from the stems and discard the stems. Finely chop the herb leaves and set aside.
3. Using a whisk, blend the olive oil, salt, and pepper into the garlic-vinegar mixture. Add more salt and pepper to taste.
4. Toss the peppers, herbs, and onion with the dressing, then add feta and toss gently. Serve at room temperature or cover and chill for up to 2 hours.

### Fierce Foods Facts

This beautiful and healthy salad provides an ample amount of antioxidants and folate to keep you healthy. Consider replacing some of the milder peppers with hotter peppers if you can handle the heat—this will help to create a healthier heart and add more anti-inflammatory spice to your life!

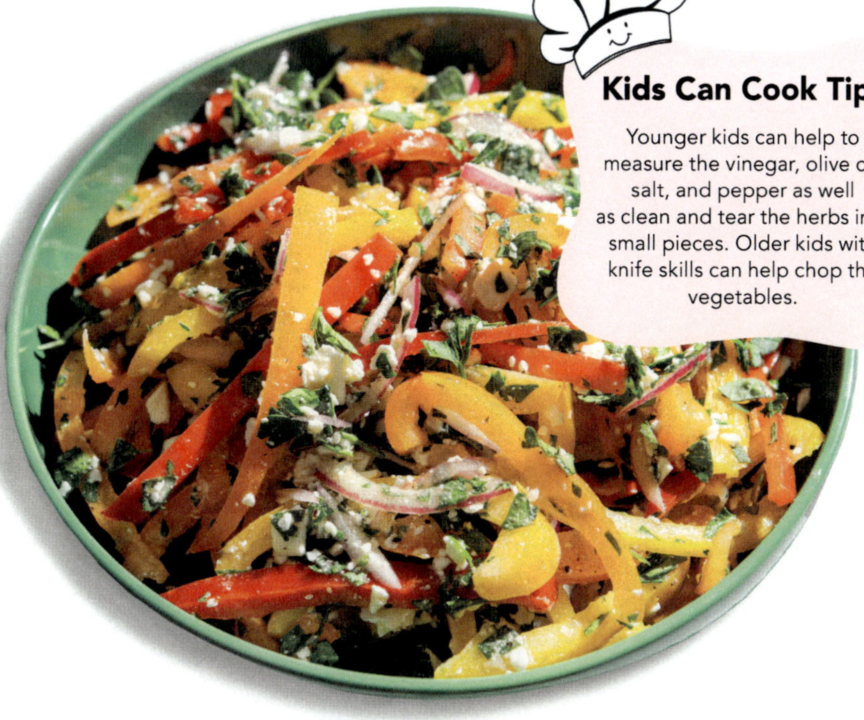

### Kids Can Cook Tips

Younger kids can help to measure the vinegar, olive oil, salt, and pepper as well as clean and tear the herbs into small pieces. Older kids with knife skills can help chop the vegetables.

Chef Cathy McKnight

# Skillet Cornbread

**Makes 12 servings:** each ~2"x2" square, 92 grams

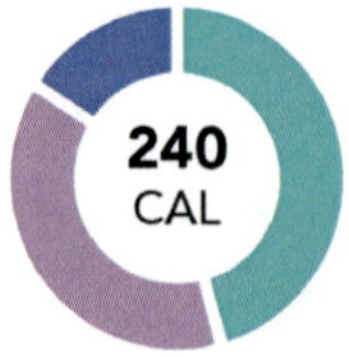


18g **Fat**
15g **Net Carb**
6g **Protein**

18g **Net Carb** with the addition of the corn

## Ingredients

1½ cups cornmeal

1 cup almond flour

2 tsp baking powder

1 tsp baking soda

1 tbsp granulated allulose sweetener

1 tsp sea salt

1 tsp smoked paprika

2 eggs

2 cups buttermilk

1 cup fresh or frozen corn (optional)

½ cup shredded cheese (optional)

½ cup scallions chopped (optional)

½ cup avocado oil

## Directions

1. Preheat the grill to 425°F. Place a 9" cast iron skillet on the grill and let it heat up while you make the cornbread batter.

2. In a large mixing bowl, add the eggs, sweetener, and buttermilk, then blend together with a whisk or an electric mixer. In a separate mixing bowl combine almond flour, cornmeal, baking powder, baking soda, salt, and smoked paprika. Add the dry ingredients to the wet ingredients slowly, and incorporate do not over mix. Fold in the corn, scallions, and/or cheese.

3. Allow the batter to set up at room temperature for 5–10 minutes before baking. Carefully remove the cast iron skillet from the grill and pour the avocado oil into the middle of the pan. Tilt the pan around in a circular pattern to oil up the sides of the pan, careful not to spill the hot oil. Pour the batter into the center of the pan with caution: it will bubble and splatter. Place the cast iron pan back onto the grill away from direct heat. Close the grill and bake for 15–25 minutes.

4. To check for doneness, shake the pan: the center should be firm. Then push a bread knife down through the middle and when it is fully cooked the knife should come out clean. When cooked, remove it from the grill and let it cool for a few minutes before serving.

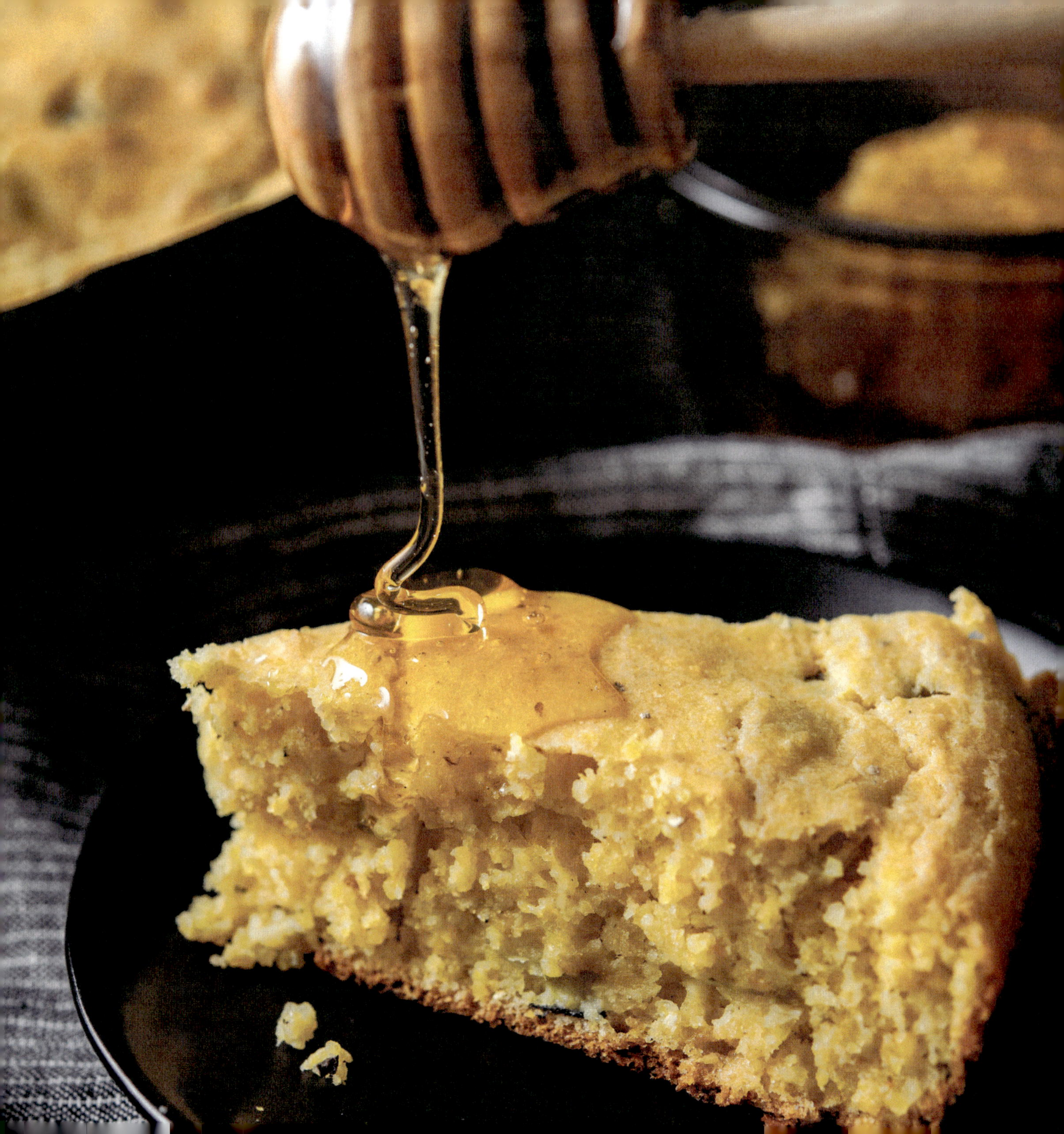

Chef Cathy McKnight

# Drop Biscuits

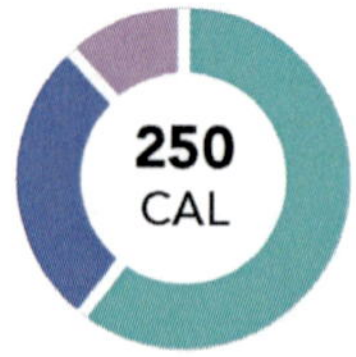


22g Fat
4g Net Carb
10g Protein

**Makes 12 servings:** 1 each, 64 grams

## Ingredients

3 cups almond flour

4 tsp baking powder

1 cup shredded cheddar cheese (optional, but highly recommended)

½ cup full-fat yogurt, unflavored

4 large eggs

4 tbsp unsalted butter, softened

1 tsp sea or kosher salt

½ cup chopped green onions or chives (optional)

## Directions

1. Preheat the oven to 400°F. In a large mixing bowl add yogurt, eggs, cheese and butter, then mix or beat with an electric mixer. Add in almond flour, baking powder, salt, and green onions (if using).
2. Let stand at room temperature for 5 minutes. Using a 2-ounce ice cream scoop, drop biscuits evenly onto a parchment-lined 18"x13" sheet pan. Bake for 10–12 minutes until the biscuits are golden brown.
3. Remove from the oven and let cool. Enjoy immediately or store in a sealed container in the refrigerator for up to a week.

### Fierce Foods Facts

Warm, fresh biscuits out of the oven are a favorite for sure! This one comes loaded with bone-building calcium, phosphorus, copper, and magnesium thanks to the almond flour and the dairy, plus plenty of fiber—all in a low-carb package!

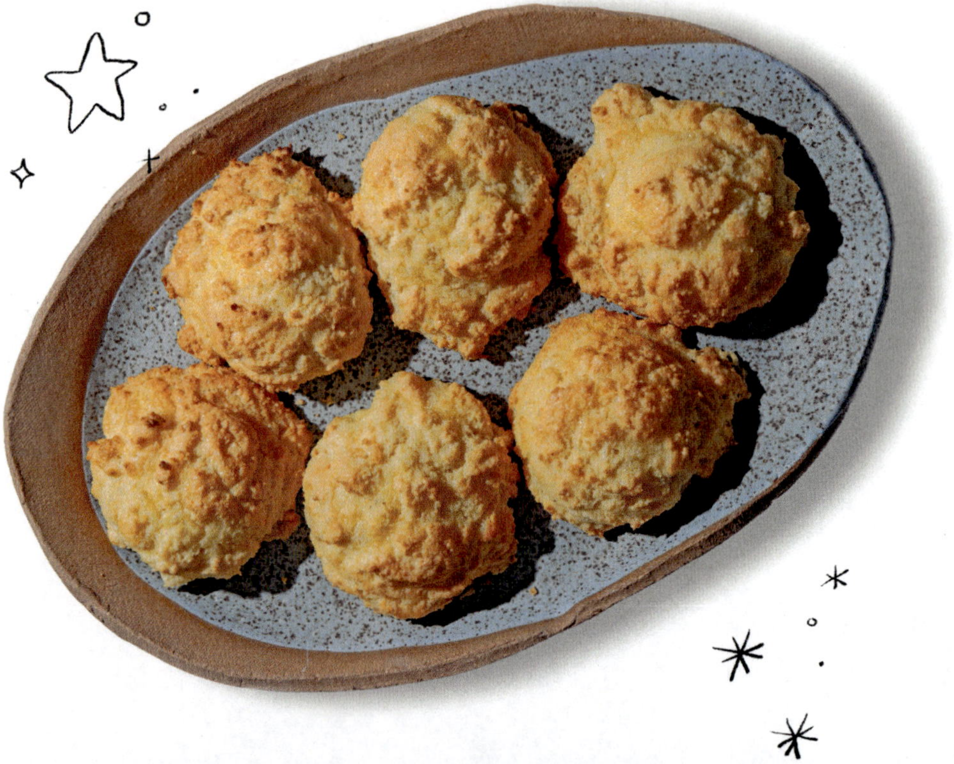

Chef Andrew Johnson

# Hushpuppies

**Makes 6 servings:** 2 puppies each, 93 grams

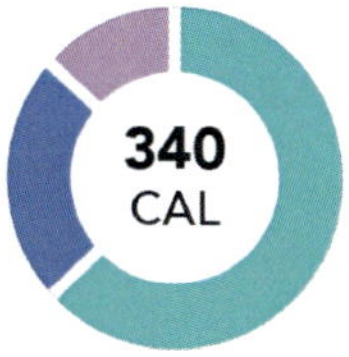


30g **Fat**
6g **Net Carb**
11g **Protein**

## Ingredients

2 cups almond flour

1 tbsp tapioca flour

2 tsp baking powder

1 tsp sea or kosher salt

½ cup buttermilk

2 large eggs

½ cup scallions, finely chopped

Avocado oil spray

## Directions

1. In a large mixing bowl, combine the almond flour, tapioca, baking powder, and salt, then add in the buttermilk and eggs. Fully incorporate the ingredients, careful not to over-mix, then fold in the scallions.
2. Let the mixture rest at room temperature for 5–10 minutes. Preheat the oven to 425°F. Spray a mini muffin tin with avocado oil spray, and then, using a small ice cream scoop or tablespoon, drop the hushpuppy batter into the muffin tin. Once all the batter is used up, spray the tops of the batter with a light coat of avocado oil spray and place in the oven for 15–20 minutes until golden brown and crispy. Enjoy immediately.

### Fierce Foods Facts

The almond flour substitutes nicely for the cornmeal in this makeover recipe, providing ample amounts of the antioxidant vitamin E and bone-building phosphorus in the process. This low-carb side hits the mark when accompanying many Southern favorites and is super easy and fast to put on the table.

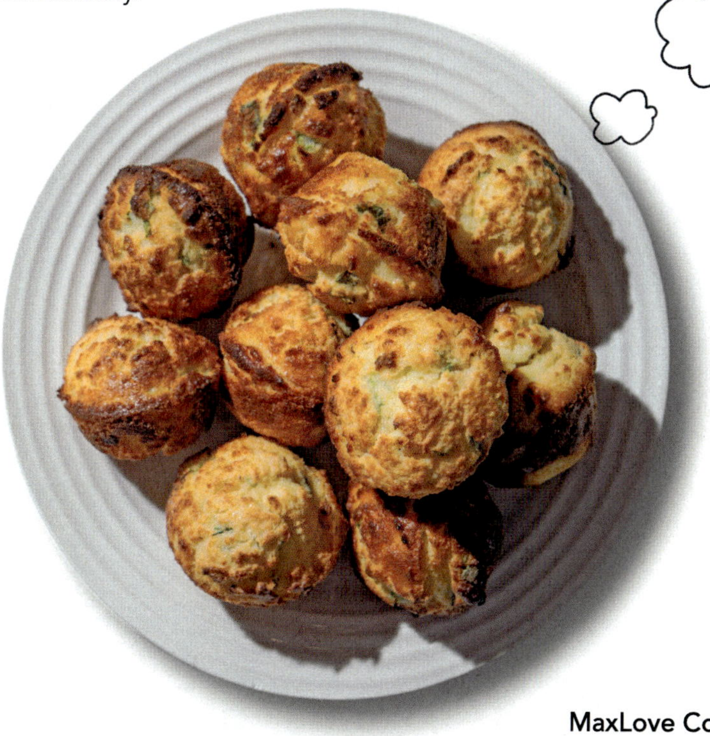

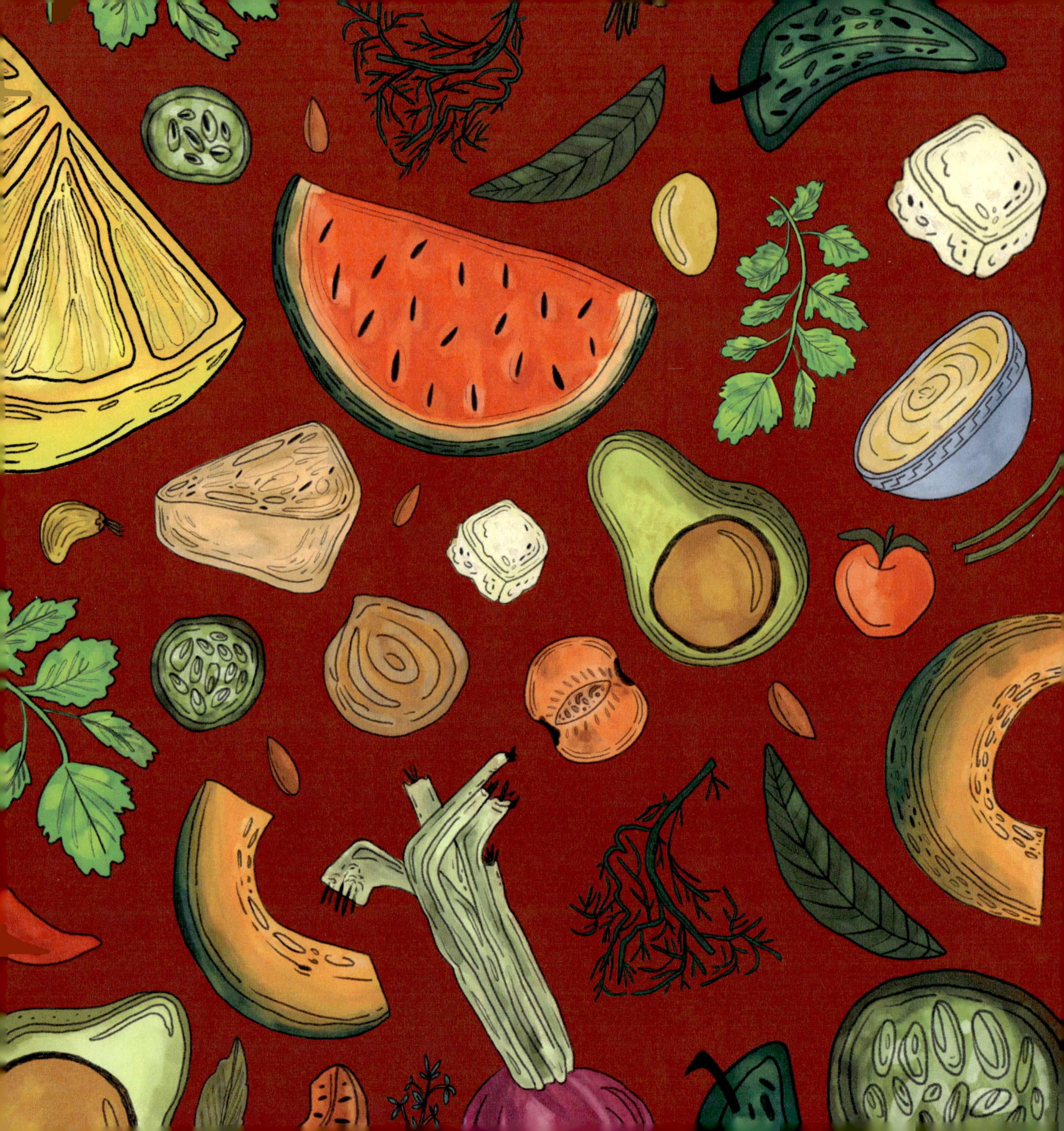

# STAPLES

# Staples



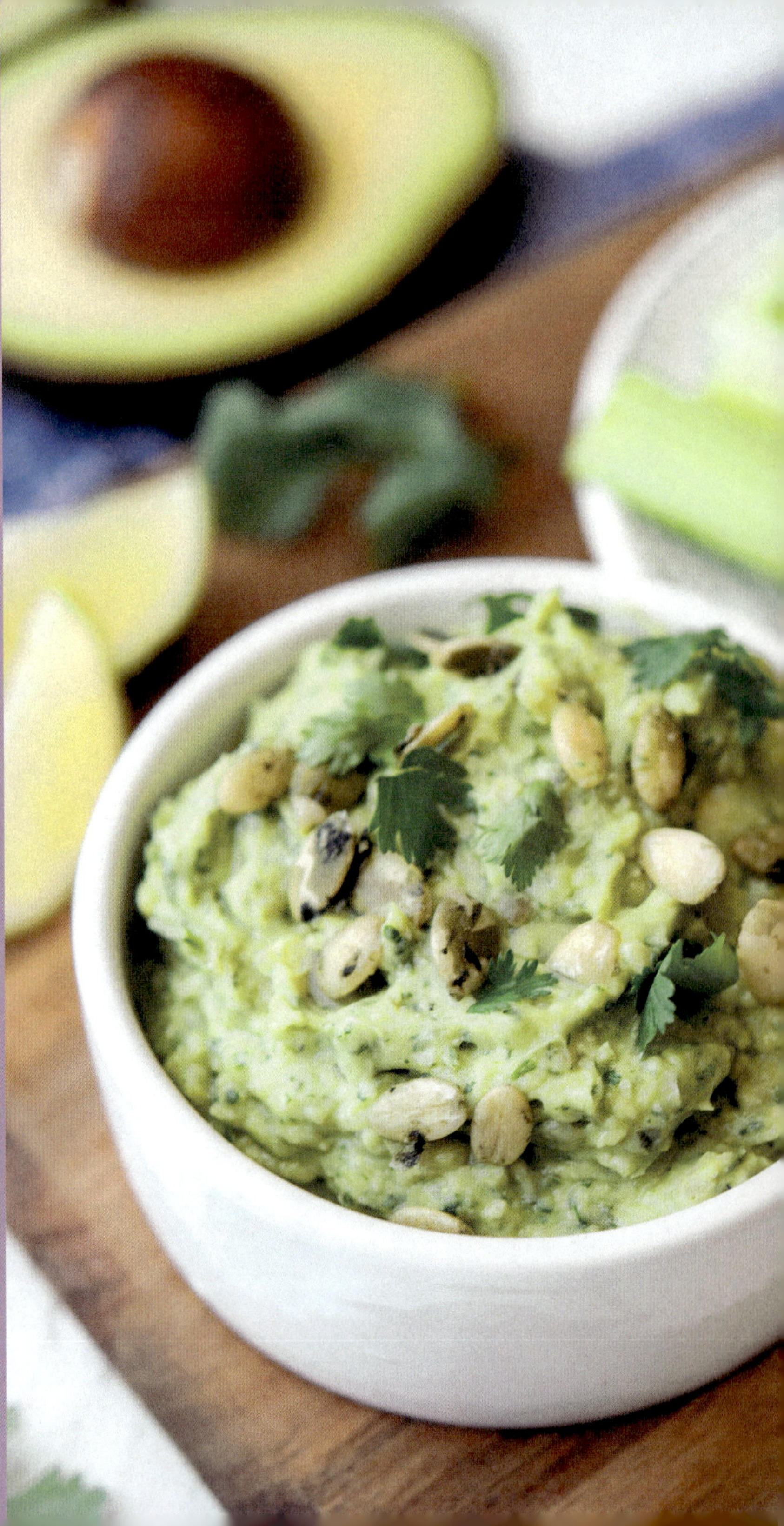

The frustrating part about purchasing pre-made staples such as broths, dips, and dressings is that they are often made with low-quality, inexpensive ingredients and then loaded with sugar to make them taste better. It doesn't serve health needs when sugar is the first ingredient on the list (and therefore the most by volume in the bottle).

There is now an abundance of evidence showing that too much added sugar is leading to serious diseases such as diabetes, heart disease, and liver disease. Newer research is also showing a link between excessive sugar intake and decreased quality of mental health. Making your own dips, dressings, and marinades at home will allow for more control of ingredients and thus ensure more nutrient density (and less sugar) in the final product.

Almost every recipe in this chapter can be batch cooked, pre-portioned and then frozen so it can be used later as a base or a staple in other recipes. This will improve nutrient quality, as well as save time and money!

Dips in this section can provide a flavorful bridge that will allow the intake of more vegetables and thus more nutrition. Adding the tangy note of lemon or the savory note of dill just prior to eating can sometimes provide a necessary distraction for someone dealing with altered taste buds affected by treatment and make eating less of a chore.

Flavorful dressings with anti-inflammatory fats can help support weight gain by providing a soothing salve for someone with mouth sores. Marinades that are bursting with herbs not only provide flavor for barbeques and roasts but also quench the undesirable carcinogenic chemicals created by cooking at high heat.

The following recipes are meant to be simple, without the need for complicated ingredients or tools. However, they are also easily customizable, as a base for different flavor profiles or also for the addition of superfoods that may provide a solution to nagging side effects.

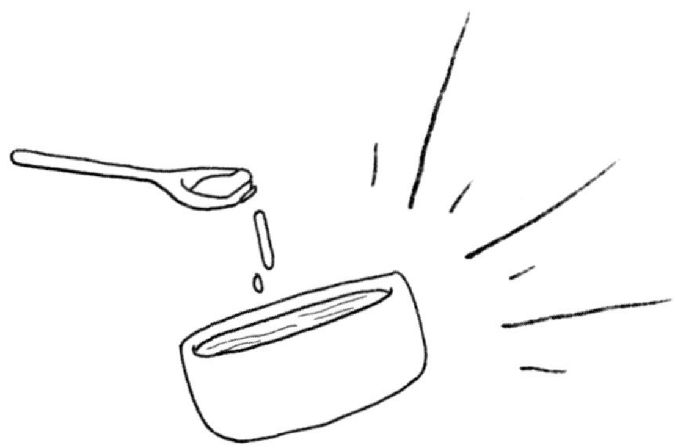

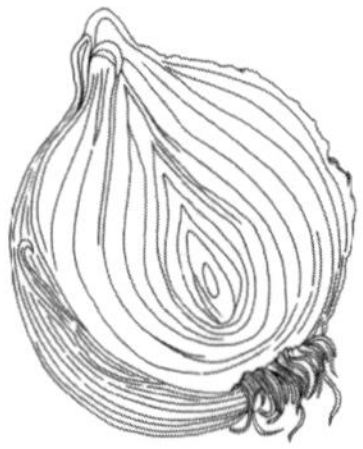

## Bone Broths

Broths often evoke warm memories of comfort food. Since bone broth usually makes up the foundation of a soup or stew, it provides many additional evidence-supported health benefits.

In one important example, studies conducted on both mice and piglets showed increased white blood cell counts after consuming beef bone marrow (the superpower nutrient inside the bones that is released upon cooking). Maintaining white blood cell counts is valuable to those undergoing oncology treatments which can be interrupted if counts fall too low.

Soups are generally loaded with soft, cooked vegetables and spices that have some culinary medicine superpowers too. For example, the addition of ginger can be useful for fighting nausea, while fresh basil can be soothing for mouth sores. Broccoli and Brussels sprouts can provide soluble fiber that helps to minimize diarrhea. Carrots and beets can provide an anti-inflammatory boost at just the right time. Potassium-loaded bok choy and tomatoes can be just what the doctor (or dietitian) ordered to help lessen swelling.

Body systems such as the skin, digestive tract, bones, joints, and brain can all benefit from the ingredients that are broken down when bones are simmered and made into a broth. When proteins are unfolded in this way they release specialty nutrients used to repair and restore different cells in the body. This broken-down protein also makes digestion easier. Glycine is one such specialty protein that is released and when consumed, can help the nervous system to relax. Glucosamine and chondroitin are other proteins that are shown to be effective at decreasing joint pain and supporting the synovial fluid that provides a cushion between the joints and the bones. Collagen, gelatin, glycine, and glutamine also are effective in repairing the gut lining, soothing and strengthening the gut barrier, and preventing increased intestinal permeability which can also strengthen the immune system.

See the following pages for instructions to create a delicious and nutritious broth that can provide a bountiful foundation for many different dishes. A thermos full of delicious bone broth or soup can provide a welcome source of comfort during short or long hospital stays.

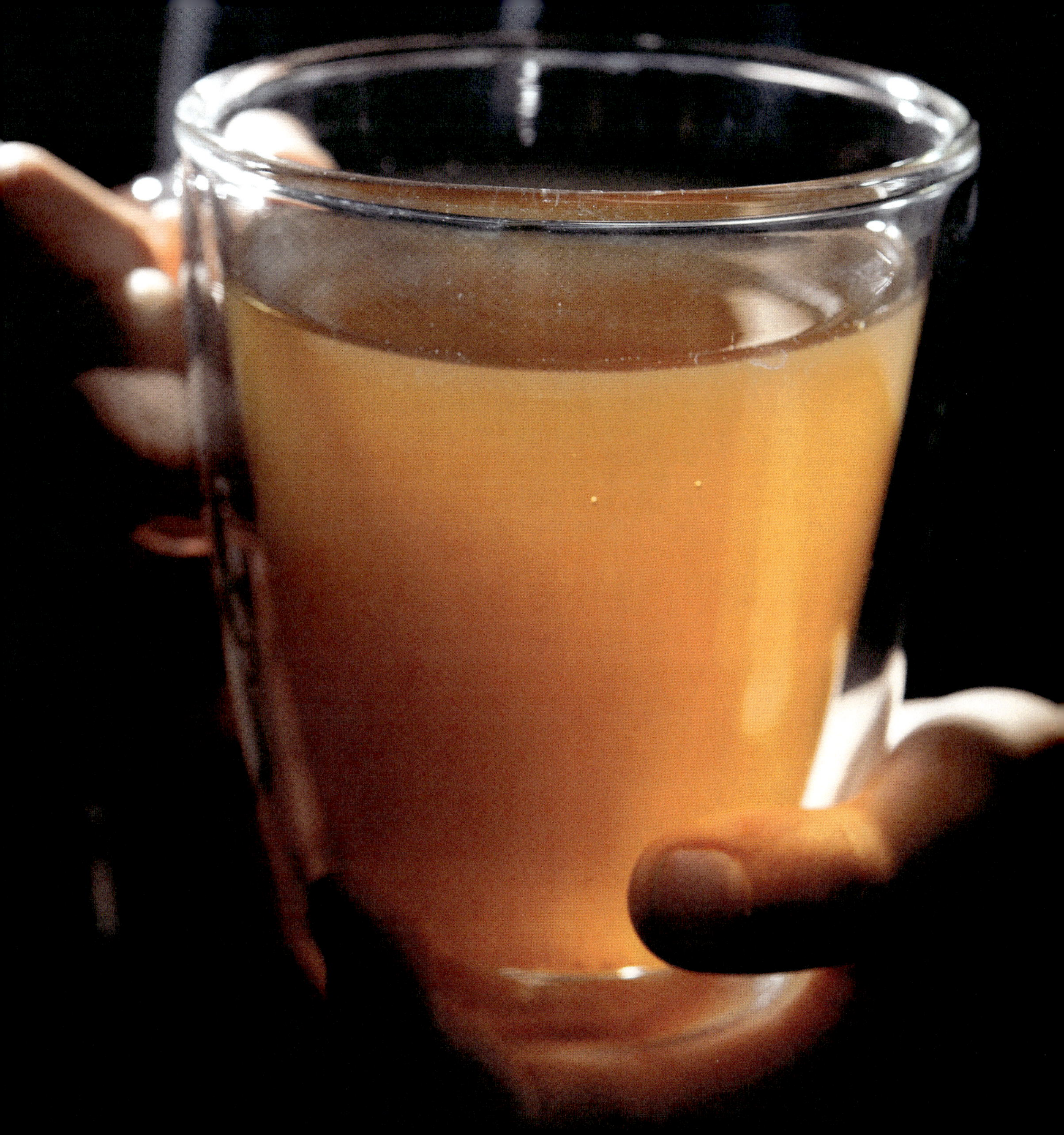

Chef Andrew Johnson

# Bone Broth

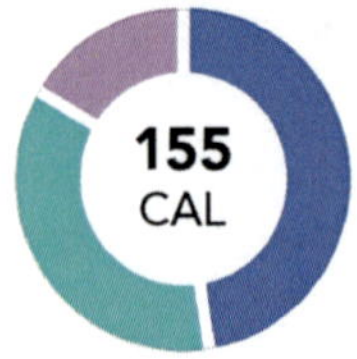


9g Fat
4g Net Carb
12g Protein

**Makes 3 quarts, 18 servings:** each 1 cup, 249 grams

## Ingredients

2½ lb of large marrow bones, beef, chicken, turkey (for best results, use bones with lots of connective tissue, e.g. chicken feet)

2 onions, rough chopped (skin on is fine)

½ lb carrots, rough chop

1 can (6 oz) of tomato paste

1–2" piece of ginger, large sliced

1–2" piece of turmeric, large sliced

3–4 cloves garlic, smashed (skin on is fine)

2 tbsp unfiltered apple cider vinegar or lemon juice

4–6 quarts water

## Directions

1. Preheat the oven to 400°F. In a large mixing bowl, toss the bones and tomato paste to evenly coat. On a parchment-lined 18"x13" baking sheet, spread out the bones in a single layer and roast in the oven for 30 minutes.
2. Remove from the oven and transfer the bones and jus into the Instant Pot or slow cooker bowl. Using the baking sheet, spread out all the vegetables in an even layer and roast in the oven for 15 minutes. When the vegetables are roasted, transfer them to the Instant Pot or slow cooker bowl, cover with water up to the max fill line, and add the vinegar or lemon juice.
3. Set the Instant Pot to manual high pressure for 120 minutes, then when complete, allow it to release steam naturally.
4. If using a slow cooker, set the temperature to high, then reduce the heat to low after the broth starts to boil and continue simmering for up to 24 hours.
5. When fully cooked, allow to cool slightly, and carefully pour the contents and liquid through a fine mesh strainer into a container. Fill your sink or a large cooler or tub with ice water, then place the container of broth in the ice bath to rapidly chill for about 1 hour. Skim the fat cap from the container of bone broth and discard.
6. Use the bone broth right away, or cover and refrigerate for up to 1 week. You can also freeze the broth in portion-sized containers for up to a year.

## Fierce Foods Facts

It is an established fact (as well as ancient wisdom) that bone broth is nutrient-dense, comforting, and immune-supporting. In fact, there is even evidence in animal studies that bone broth, when properly made, can increase white blood cell counts!

The addition of ginger and turmeric can also aid with stimulating appetite and calming nausea for those impacted by oncology treatments. Grass-fed bones also help to provide an anti-inflammatory healthy source of fat with an excellent source of collagen-based protein, helpful for skin, joints, nails, and bones.

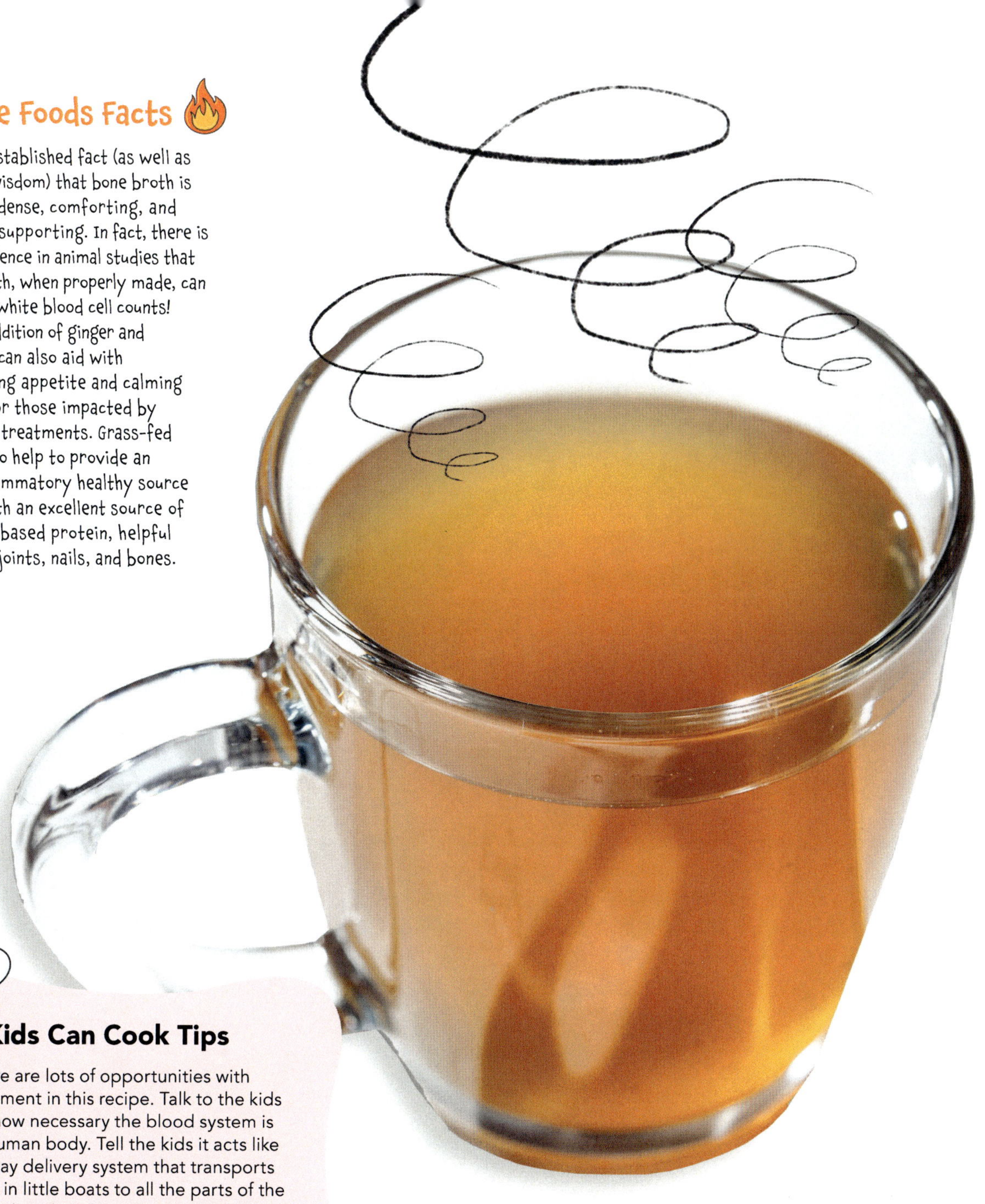

## Kids Can Cook Tips

There are lots of opportunities with measurement in this recipe. Talk to the kids about how necessary the blood system is to the human body. Tell the kids it acts like a highway delivery system that transports nutrients in little boats to all the parts of the body. Explain that the nutrients in the bone broth help to support a strong blood system.

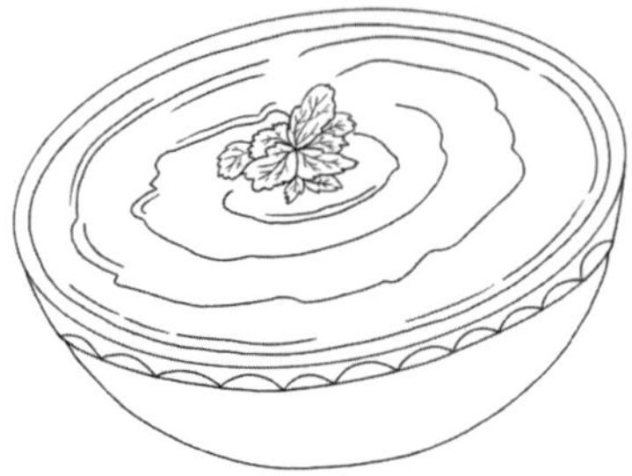

## Dressings and Dips

As stated previously, store-bought dressings and dips can be full of unwanted ingredients and too much refined sugar. Homemade dips like those created by our amazing chefs are flavorful and nutrient-dense. They can be made in advance, saving time and money.

Several of the recipes in this chapter are designed to be made in large batch cook sections and frozen into ice cube trays for just the right serving size for future meals. This is a great way to preserve potassium-packed citrus fruits or cancer-fighting polyphenol-filled herbs for use when they are no longer in season.

The creamy moisture of dips and dressings provides a welcome solution to those who have mouth sores, low saliva production, or taste alterations due to treatment. They also provide a tasty bridge that encourages the consumption of the recommended 8+ servings of daily fruits and vegetables. The addition of anti-inflammatory fats can help with weight gain, quickly adding calories to assist if someone doesn't feel up to eating large amounts of food.

Dressings and dips often contain a concentrated mix of fresh and dried herbs that can be used for culinary medicine purposes. For example, turmeric, garlic, and basil are anti-inflammatory but also have anti-bacterial functions too. Consider using the delicious Basil Cream Pesto with chicken or fish to help bring relief. Flax and chia are called "mucilaginous" herbs, meaning that they can soothe and protect inflamed internal tissues, especially in the GI tract.

Ginger, garlic, lemon balm, and parsley are called "carminative" herbs that can reduce gas, lessen abdominal cramps and increase motility in the GI tract, preventing constipation.

Enjoy the flavorful dressings, dips, and marinades in this chapter by making some today and storing some for later too!

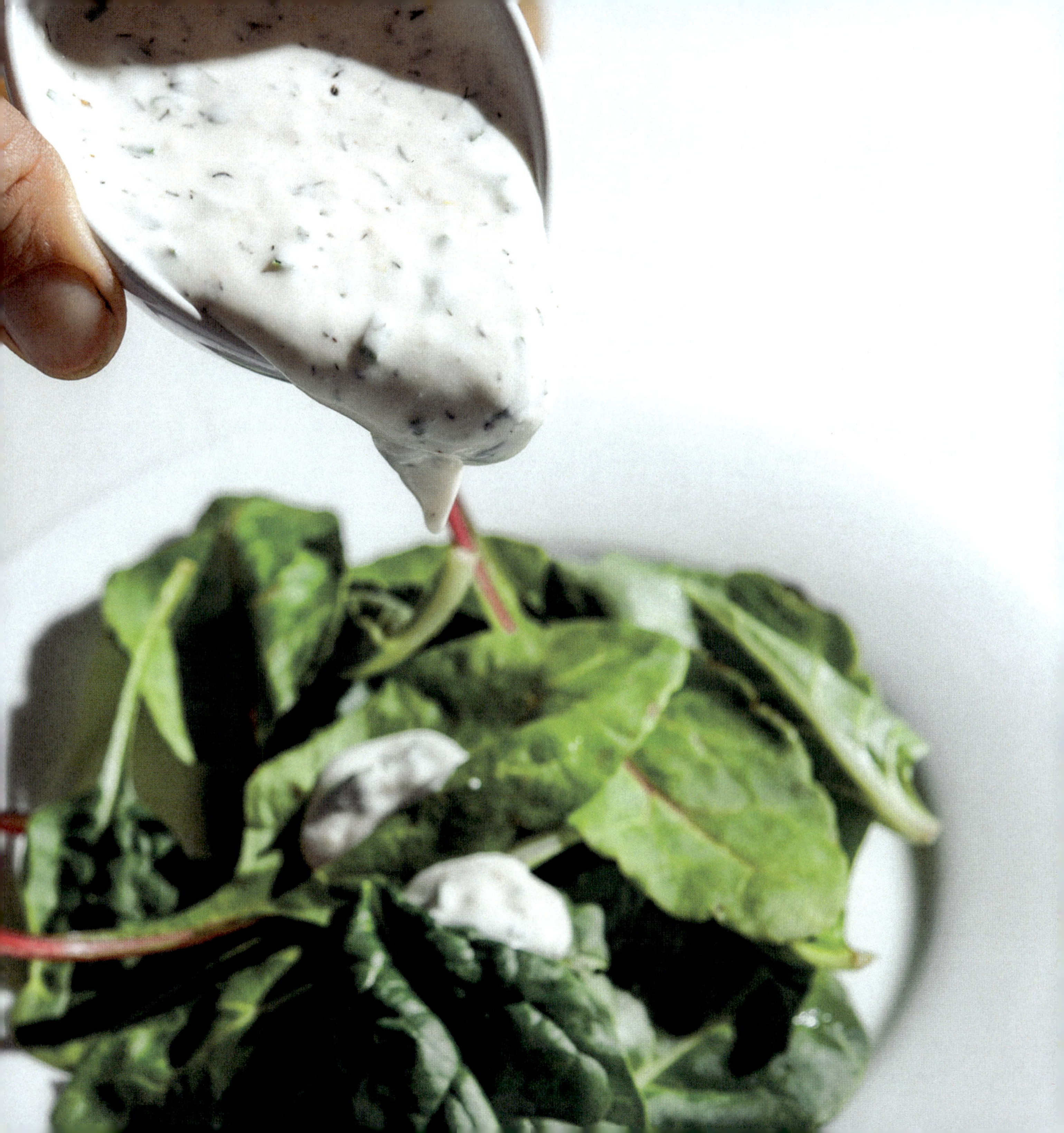

Chef Alexia Hall, RDN

# Avocado Pepita Dip

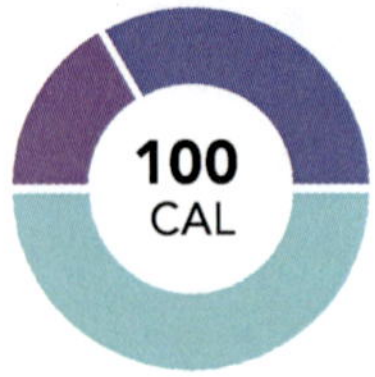


9g **Fat**
2g **Net Carb**
3g **Protein**

**Makes 8 servings:** each ~2 tablespoons, 55 grams

## Ingredients

2 large avocados, pitted and sliced

1 cup cilantro, packed (mostly leaves, some small stems are okay)

½ cup pepitas

1 jalapeño, seeded and roughly chopped (or ¼ tsp red pepper flakes)

2 cloves garlic, roughly chopped

3 tsp lime juice, separated

2 tbsp water

1 tsp fine grain sea salt

Freshly ground black pepper to taste

## Directions

1. Toast the pepitas in a skillet over medium heat until they are fragrant and slightly brown. If using sprouted pepitas, it's okay to skip this step as they already have the desired crunch.
2. Transfer to a bowl and set aside. In a food processor or blender, combine the avocado, cilantro, jalapeño, garlic, and salt. Blend to desired consistency. Add the pepitas and blend until chopped. Add 2 teaspoons of the lime juice, then pulse a few more times (you may add more to reach desired taste).

**Pro Tip:** To store, use the remaining teaspoon of lime juice to sprinkle over top of the dip so that it doesn't turn brown, and cover tightly in the refrigerator. Use within 3 days.

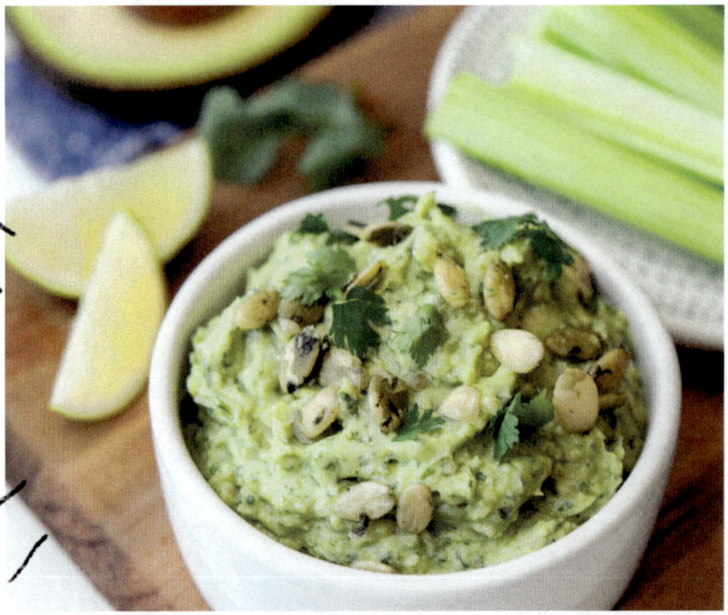

Chef Andrew Johnson

# Basil Pesto Cream Sauce

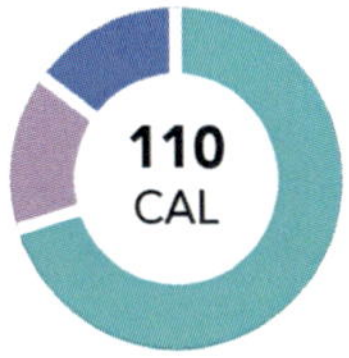


10g Fat
2g Net Carb
2g Protein

**Makes 20 servings:** each ~2 tablespoons, 30 grams

## Ingredients

1½ cups fresh basil leaves

½ cup pine nuts (or cashew nuts)

2–3 cloves fresh garlic

½ cup extra virgin olive oil

1 cup parmesan cheese, grated and divided

1 cup half and half or non-dairy option (e.g. Nutpods)

⅛ tsp dried red pepper flakes (optional)

Salt and freshly ground black pepper to taste

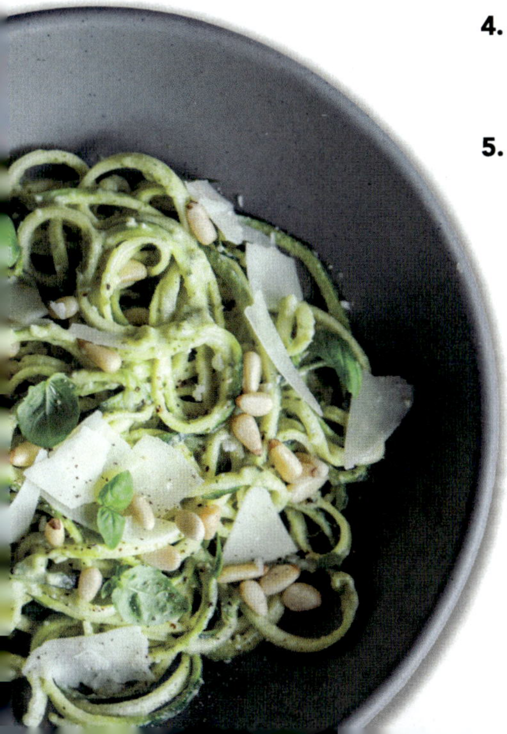

## Directions

1. Fill a saucepot halfway with water and bring to a boil. In a medium mixing bowl, fill with ice and water Remove the stems from the basil leaves, toss the basil in the saucepot, and blanch for 15 seconds. Remove the basil from the boiling water and shock it in the ice water bath.
2. In a food processor, finely chop the basil, pine nuts, and garlic. With the food processor running, slowly drizzle olive oil through the feeder and continue to process until fully incorporated. Add ½ cup of grated parmesan to the food processor. Taste and add salt and pepper.
3. Transfer the finished basil pesto to a bowl or a small jar. The pesto can be made up to 3 days in advance, but be sure to top the pesto with olive oil to minimize browning/oxidation.
4. In a medium saucepan, bring half and half to a boil. Lower the heat to medium and whisk in the pesto and remaining ½ cup of parmesan. Taste and season with salt and pepper.
5. Toss the pesto cream sauce with your favorite pasta or vegetable noodles. Garnish with a few pine nuts, fresh basil leaves, and shaved parmesan.

**Pro Tip:** For an extra zing, add 1 teaspoon of lemon zest to the pesto mixture.

Chef Andrew Johnson

# Dairy-Free Ranch Dressing

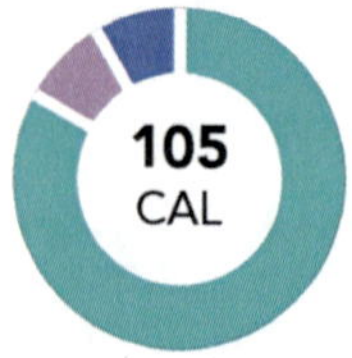


11g Fat
1g Net Carb
1g Protein

**Makes 8 servings:** each ~2 tablespoons, 36 grams

## Ingredients

½ cup plain unsweetened yogurt (full fat Greek or vegan yogurt)

½ cup mayonnaise

¼ –½ cup full fat milk (or unsweetend non-dairy alternative)

1 lemon, zested and juiced

1 tbsp dill, chopped

1 tbsp parsley, chopped

1 tbsp chives, chopped

1 clove garlic, finely minced

Salt and pepper to taste

## Fierce Foods Facts

This flavorful ranch dip is the bridge needed to help funnel more veggies into the mouths of both kids and adults! Feel free to use full cow's milk dairy if not intolerant, though both provide needed calcium. Fresh herbs offer a concentrated source of antioxidants which provide a nice boost for immune systems!

## Directions

1. In a medium-sized mixing bowl, add the yogurt, mayo, lemon juice, garlic, salt, pepper, and fresh herbs. Whisk until smooth, then add the milk gradually, a little at a time. Stop whisking to assess the viscosity. Continue adding milk until you have reached your desired consistency.
2. Enjoy immediately or store in a mason jar with a lid. Refrigerate for up to a week.

## Kids Can Cook Tips

Little fingers are perfect for tearing fresh herbs into small pieces. Younger kids will also enjoy measuring the remaining ingredients and taste testing for adequate salt and pepper!

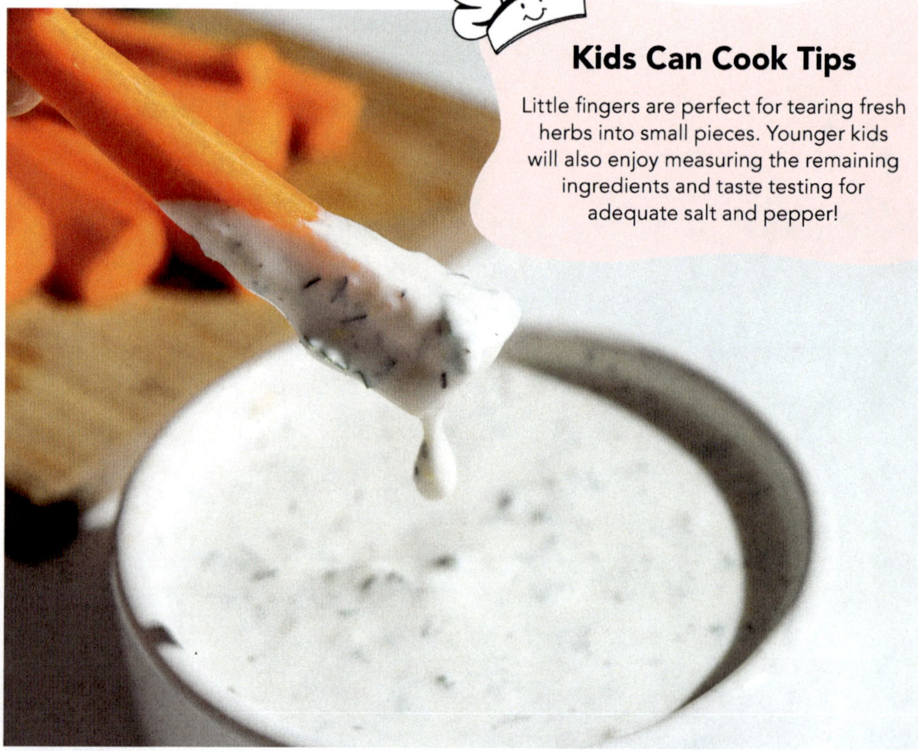

Chef Cathy McKnight

# Brown Butter

**Makes 24 servings:** each 1 teaspoon, 5 grams

50 CAL

5g Fat
0g Net Carb
0g Protein

## Ingredients

1 stick high-quality unsalted butter (8 tbsp)

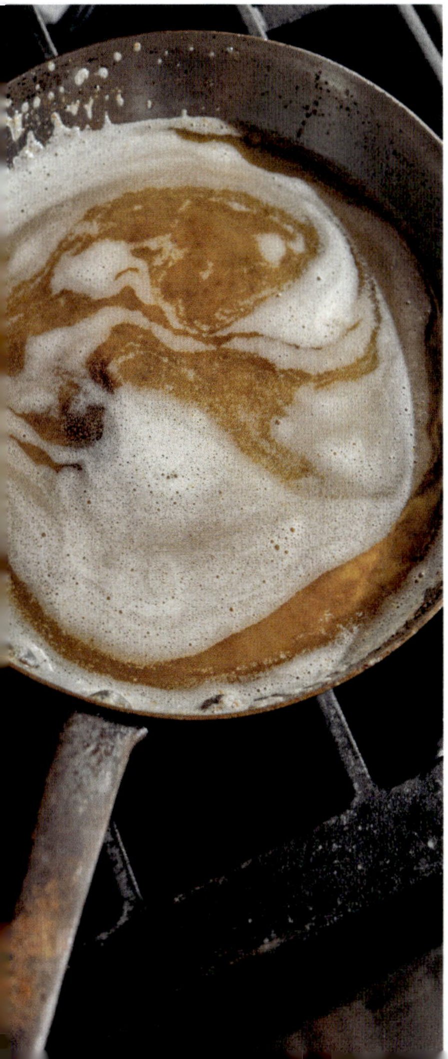

## Directions

1. Use a heavy-bottomed sauté or saucepan with at least a 2-cup capacity, and heat to medium. Slice the butter into 8 equal pieces, then add to the pan in a single layer.
2. Whisk frequently. The butter will foam: this is normal and why you need a larger pan to cook it. Watch for brown specks on the pan bottom. These are the cooked milk solids.
3. The foam will recede as more brown specks form. Reduce the heat if it is browning too quickly. It should take about 6–7 minutes to finish the process. Remove from the heat and pour into a glass bowl to stop the cooking process.
4. Store in a glass mason jar on the countertop for up to 5 days, or in the refrigerator for up to 2 weeks.

**Pro Tip:** Browned butter goes to black butter very quickly, so don't hurry the process. You'll be rewarded with a delicious, nutty butter that enhances many dishes.

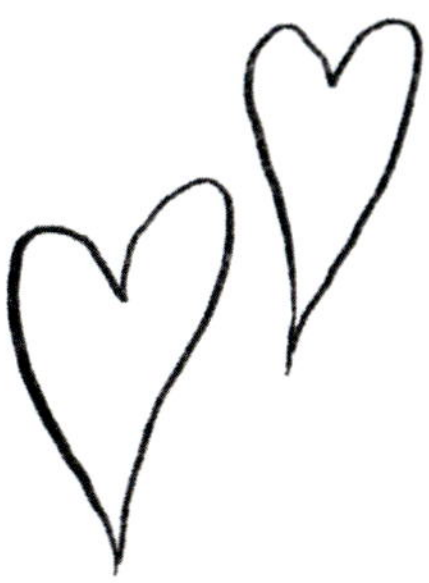

### Fierce Foods Facts

Grass fed dairy provides a higher anti-inflammatory omega 3 fat concentration than dairy from cows that are grain fed. This brown butter sauce is a useful tool for those following a ketogenic diet or very low carbohydrate diet, providing excellent flavor and nutrition that can be added to any meal.

Chef Cathy McKnight

# Peach Habanero Barbecue Sauce with Chicken Drumsticks

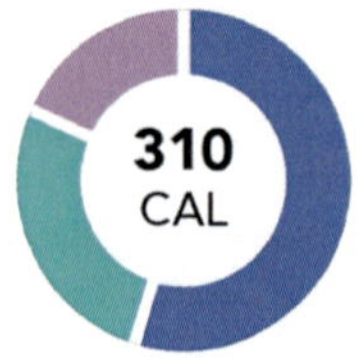


15g Fat
10g Net Carb
32g Protein

**Makes 4 servings:** each ~4 ounces chicken and 2 tablespoons sauce, 167 grams

## Ingredients

5 medium peaches

16 oz Medjool dates (approx. 2 cups), pitted and chopped

4 medium habanero peppers, seeds removed (use 2 for milder heat)

3 tbsp smoked chipotle chili paste

2 tsp salt

1 lemon (approx. 3 oz), juiced

16 oz apple cider vinegar

¼ cup organic sugar or alternative sweetener (optional)

1 lb chicken drumsticks, skin on

2 tbsp avocado oil

½ tsp garlic powder

½ tsp sea salt

¼ tsp pepper, freshly ground

## Directions

1. Fill a large stock pot with water and bring it to a boil. While the water is boiling, fill a large bowl with ice and just enough water to cover the ice. Once the water boils, drop in the peaches whole, one at a time, using a slotted spoon. Boil for 2 minutes, then remove with a slotted spoon and place in the cold water.
2. If the peach was ripe the skin will now slip right off. Do this with all of the peaches until they are all peeled. Cut the peaches in half and remove the pits, then set them inside a medium saucepan that will fit all the peaches.
3. Add the chopped dates and the habaneros to the saucepan, then add the chipotle paste, salt, lemon juice, apple cider vinegar, and sugar, and stir well. Bring the pan to a low boil and then to a simmer. Watch the heat—do not let the peaches scorch. Simmer for 3–4 hours until the peaches fall apart when stirred well with a spoon.
4. Let the mixture cool, and store in glass mason jars until ready to use (this recipe makes 6 pints).
5. Pour ½ cup barbecue sauce into a small bowl. Rinse the chicken drumsticks and pat dry. Sprinkle with salt, pepper, and garlic powder, then drizzle with avocado oil.

6. Cook the chicken drumsticks for approximately 30–35 minutes on a grill at 375-400°F, flipping about every 5 minutes and applying the sauce for the last 5–10 minutes. The internal temperature should be 175°F when done.
7. When fully cooked, remove the chicken from the grill and let rest for a few minutes before serving. Consider pairing with a green salad or fresh vegetables or cauliflower rice.

### Fierce Foods Facts

This tangy backyard barbecue dish just screams summer. Wouldn't it be nice to have the entire summer's low-sugar barbecue sauce all bottled and ready to serve? Chicken drumsticks provide more than 50% of just about every B Vitamin and have a nice amount of brain and heart health-supporting choline. This recipe also provides selenium, phosphorus, and zinc, helpful for strong bones and thyroid function.

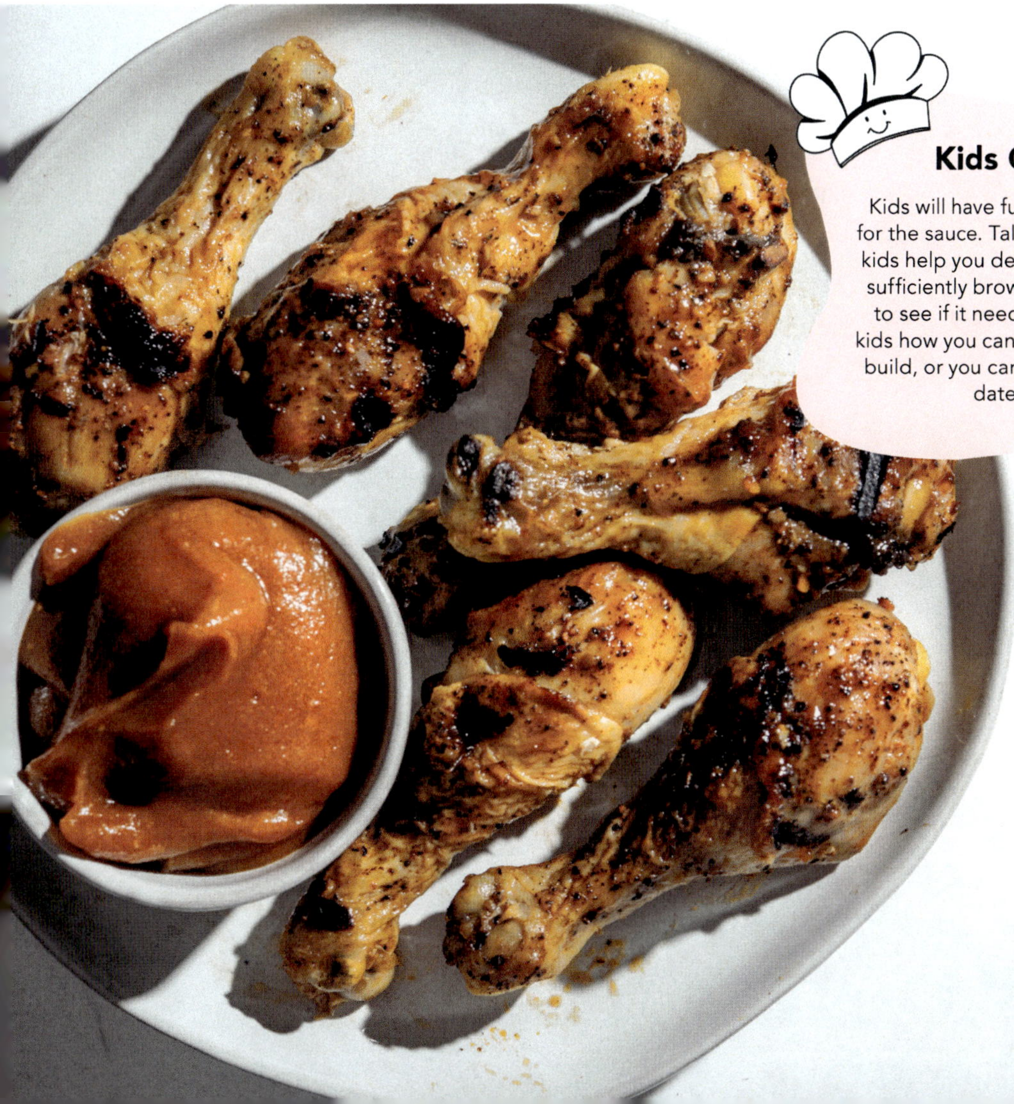

### Kids Can Cook Tips

Kids will have fun measuring the ingredients for the sauce. Talk through the colors and have kids help you decide when the drumsticks are sufficiently browned. Have them "taste test" to see if it needs more spice...or less! Show kids how you can start with a little chipotle and build, or you can use more peach, vinegar, or dates to cool it down.

Chef Andrew Johnson

# Roasted Beet Hummus

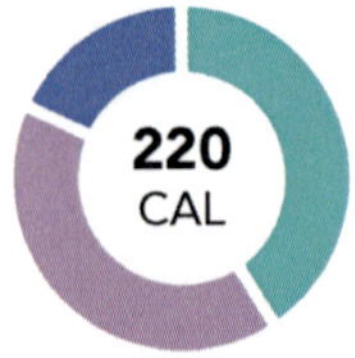


**Makes 6 servings:** each ~¼ cup, 120 grams

14g **Fat**
14g **Net Carb**
6g **Protein**

## Ingredients

1 small roasted beet (approx. ~½ cup)

1 can (15 oz) garbanzo beans (chickpeas)

1 large lemon, zested and juiced

¼ tsp salt

¼ tsp black pepper

2 large cloves garlic, minced

2 heaping tbsp tahini

¼ cup extra virgin olive oil

### Fierce Foods Facts

This healthy brilliant-colored dip is loaded with protein and fiber to keep the hungry snack attack at bay during the summer holidays. It comes with a nice amount of folate and choline as well as vitamin K, helpful for strong red and white blood cells. It's a great way to encourage snacking on veggies too!

## Directions

1. Remove the beet tops to within 2" of the beet. Scrub any dirt off the beets, leaving the skin intact.
2. Place each beet on its own large sheet of foil, then drizzle 1 teaspoon olive oil and ¼ teaspoon salt over each beet and coat to cover the whole beet. Wrap in a foil packet, place on a cookie sheet, and roast for 55 minutes at 400°F.
3. Remove from oven and cool slightly. While still warm, remove the skin from the roasted beets by rubbing them gently with a coarse kitchen towel. The skins will come off very easily. Warning: This will stain your towel and hands easily but will wash off with very hot water.
4. Once your beet is cooled and peeled, quarter it and place it in your food processor. Blend until only small bits remain. Add remaining ingredients except for olive oil and blend until smooth.
5. Drizzle in olive oil as the hummus is mixing. Taste and adjust seasonings as needed, adding more salt, lemon juice, or olive oil if needed. If it's too thick, add a bit of water. This will keep in the fridge for up to a week.

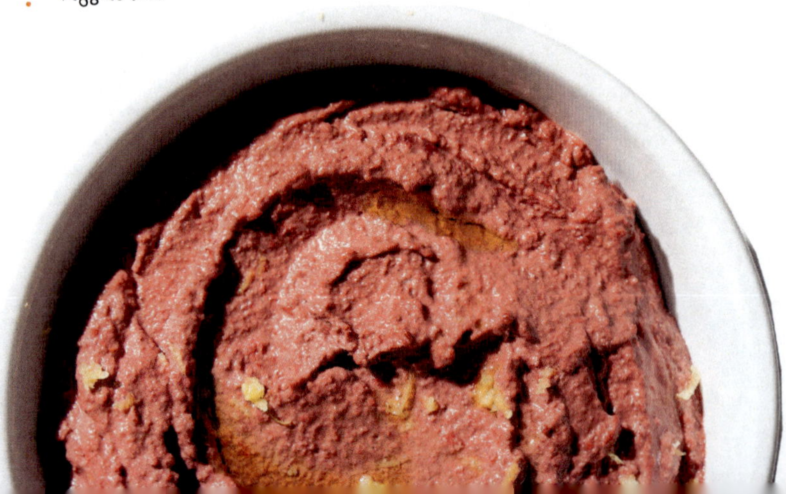

### Kids Can Cook Tips

Forget the food processor and let the kids use their muscles while using a potato masher to smash the roasted beets and garbanzo beans. Have them help taste seasonings and decide together whether it needs more lemon, salt, pepper, or garlic.

Chef Cathy McKnight

# Roasted Cherry Tomatoes

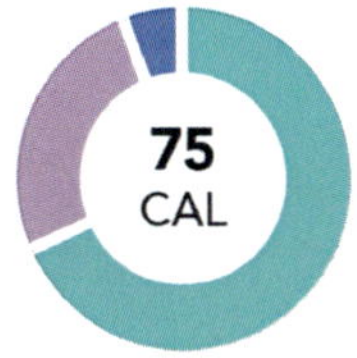


7g **Fat**
3g **Net Carb**
1g **Protein**

**Makes 16 servings:** each ~¼ cup, 68 grams

## Ingredients

2 lb cherry tomatoes, left whole

4 garlic cloves, smashed

8 tbsp extra virgin olive oil

2 tbsp red wine vinegar

2 tbsp fresh thyme, leaves only

1 tbsp fresh oregano, leaves only

2 tbsp Lakanto golden monk fruit sweetener

2 tsp coarse salt

1 tsp coarse pepper

## Directions

1. In a medium-sized glass bowl, mix together the garlic, olive oil, vinegar, sweetener, and salt. Whisk to combine until the sweetener and salt are dissolved, then add the herbs.
2. Place the washed cherry tomatoes on a half sheet pan and pour the oil mixture over them. Toss the tomatoes to evenly coat with the mixture.
3. Bake for 75 minutes at 325°F. Remove from the oven and let cool on the pan. Scrape every little juicy bit into a glass jar and refrigerate for up to 5 days. Use on pasta, pizza, scrambled eggs, and more!

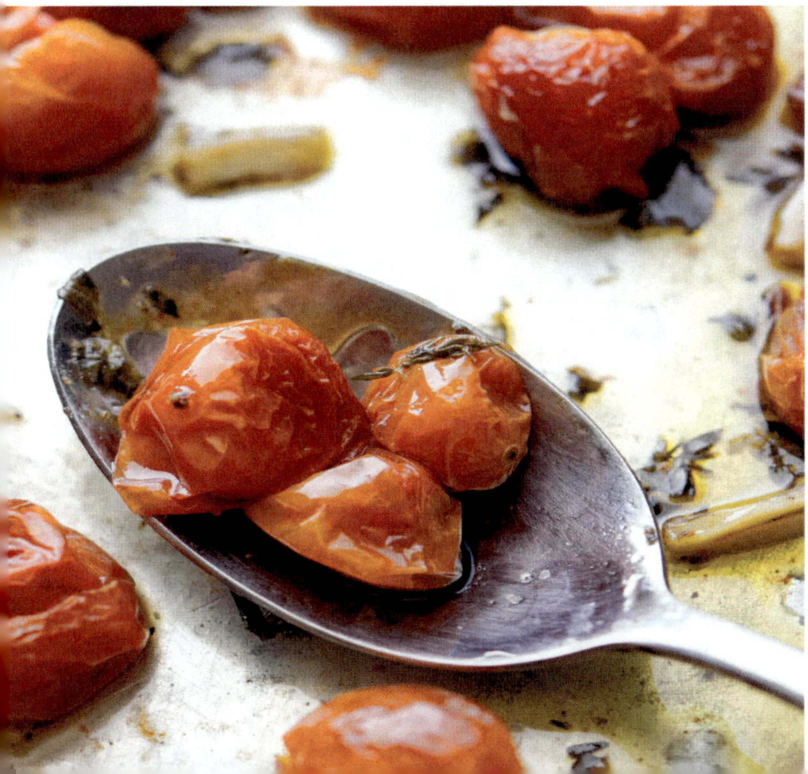

### Fierce Foods Facts

Tomatoes are an important source of potassium, a mineral that helps to conduct electrical impulses throughout the body, which is especially important for the heart. Roasted tomatoes also release lycopene in an easily absorbable raw form, which is a carotenoid that may improve cancer risk.

Chef Cathy McKnight

# Mason Jar Vinaigrette

**Makes ~7 servings:** each ~2 tablespoons, 26 grams

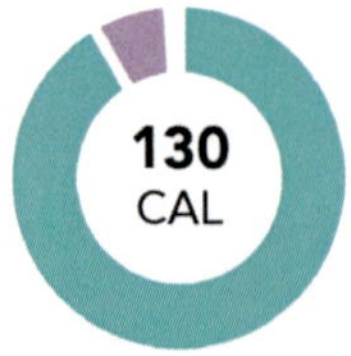


14g **Fat**
1g **Net Carb**
0g **Protein**

## Ingredients

**Base Ingredients**

1 large shallot, peeled and minced

1 clove garlic, minced

½ tsp Dijon mustard

4 oz extra virgin olive oil

4 tbsp red wine vinegar

1 tsp honey or Pyure Hunny

Salt and fresh cracked pepper to taste

**Lemon Vinaigrette**

1 tsp lemon zest

2 tbsp fresh lemon juice in place of 2 tbsp of red wine vinegar

**Bacon Vinaigrette**

1 tbsp bacon fat in place of 1 tbsp olive oil

**Balsamic Vinaigrette**

4 tbsp balsamic vinegar in place of 4 tbsp red wine vinegar

## Directions

Add all ingredients to a mason jar, then shake vigorously to mix.

**Pro Tip:** Add 1 teaspoon fresh minced lemon verbena or thyme for a more herbaceous taste.

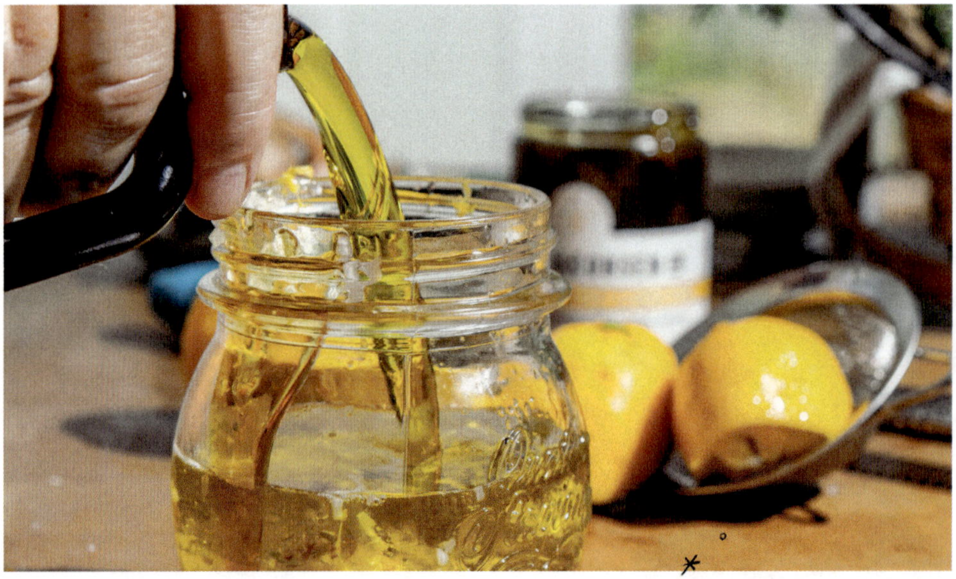

### Fierce Foods Facts

Making your own salad dressing is a snap! Almost every store-bought dressing is loaded with undesired extra sugar, and making your own flavorful vinaigrette leaves you in control of how much sugar you eat! This recipe also provides monounsaturated fat from the olive oil, which is helpful to support healthy cholesterol and decrease inflammation.

Chef Cathy McKnight

# Sausage Gravy

**Makes 8 servings:** each ~⅔ cup, 140 grams

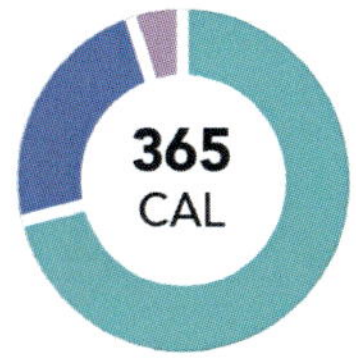


34g Fat
2g Net Carb
11g Protein

## Ingredients

1 lb ground breakfast sausage, no casings

1–2 cups bone broth or low-sodium chicken stock

1 cup heavy cream

¼ cup shallots, finely minced

1 tbsp fresh thyme or sage

⅛ tsp red pepper flakes

½ tsp xanthan gum

Sea or kosher salt and pepper to taste

## Directions

1. In a large sauté pan over medium-high heat, add the sausage and cook, breaking the sausage into small chunks with a wooden spoon. When there is a bit of pink still left in the sausage add the shallots to the pan. Continue cooking until it is cooked through and the shallots are translucent. Drain off excess fat.
2. With a blender or hand blender add the xanthan gum and 1 cup of chicken stock and mix into a slurry. Place the pan back on the stove on low-medium heat, then add the xanthan gum slurry, black pepper, and fresh herbs. Simmer, stirring frequently, until the mixture thickens to a gravy-like consistency.
3. Remove the pot from the stove and allow it to cook slightly. When it has cooled a bit, temper in the heavy cream by vigorously stirring the pot and slowly adding the heavy cream into the coolest side of the pan (in order to not curdle the cream). Bring mixture to a simmer, stirring frequently. Turn heat to low and simmer until gravy has thickened to the desired consistency, you can add more chicken stock if the gravy is too thick, or cook it longer to thicken it.
4. Remove from heat, taste, and add salt and pepper if needed. Serve over **Drop Biscuits** or your favorite toast.

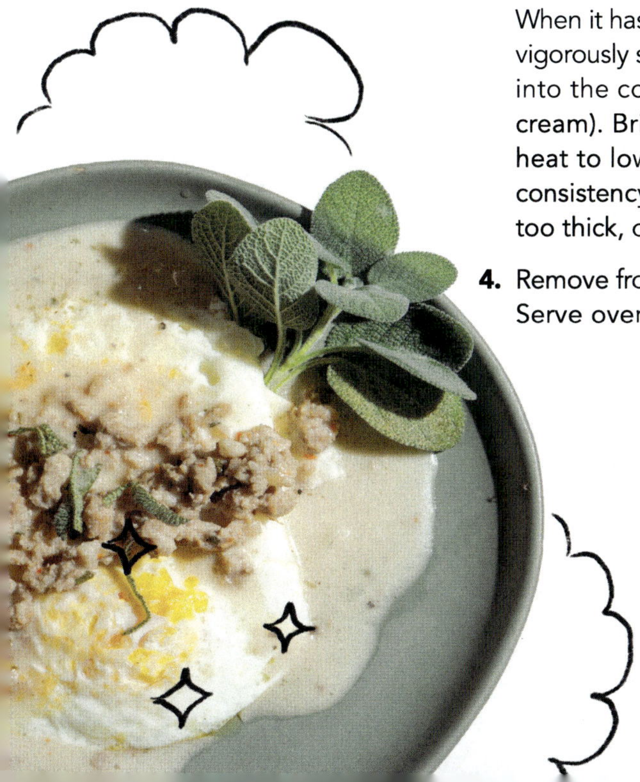

### Fierce Foods Facts

This breakfast favorite comes with ample selenium and zinc, helpful for a strong immune system. Serve over the **Drop Biscuits** for a low-carb breakfast that is well-rounded in nutrients.

Chef Andrew Johnson

# Sugar-Free Teriyaki Sauce

**Makes 8 servings:** each ~2 tablespoons, 80 grams

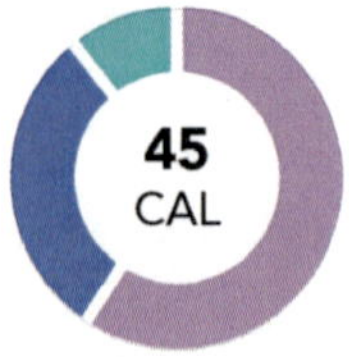


1g **Fat**
6g **Net Carb**
3g **Protein**

## Ingredients

1 cup soy sauce or coconut aminos

1 orange, zested

2 oranges, juiced

1 lime, juiced

2–3 drops sesame oil

1 tbsp ginger, grated or finely minced

1 tbsp garlic, grated or finely minced

1 tsp Lakanto gold or brown monk fruit sweetener

1 tbsp arrowroot powder

½ cup chicken, beef, or vegetable stock

## Directions

1. In a small saucepan, add soy sauce, zest, orange and lime juice, sesame oil, ginger, garlic, and sweetener. Bring the pot to a boil and then reduce to medium heat. In a small bowl, add the arrowroot powder and stock, stirring until the slurry is smooth and there are no lumps.

2. Add the slurry to the saucepan and stir. Cook on medium heat for 8–10 minutes, or a bit longer if you want a sauce with a thicker consistency. The sauce is complete when it coats the back of a spoon. Let cool and use immediately or seal in a glass jar. Store in a refrigerator for up to 5 days, or freeze for later use.

### Fierce Foods Facts

This flavorful sauce comes with a nice dose of immune-supporting and skin-brightening vitamin C thanks to all of the citrus, ginger, and soy. Some studies have even shown that a nice dose of vitamin C can improve mood and behavior!

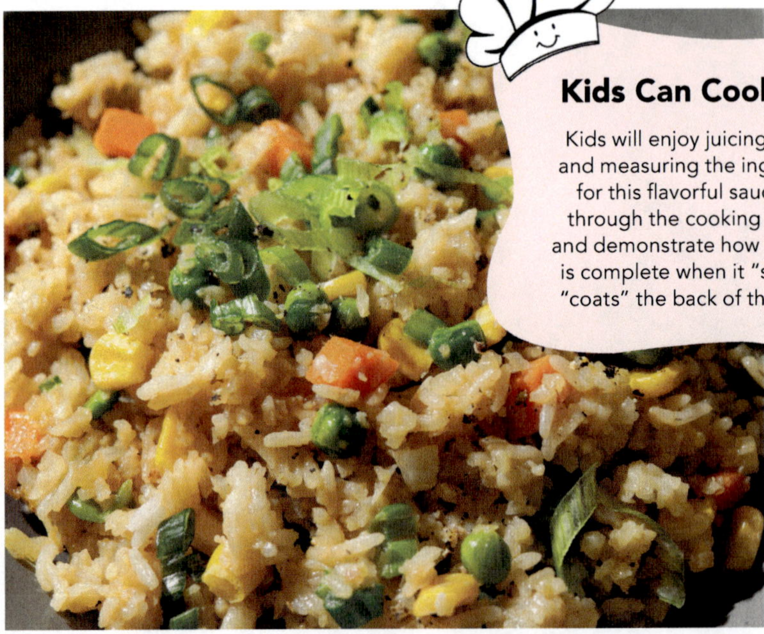

### Kids Can Cook Tips

Kids will enjoy juicing the fruit and measuring the ingredients for this flavorful sauce. Talk through the cooking process and demonstrate how the sauce is complete when it "sticks" or "coats" the back of the spoon.

Chef Andrew Johnson

# Summer Fruit Kabobs with Yogurt Dipping Sauce

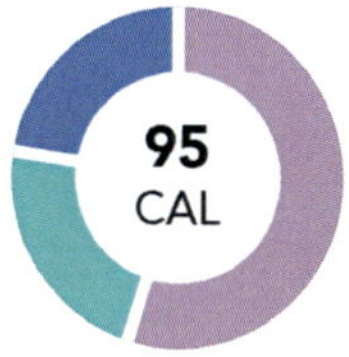


4g **Fat**
10g **Net Carb**
4g **Protein**

**Makes 6 servings:** each ½ cup veggies and 2 tablespoons dip, 141 grams

## Ingredients

### Kebabs

1 cup cucumber, ¾ half-moons and ¾ rounds

1 cup watermelon, 1" cubes

1 cup cantaloupe, 1" balls

½ cup jicama, ½" thick square slices

1 lemon, zest and juice

1 tsp Tajin seasoning

### Dipping Sauce

1 cup yogurt or non-dairy alternative (e.g. Forager or Kite Hill), unflavored

½ cup crumbled feta cheese or non-dairy alternative (e.g. VioLife Vegan Feta)

1 cup fresh cilantro, basil, lemon verbena, and/or mint

1 lemon, zest and juice

Salt to taste

## Fierce Foods Facts

Light, fresh, and easy, these kabobs are flavorful even without the dipping sauce! They make an excellent substitute for chips and crackers and provide so much more nutrient density along with some needed hydration for those hot days!

## Directions

1. Cut all of your fruit and vegetables into the desired shapes and place each in a small or medium bowl for kebab assembly.
2. Using 8" bamboo skewers, assemble kebabs in the following order: cucumber round, watermelon cube, cantaloupe ball, jicama slice, cantaloupe ball, jicama slice, watermelon cube, and cap the kebab with a cucumber half-moon.
3. Repeat with the rest of the kebabs and place them on a baking sheet or serving trap. Sprinkle the prepared kebabs with lemon juice, lemon zest, and Tajin.
4. In a food processor or blender add the yogurt, feta, fresh herbs, and lemon, then blend until smooth, adding salt to taste. Pour into a serving bowl and top with a couple of fresh herb leaves and a sprinkle of Tajin.

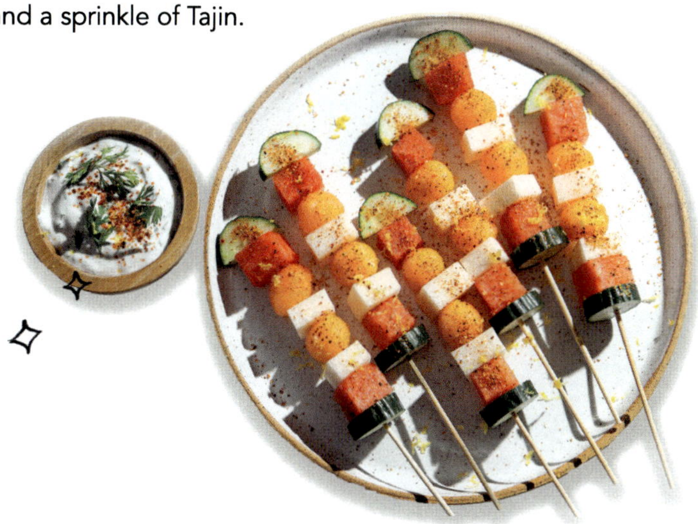

Chef Andrew Johnson

# Tzatziki Sauce

**Makes 12 servings:** each ~¼ cup, 60 grams

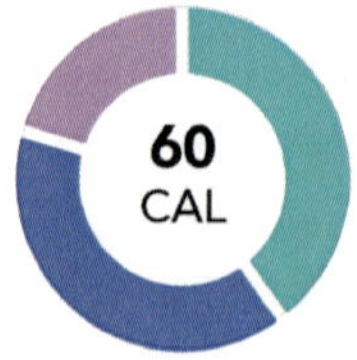


4g **Fat**
2g **Net Carb**
4g **Protein**

## Ingredients

1 cup cucumber, finely chopped and drained

2 cups plain Greek yogurt or vegan alternative (e.g. Forager or Kite Hill)

2 tbsp extra virgin olive oil

4 tbsp fresh dill, finely chopped

1 lemon, zested and juiced

1 medium garlic clove, minced

Sea salt and black pepper to taste

## Directions

1. Finely chop the cucumber and pat it dry with paper towels or clean kitchen towels. In a large mixing bowl, add yogurt, olive oil, dill, lemon, and garlic and mix well. Then, fold in the cucumber and season with salt and pepper.
2. Eat immediately or refrigerate until it is time to enjoy. This recipe can be refrigerated in a sealed container for up to a week. Serve with pita bread, snap peas, and/or large julienned vegetable fingers such as carrot, cucumber, bell peppers, or jicama.

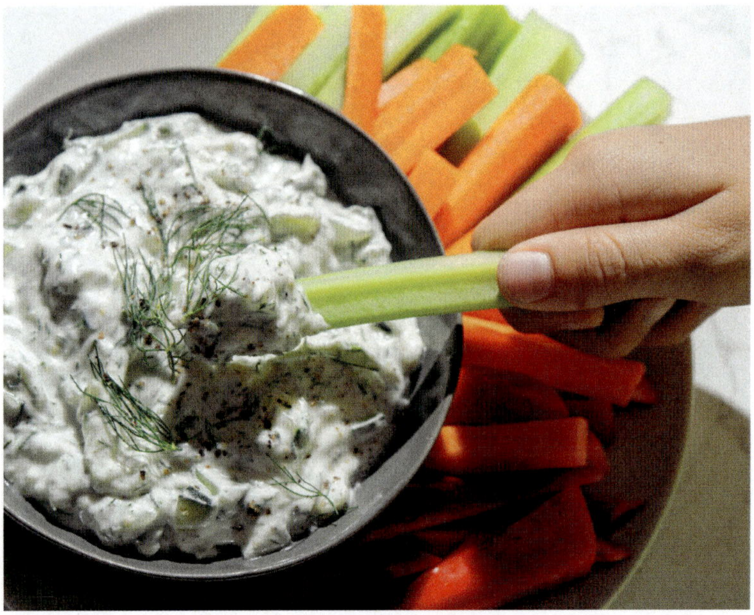

### Fierce Foods Facts

Fun nutrient-dense dips provide the perfect bridge to eating even more vegetables! And this one provides some calcium for growing strong bones as well!

### Kids Can Cook Tips

Make the cucumber sushi and use the hollowed-out portions of the whole cucumber to make this dip

Chef Andrew Johnson

# Tofu French Onion Dip

**Makes 16 servings:** each ~¼ cup, 69 grams

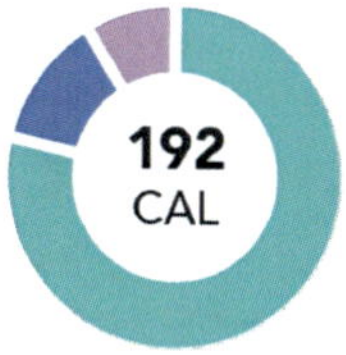


20g Fat
2g Net Carb
3g Protein

## Ingredients

2 medium-large white or yellow onions, small diced

½ cup olive oil

1 cup mayonnaise

16 oz silk tofu or 1 pt unflavored yogurt (dairy or non-dairy alternative)

1 bunch chives, minced

1 tbsp lemon pepper

1 tsp sea salt

1 lemon, zested (optional)

## Directions

1. On high heat, add olive oil to a medium sauce pot, and when hot, add onion. Once a good sizzle starts happening, reduce the heat to low-medium, then stir frequently and continue to slowly caramelize the onions.
2. Cooking the onions slow and low will optimize the flavor (you are basically making confit onions). This step may take 30–60 minutes.
3. The onions are done cooking when they are dark golden brown and not burnt. Once done cooking, remove from heat and allow to cool.
4. In a food processor, blender, or by hand with a whisk, fully blend the mayonnaise, tofu, or yogurt, choves, and spices. Fold in the onion confit into the creamed mixture and garnish with freshly chopped herbs and lemon zest.

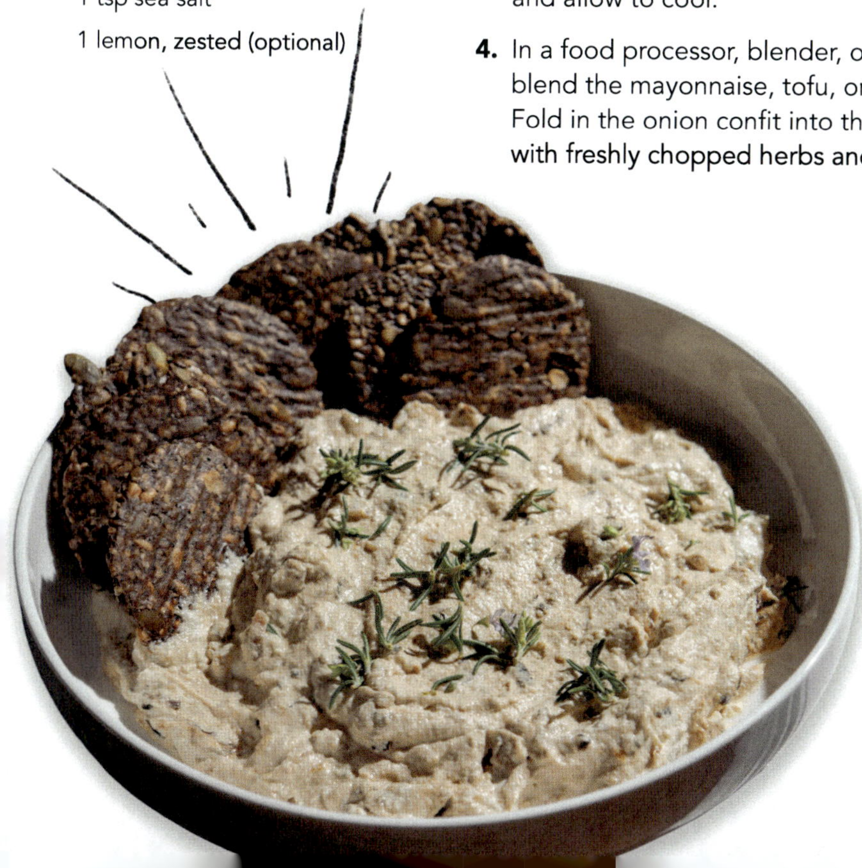

Chef Andrew Johnson

# Grilled Peach Salsa

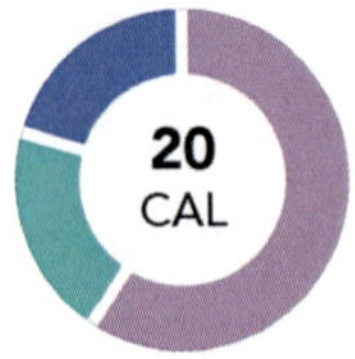


1g Fat
3g Net Carb
1g Protein

**Makes 12 servings:** each ~¼ cup, 67 grams

## Ingredients

2 cups peaches, (approx. 2 large, firm to slightly ripe)

2 cups cherry tomatoes, cut in half

¼ cup scallions, green and white parts, finely chopped

¼ cup cilantro or parsley, chopped

1 each lime, zested and juiced

1 each jalapeño, small dice (remove ribs and seeds for less heat)

1 clove garlic, minced

1 tsp olive oil

½ tsp black pepper

Salt to taste

## Directions

1. Preheat the grill to medium-high. Cut the peaches in half and remove the pits. Place the peaches on the grill and cook for 5–7 minutes. Remove the peaches from the grill and let them cool.
2. Chop the grilled peaches into a medium dice. In a glass or ceramic mixing bowl, gently combine peaches, tomatoes, scallions, fresh herbs, lime juice, jalapeño, garlic, olive oil, salt, and pepper.
3. Enjoy immediately or refrigerate before serving (best within 3 days).

### Fierce Foods Facts

This salsa is bursting with summer flavor and will provide a whole serving of fruits and vegetables as well as provide a bridge for more when used as a dip. The peaches, jalapeños, and tomatoes are a great source of vitamins A and C along with other antioxidants to support immunity.

### Kids Can Cook Tips

This recipe provides lots of knife skill practice opportunities for older kids. Talk about color and flavor with the younger kids. Make a game out of taste testing the individual ingredients and then how the tastes change when all are combined.

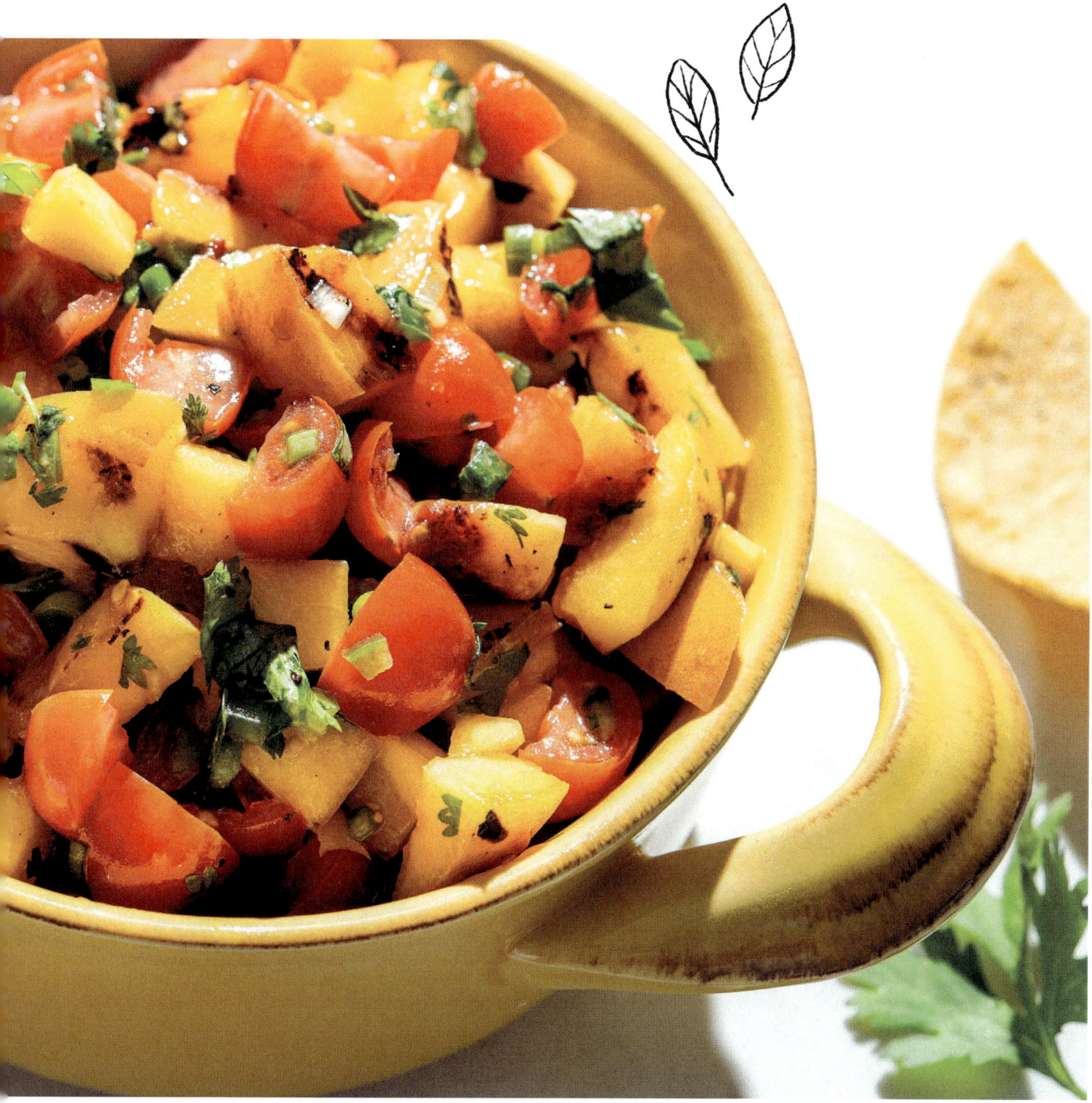

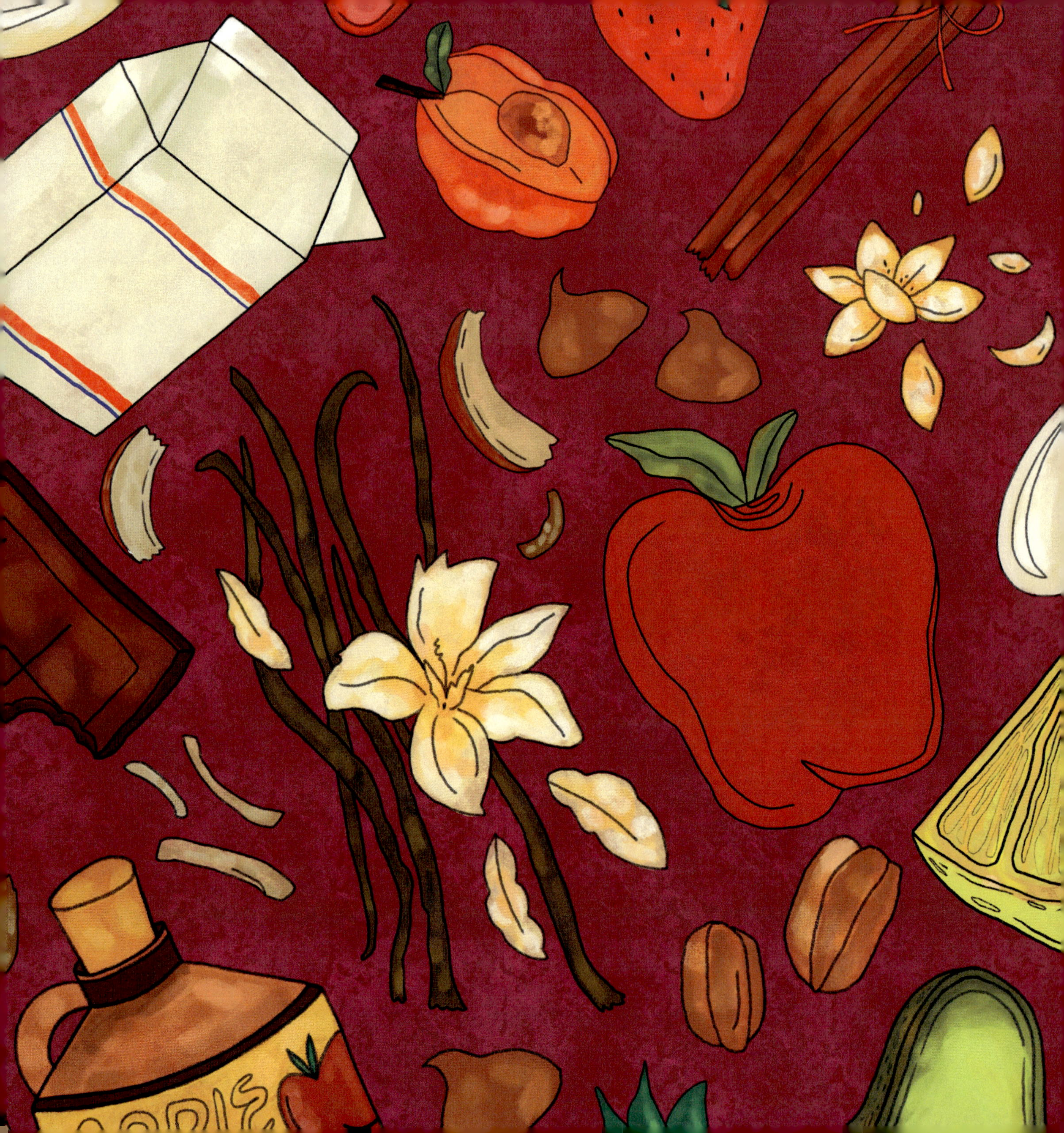

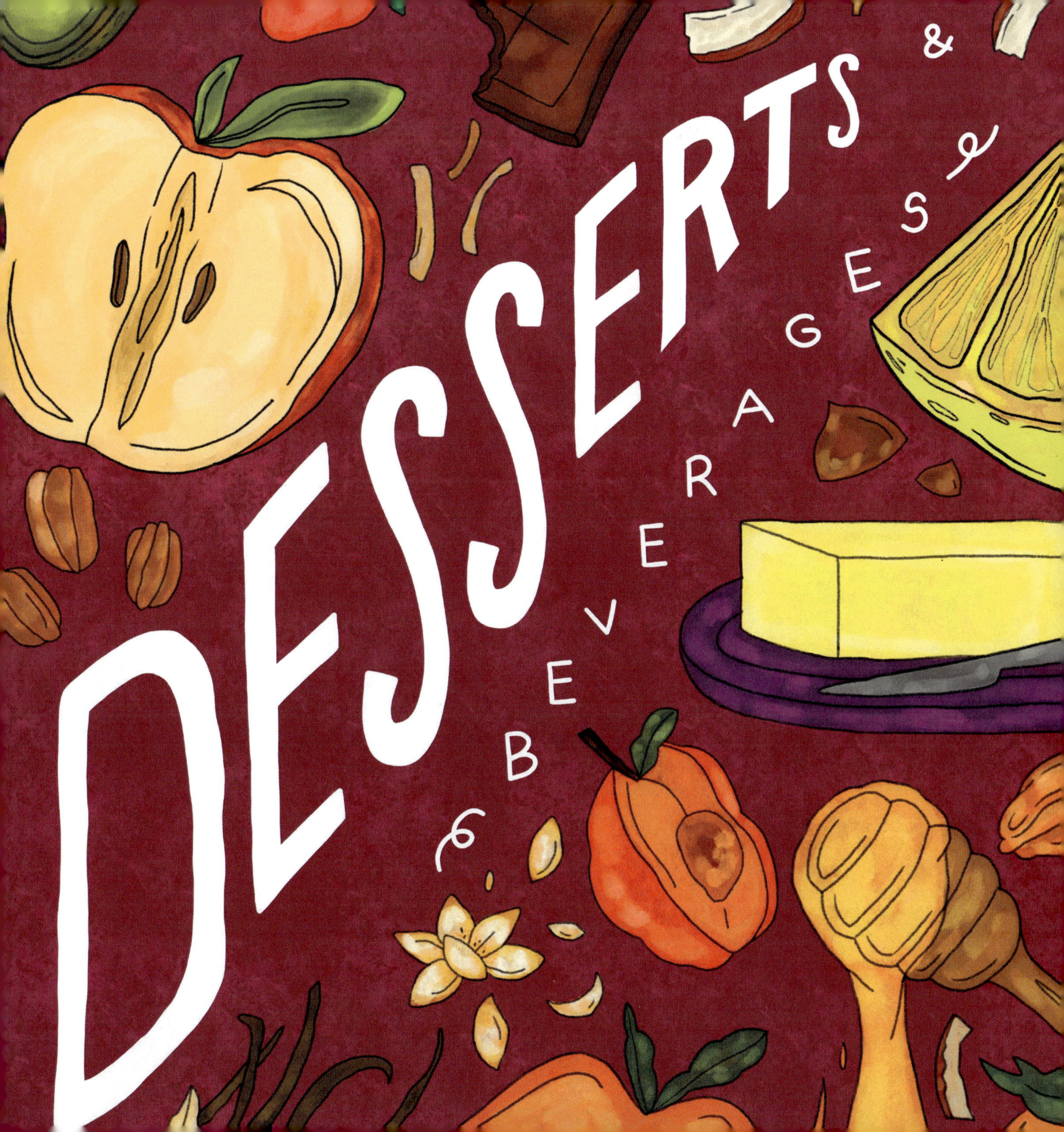
DESSERTS &
& BEVERAGES

# Desserts and Beverages



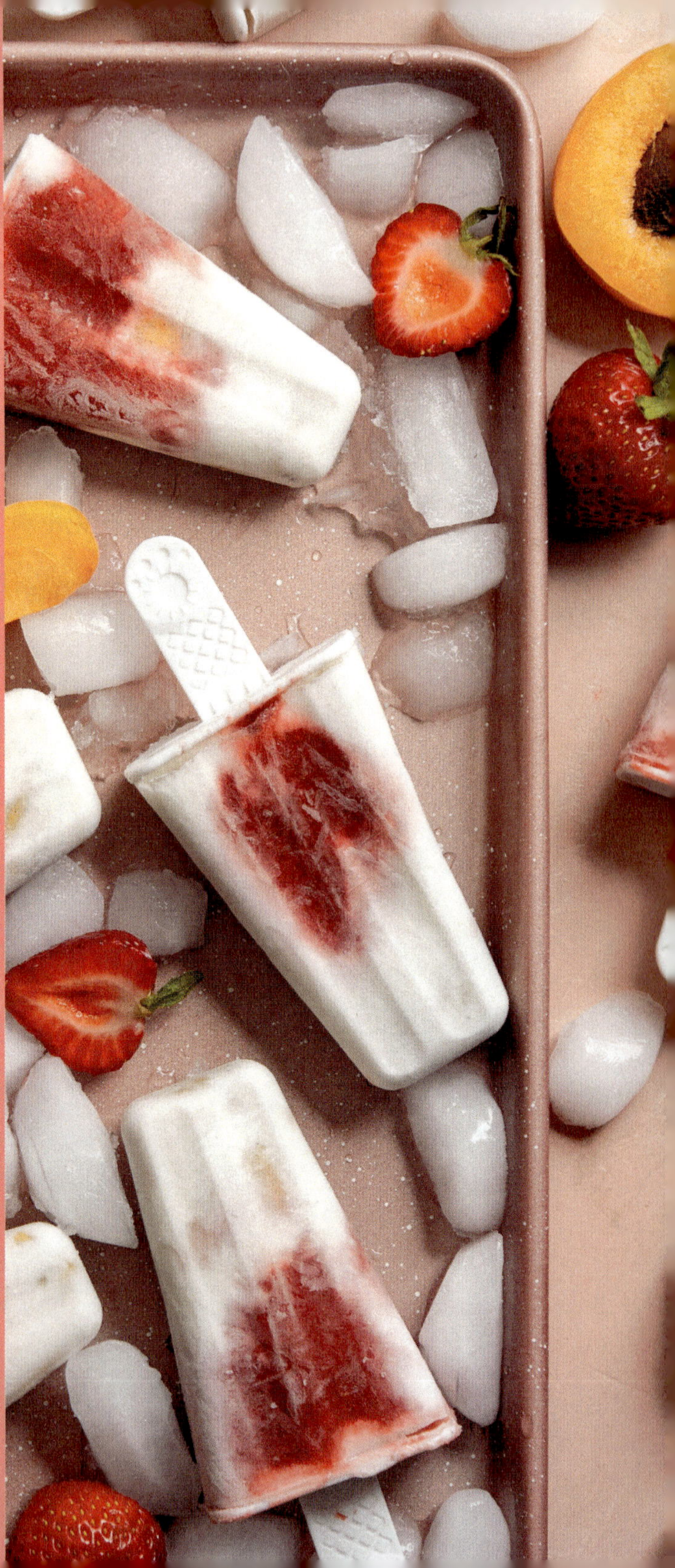

It's clear that high blood glucose increases inflammation which negatively impacts our ability to fight most cancers. The good news is that it's easier than ever to kick sugar to the curb. There are now quite a few amazing alternative sweeteners on the market that work well in so many different treats. These days, we get to have our sugar-free cake and eat it too.

So, what makes a great sugar alternative? First, it has to have as minimal an effect on blood sugar as possible. Second, we want it to be 100% safe, including not upsetting our kids' (or our) tummies. Many sugar alcohols like maltitol, can cause "digestive problems" when consumed even at suggested serving sizes. Third, we want the sugar alternative to taste like sugar. What's the point of sweetening something if it has a bad aftertaste?

**With all this in mind, here are our top five sugar alternatives:**

### 1. Allulose

Allulose delivers a mere fraction of the calories when compared to table sugar. It is absorbed in the small intestine but it isn't metabolized and the kidney is able to excrete Allulose almost intact, reducing its affect on blood sugar to nearly zero.

Studies show it's totally safe and has little impact on tummies when consumed in normal amounts. What does this mean? For a100-pound child, there shouldn't be any GI issues with up to 18 grams of allulose consumed at a single time.

Finally, allulose tastes like real sugar. It comes in granulated, powdered, and syrup forms. It really is the most sugar-like alternative sweetener on the market.

Allulose provides a cake-like texture and works well for both caramels and custards as it caramels and browns easily.

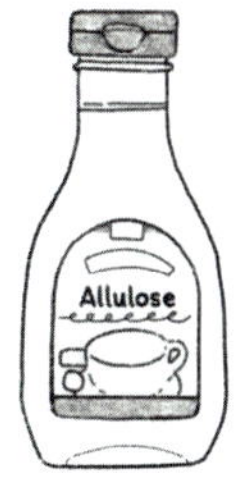


**Allulose**

### 2. Erythritol

Definitely second place but it has its drawbacks. Erythritol has zero glycemic impact (most of it passes through the small intestine unmetabolized) and has been found to be very safe, even in large amounts.

In one study, 50 grams consumed by young adults at one meal did cause some GI distress. But this is a level that is unlikely to be consumed at one time. Most products containing erythritol are in the 5–20-gram range.

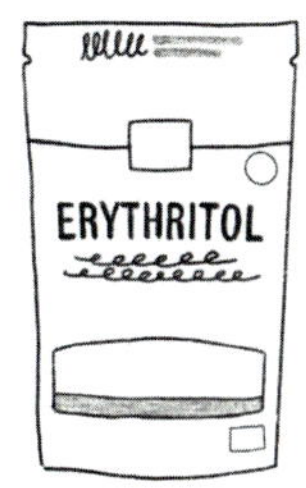


**Erythritol**

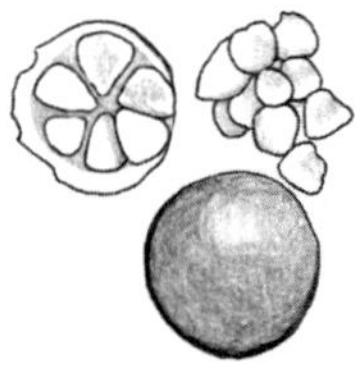

*Monk Fruit*

So, how does it taste? In chocolate bars, ice cream, and beverages, it tastes just like sugar. But erythritol has what food scientists call a "cooling effect," i.e., it feels cool on the tongue. This is great for cold things, but not so great for baked goods or hot chocolate.

Erythritol also can re-crystallized as it cools making it a good choice for crispy applications like cookies or bars.

### 3. Monk Fruit

The natural food industry loves this one because it's "natural." But here, we just care about science. It's practically as processed as other alternative sweeteners like allulose and erythritol, and just as safe.

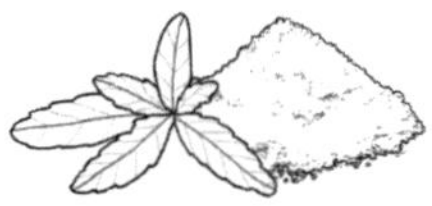

*Stevia*

So, what we really care about is glycemic impact (it's zero; yay!), the potential for GI distress (extremely low; yay!), and taste. It's hard to judge the taste of monk fruit because it's almost always mixed with erythritol or stevia.

For example, the three most popular monk fruit sweeteners on the market (Lakanto, Splenda Monk Fruit, and Monk Fruit in the Raw) all have way more erythritol than monk fruit. These sweeteners work really well for many recipes, and they're great zero-glycemic options. Just don't expect to be consuming mostly monk fruit.

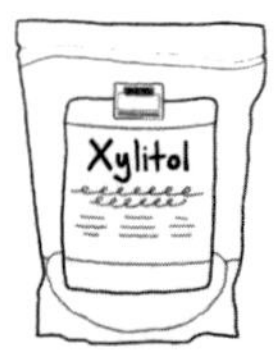


*Xylitol*

Note that monk fruit requires a bulking agent and not all use erythritol so be sure to read the nutrition facts label when using. It does not caramelize or brown by itself.

### 4. Stevia

This has long been the most popular "natural" sugar alternative. It's still pretty popular as you can find it in sodas, chocolate, ice cream, and many other products. Like our first four sugar alternatives, stevia has zero glycemic impact and is quite safe.

The big issue with stevia is taste. Pure stevia extract is 200 times sweeter than sugar but it has an astringent aftertaste. Food engineers have been able to make stevia taste much better over the years but it's still noticeably different from sugar.

Stevia also does not caramelize or brown by itself.

### 5. Xylitol

It's last on the list for two reasons:

First, it's not zero glycemic. It's very low (around 7 on a scale where straight glucose is 100), so it's still a good sugar alternative.

Second, and more importantly, it can cause upset tummies at lower amounts than its sugar alcohol cousin, erythritol. It's been shown to be quite safe, beneficial for dental health, and the taste is closer to sugar than erythritol, stevia, or monk fruit.

But it's the potential GI distress that knocks this one down the list. If you see it listed in a product, give it a try but don't overdo it. It's also toxic to dogs.

This chapter will provide a wide variety of treats to help celebrate special occasions while still keeping your family on track with their anti-inflammatory goals.

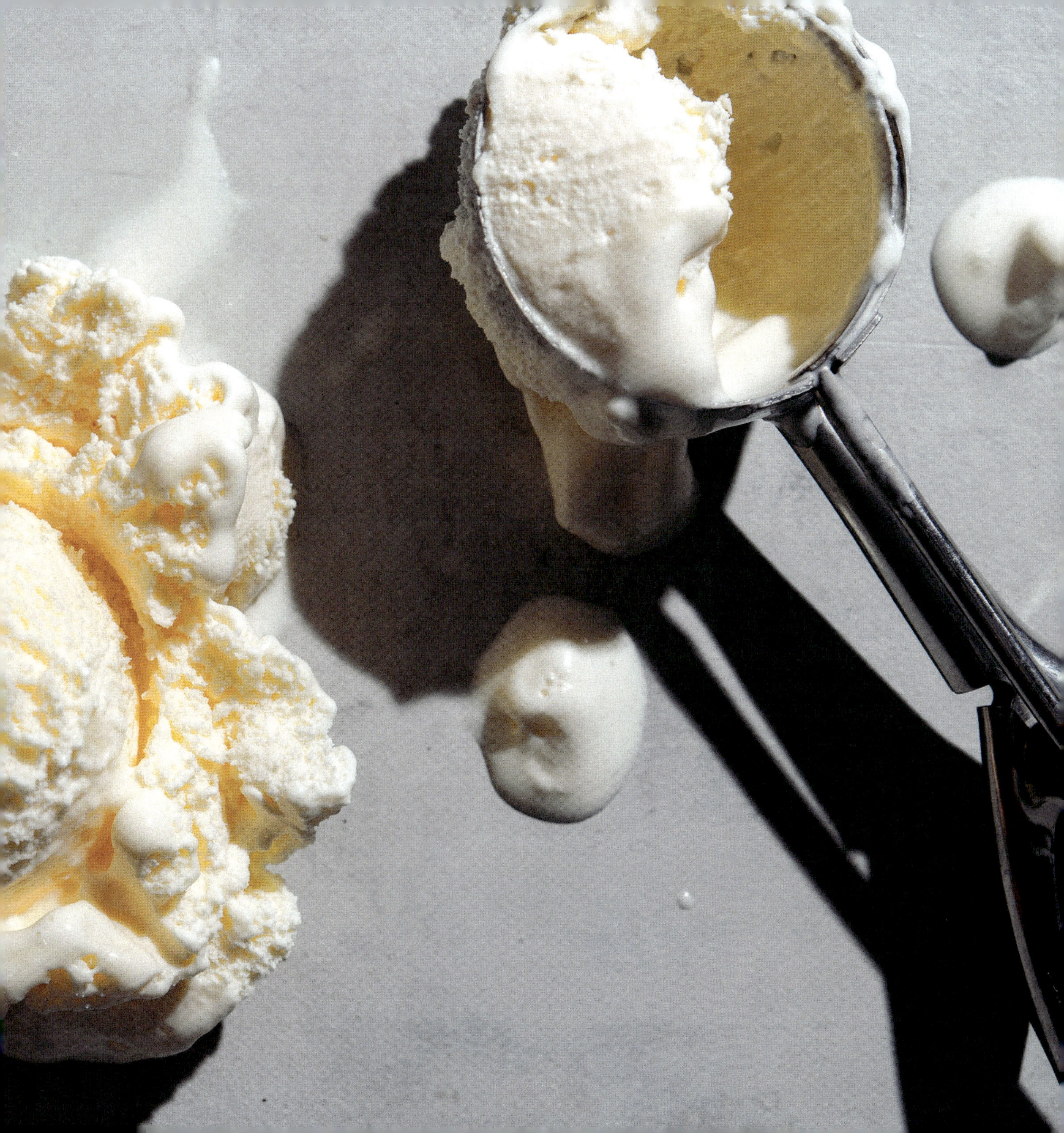

## Cakes and Frostings

Birthdays and other celebrations fall a little flat without a beautiful cake to blow out the candles on, so we have you covered in this area too!

The NSNG Brownie Bakes are amazingly dense and will compete with any fudgy chocolate brownie out there. The base frosting with four possible variations is also sugar-free and dreamy as can be.

For those that might like to have a little more sparkle and pizazz, there are several sugar-free confetti sprinkles available at specialty online markets, and they are sure to be a big hit at parties for any occasion. Also, consider using the cream cheese frosting in this chapter to bump up calcium contents too.

Want to go a simpler route? Decorating a cake with a light glaze made with flavors that pop, such as lemon or lime, works equally well. Grate a little lemon or lime on top of that for an added splash of color. Combining a little powdered erythritol with lemon and water makes a beautiful glaze for the lemon zucchini coconut bread.

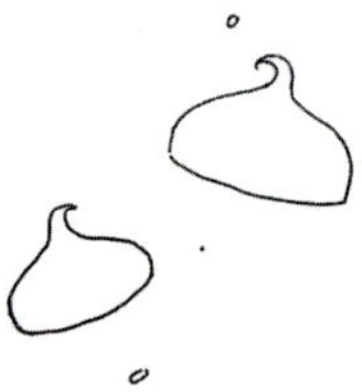

Other beautiful garnishes include fresh edible flowers like nasturtium and pansy, or consider decorating with some low glycemic fruit like kiwi, blueberries, and strawberries. A light dusting of powdered monk fruit and erythritol or cacao powder in a fun design with a stencil is also a great way to get that wow factor.

So go ahead, have your cake and eat your frosting too with this chapter's conscious and delicious recipes!

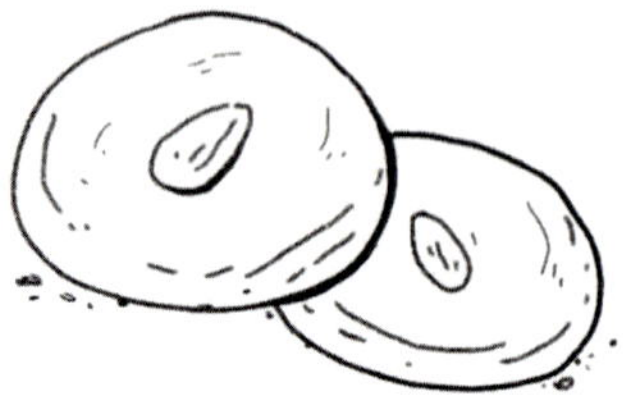

## Cookies

Eating intuitively means listening to your body's wants and needs—and sometimes your body just might be telling you it wants a sweet treat! However, with today's manufactured and ultra-processed foods that are specially engineered to hijack some of those natural messages your body sends, they could fool us into thinking we actually need more and more of that sweet stuff. There is an emerging view in the areas of sugar science that refined sugars and ultra-refined flours are addictive and the more we consume them, the more we crave them.

So what is a person to do in this sugar-fueled world that we live in? The answer lies in giving your body nutrient-dense real, whole food that it can make sense of and that doesn't trick the brain into overconsuming. The nutrients in whole food provide messages and instructions to the brain. Giving the body quality nutrients results in the brain feeling satisfied and allows normal chemical messaging to take place. Giving ultra-processed and nutrient-deficient food confuses the body and makes it think it hasn't been fed. This leaves us wanting more.

We definitely want to start with improving the actual sugar profile of the food (as discussed in the previous section), but we can definitely kick up the nutrition in the flour and grain department too. Replacing all or part of refined grain flours with nutrient-dense nut, seed, and coconut flours provides a low net carbohydrate binder for cookies, cakes, tarts, and pies while providing quality fats, higher protein contents, and more vitamins, minerals, and fiber, which in turn keeps us satiated.

Almond flour contains protein, quality fat, vitamin E, manganese, and zinc. Coconut flour is also high in protein and fiber, as well as medium chain fats which are especially helpful if someone needs to gain weight. Rotating the use of a variety of nut and seed flours provides a nice array of different nutrients. Using quality fats such as grass-fed butter and avocado, as well as seeds of flax, pumpkin, and hemp can also help increase the Omega 3 anti-inflammatory component of our sweet treats. And of course, using a nutrient-dense and low-glycemic fruit is always a great way to satisfy a sweet tooth craving.

The recipes that follow in this section include one of Max's favorite cookies—the jam thumbprint. This cookie provides a very low net carbohydrate per two-cookie serving, providing just 3.6 net grams of carbohydrates along with almost 3 grams of gut-loving fiber. It also has 4 grams of protein and a nice 2-to-1 ratio of Omega 6 to Omega 3 fats. It is a good source of vitamins E and C, as well as zinc and manganese. The traditional jam thumbprint cookie made with regular refined wheat flour and refined sugar has a totally different profile, coming in at over 20 grams of low-quality carbohydrates per serving, with over 10 of those coming from refined sugar. It also contains less than 1 gram of fiber with no appreciable vitamins and minerals other than the iron and folic acid that wheat flour must be fortified with. And you can easily get the daily iron needed just by eating a serving of animal protein for dinner.

So join us for a high-quality dessert—your taste buds (as well as the rest of you) will thank you later!

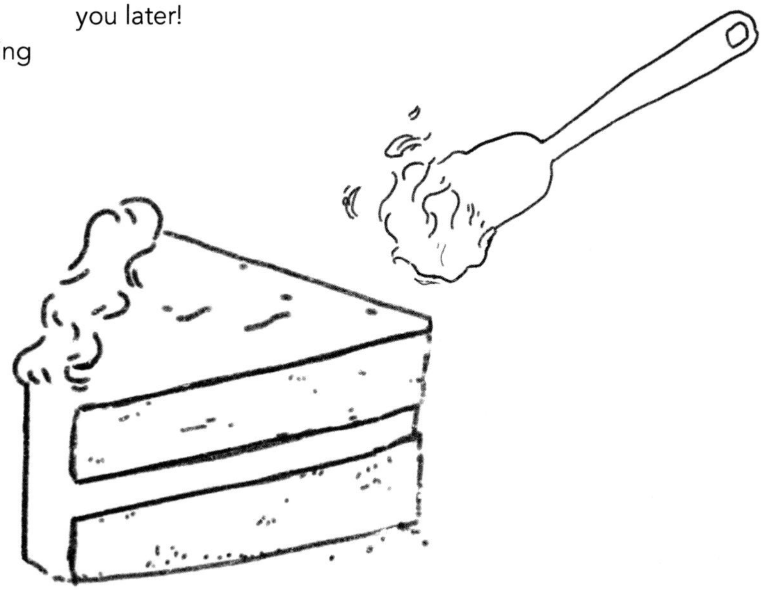

Chef Andrew Johnson

# Cakes, Cupcakes, and Muffins

**Makes 12 servings:** 1 cupcake/muffin each, or 2" x 2" squares, grams vary

## Ingredients

### Base Dry Ingredients

2 cups almond flour

½ cup tapioca flour

1 tsp baking powder

1 tsp baking soda

¼ tsp salt

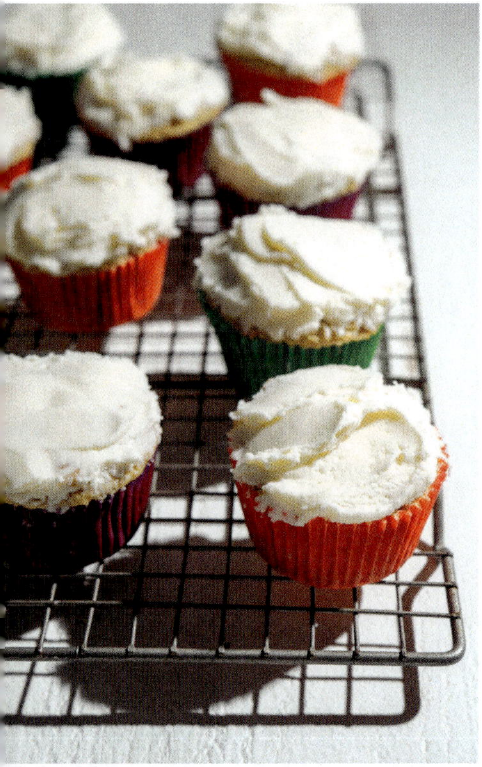

## Directions

1. Preheat the oven to 350°F. Grease two 9" springform pans, two 9" baking pans with parchment, or a 12-count muffin pan (line with muffin paper if you prefer).
2. In a medium mixing bowl, sift together the dry ingredients. In a large mixing bowl, incorporate the wet ingredients using a whisk or an electric mixer. Add the dry ingredients and mix until combined, careful not to overbeat the batter. Next, fold in the flavor additions.
3. Pour cake batter into the pans, or scoop the batter into the muffin tin with an ice cream scoop (approximately ¾ full in each muffin well). Bake for 15–20 minutes, and test for doneness by pushing a butter knife through the middle of the biggest part of the cake. It should come out clean.
4. Remove from the oven and let cool. Once cool, you can decorate with a frosting of your choice.

**Pro Tip:** Chef Andrew prefers the finished result using allulose as the sweetener, but keep in mind that the cake will be browner in color. If you would like the cake lighter in color, use the erythritol sweetener.

### Fierce Foods Facts

We have you covered with many flavor variations for all of your holiday and celebratory baking. The almond flour in place of the white flour provides a low-carb and nutrient-dense option, meeting almost 30% of the daily needs for vitamin E, an important antioxidant and helpful for the immune system. The almonds provide a nice amount of bone-building minerals such as phosphorus, selenium, and zinc as well.

### **Blueberry** *(92 grams)*

1½ cup allulose or 1 cup erythritol

½ cup butter, soft

3 large eggs

¼ cup milk

½ cup fresh or frozen blueberries, dredged in tapioca flour

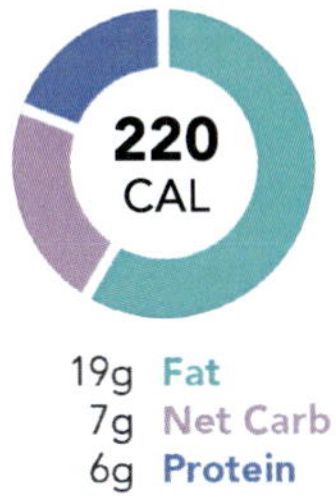
220
CAL
19g Fat
7g Net Carb
6g Protein

### **Vanilla** *(92 grams)*

1½ cup allulose or 1 cup erythritol

½ cup butter, soft

4 large eggs

½ cup milk

1 tbsp vanilla extract

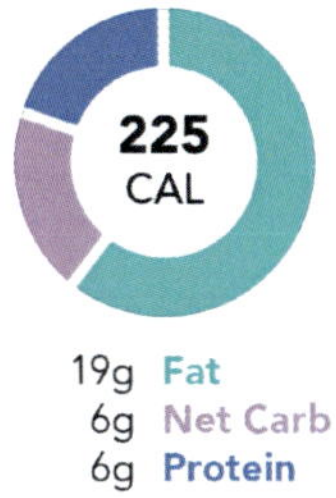
225
CAL
19g Fat
6g Net Carb
6g Protein

### **Chocolate** *(96 grams)*

1½ cup allulose or 1 cup erythritol

½ cup butter, soft

4 large eggs

½ cup milk

1 tsp vanilla extract

1 cup cocoa powder

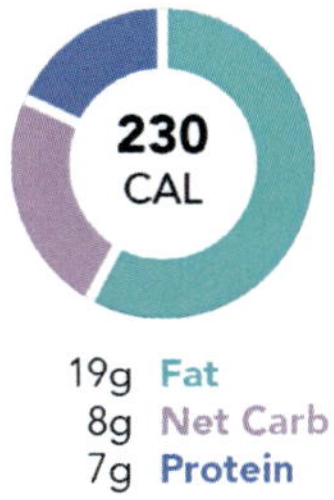


### **Lemon** *(94 grams)*

1½ cup allulose or 1 cup erythritol

½ cup butter, soft

4 large eggs

½ cup milk

1 tbsp lemon extract

1 tbsp lemon zest

1 tbsp poppy seeds (optional)

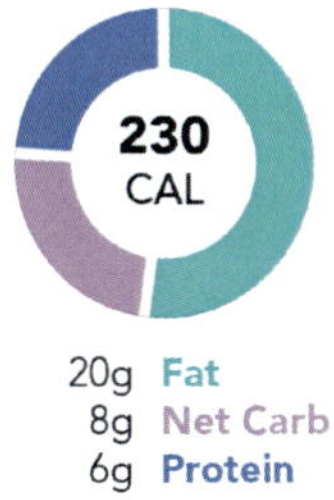


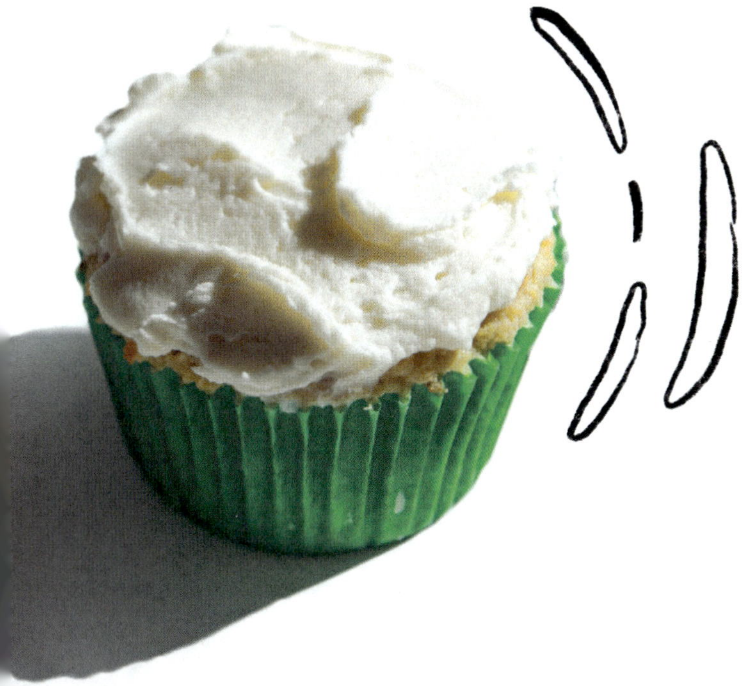

### **Pumpkin** *(104 grams)*

1½ cup allulose or 1 cup erythritol

1 cup pumpkin purée

3 large eggs

½ cup almond butter

1 tbsp pumpkin pie spice

½ cup chopped walnuts

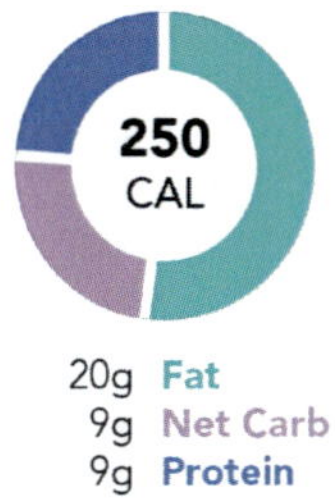

Chef Andrew Johnson

# Frosting

85 CAL

8g Fat
0g Net Carb
0g Protein

**Makes frosting for 12 cupcakes or 1 cake:** 2 tablespoons per serving, 58 grams

## Ingredients

### Base Frosting Ingredients

3 cups sugar-free powdered sugar

½ cup butter softened

1 tsp vanilla extract

### Fierce Foods Facts

You don't have to skip out on dessert if following a low-carb diet. The introduction to the desert chapter includes recommendations for acceptable sugar-free baking ingredients. Feel free to use edible flowers, Lily's sugar-free sprinkles, or sugar-free chocolates to further doll up your celebratory cake! We used Lakanto brand sugar-free powdered sugar to make these frostings.

## Directions

1. In a large mixing bowl, add sugar and butter. Whisk or beat with an electric mixer until smooth, then add vanilla extract and incorporate.
2. Add in your flavors and continue beating until you achieve optimal consistency. For a thinner consistency, add more milk.
3. The finished frosting can be used immediately or stored in the refrigerator for up to a week.

### Chocolate

½ cup cocoa powder

1–2 tbsp milk of choice

95 CAL

8g Fat
1g Net Carb
1g Protein

### Cream Cheese

8 oz cream cheese softened

1–2 tbsp milk of choice

1 tsp lemon extract (optional)

1 tsp lemon zest (optional)

150 CAL

13g Fat
1g Net Carb
2g Protein

### Vanilla

1–2 tbsp milk of choice

85 CAL

8g Fat
0g Net Carb
0g Protein

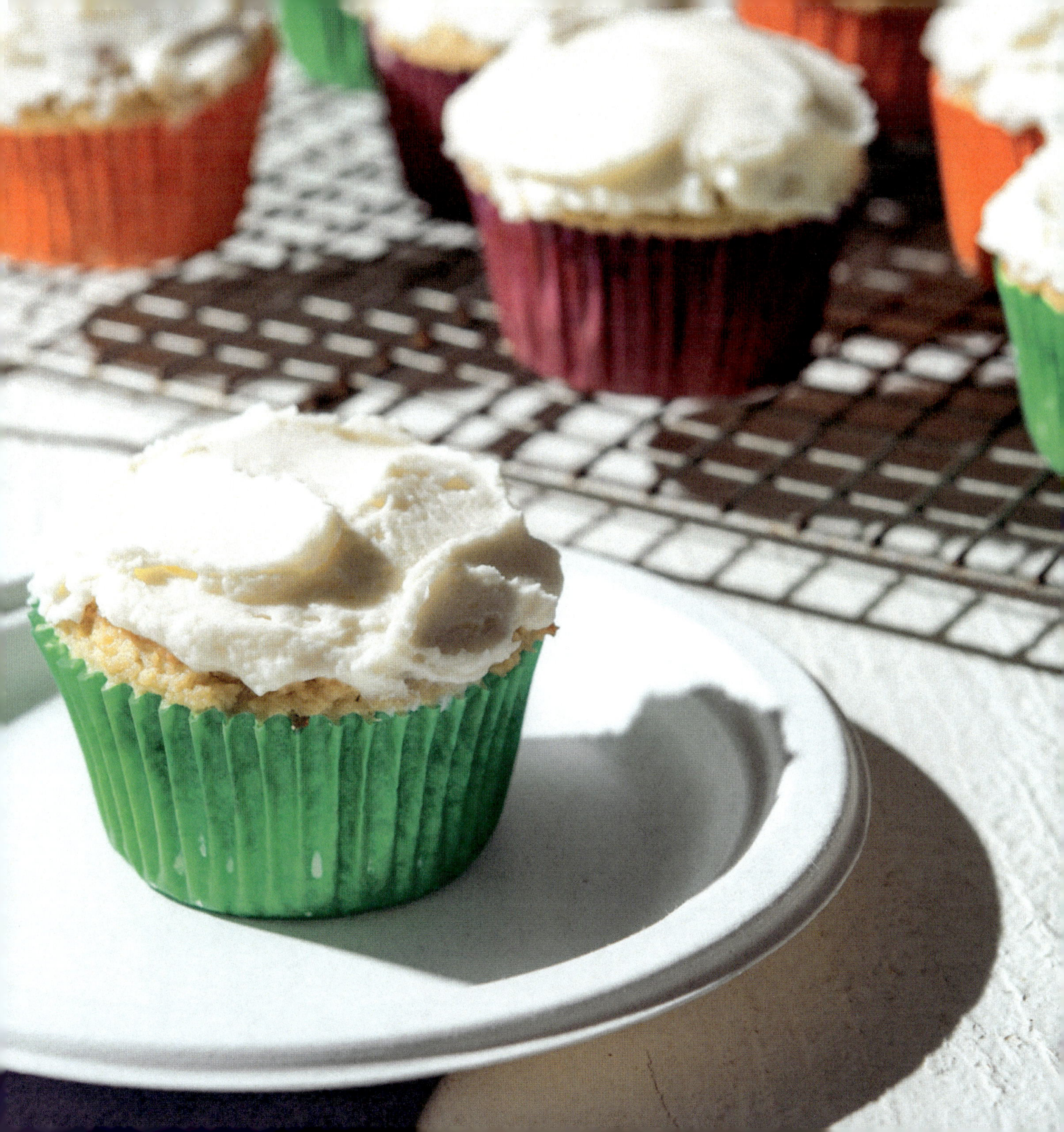

Chef Cathy McKnight

# Chavocado Pudding

**Makes 6 servings:** ¾ cup each, 184 grams

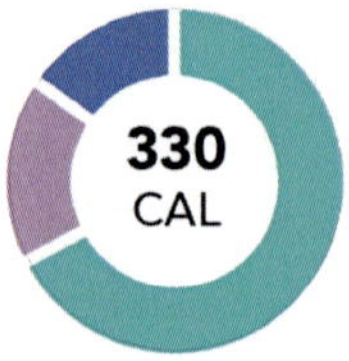


28g **Fat**
7g **Net Carb**
6g **Protein**

## Ingredients

2 cups avocado pulp

8 oz full-fat coconut milk from a can

½ cup cacao powder

1 tbsp vanilla extract

1 tsp sea salt

¼ cup Lakanto gold monk fruit sweetener

6 tbsp Lily's semi-sweet chocolate chips

## Directions

1. Using a food processor, add all of the ingredients to the base and pulse for 30 seconds. Select the continuous speed option and process for another minute.
2. Pour pudding into six 4-ounce glass jars. Top each with 1 tablespoon of chocolate chips (optional).

### Kids Can Cook Tips

Have kids help squish the avocado out of its shell, measure the rest of the ingredients, and divide the servings.

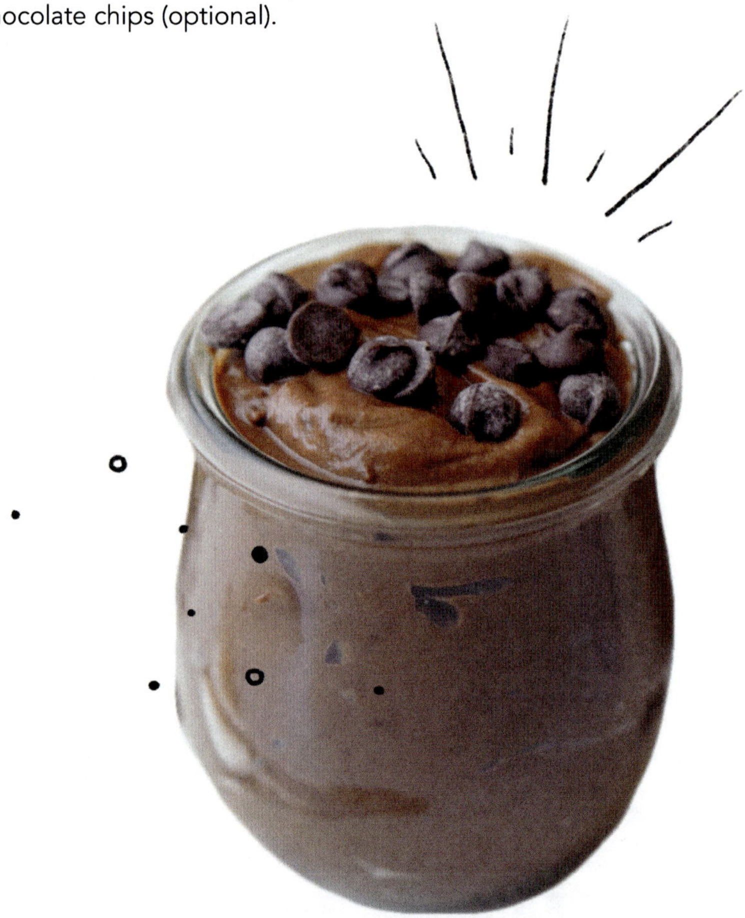

### Fierce Foods Facts

When you want a sweet treat, this is one healthy way to satisfy that craving. Avocados provide heart-healthy fat while the cacao powder is densely packed with minerals like iron and magnesium, which support blood pressure, stress release, and mood.

Chef Andrew Johnson

# Easy Peach Crisp

**Makes 10 servings:** ½ cup each, 128 grams

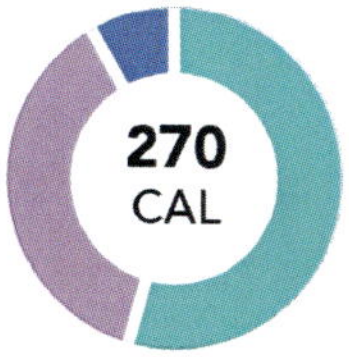


22g Fat
15g Net Carb
3g Protein

## Ingredients

6 ripe peaches, pitted and roughly chopped

2 tbsp tapioca flour

1 tsp vanilla extract

½ tsp cinnamon

½ tsp nutmeg

¼ tsp chili powder (optional)

**Topping:**

1 cup raw pecans

½ cup blanched almond flour or almond meal

¼ cup maple syrup, agave, or honey

½ cup coconut oil or butter, melted

½ tsp sea salt

## Directions

1. Preheat the oven to 350°F. In a large mixing bowl add peaches, vanilla extract, cinnamon, nutmeg, and chili powder (optional), and toss to evenly coat. Then sprinkle in the tapioca flour and toss to fully incorporate, adding a bit more tapioca flour if the peaches are not all coated.

2. In a greased 2–3 quart casserole baking dish add the peach mixture. In a food processor add the pecans and pulse until roughly chopped, then add the almond flour and pulse again. Add the salt, maple syrup, and melted oil or butter, and pulse until it creates a slightly wet dough. Take the topping and spread it evenly over the baking dish with the peaches. Bake for 40–45 minutes. Enjoy immediately or refrigerate for up to a week.

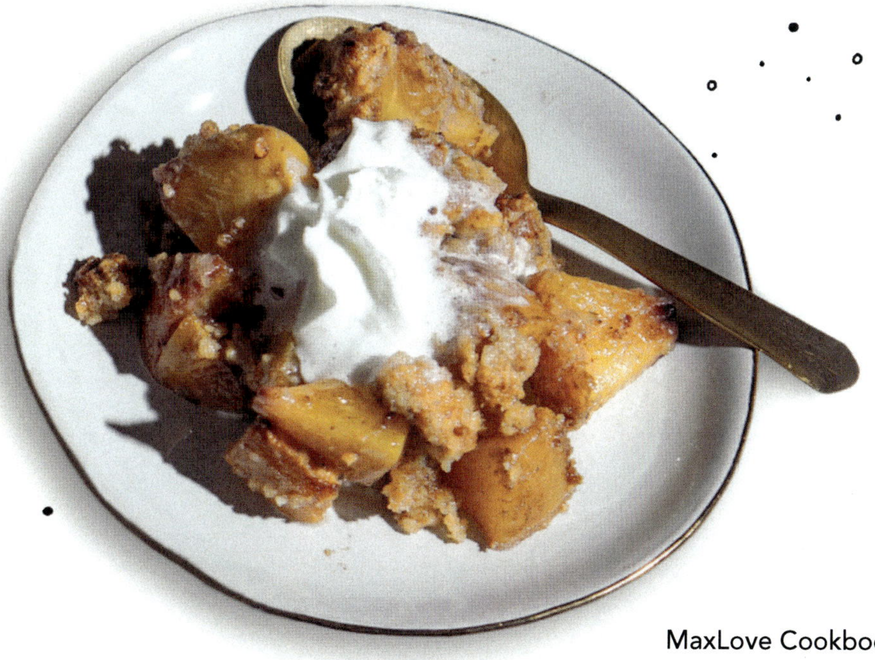

Chef Audra DiPadova Wilford

# Almond Cookies

**Makes 24 servings:** 1 cookie each, 23 grams

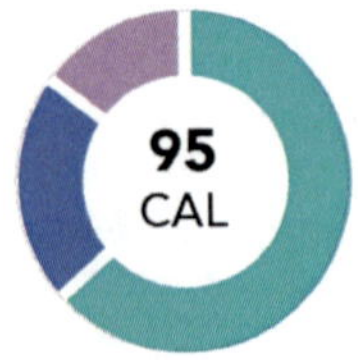


9g **Fat**
2g **Net Carb**
3g **Protein**

## Ingredients

2 egg yolks

¼ cup xylitol honey

¼ cup erythritol-stevia blend

¼ cup coconut oil or clarified butter, warmed

1 tsp vanilla extract

1 tsp almond extract

2 cups finely ground blanched almond flour

1 tsp salt

1 tsp baking soda

¼ cup Lily's sugar-free chocolate chips

¼ cup sliced raw almonds

## Directions

1. Using a whisk, blend all the wet ingredients (egg yolks, honey, stevia, coconut oil, and vanilla and almond extracts), then add the remaining dry ingredients (almond flour, salt, baking soda, and Lily's chocolate chips). Mix until incorporated.
2. Using a cookie scoop or 2 teaspoons, form dough into round balls, about 1" across. Place dough balls onto a baking sheet and flatten slightly with the palm of your hand or the back of a spoon.
3. Consider placing sliced almonds across the top of each cookie for decoration. Bake at 350°F for about 15 minutes or until golden brown.

### Fierce Foods Facts

This low-sugar treat is a surefire way to please any sweet tooth! The added fiber, protein, and vitamin E are a super bonus!

### Kids Can Cook Tips

Kids love to make cookies and will enjoy measuring and mixing the ingredients as well as forming the balls and decorating the top of each cookie with the almond slices.

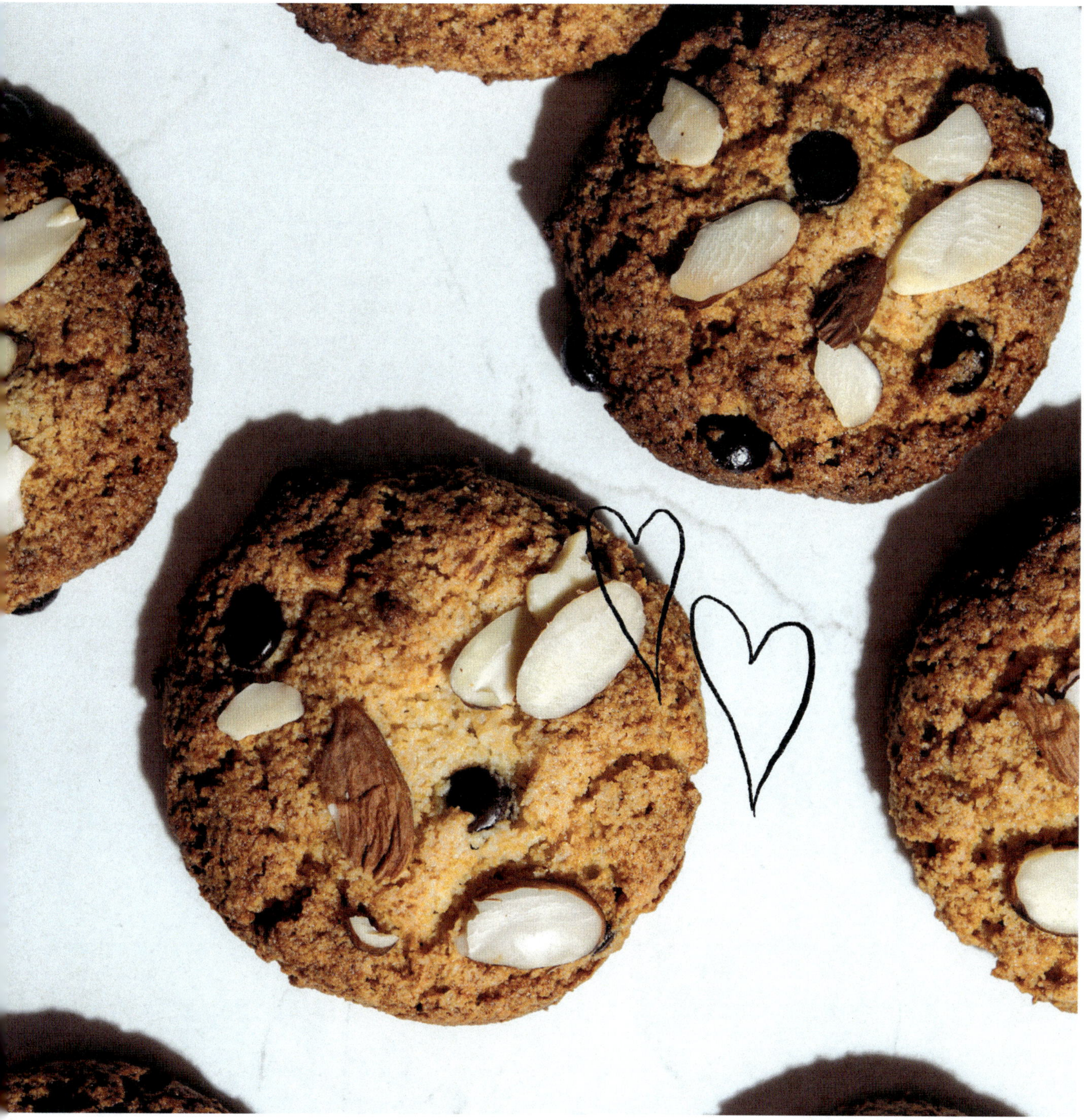

Chef Cathy McKnight

# Gingerbread Cookies

**Makes 24 servings:** 1 cookie each, 20 grams

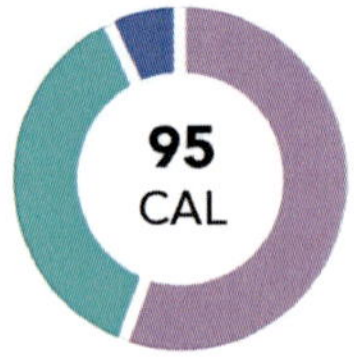


6g **Fat**
9g **Net Carb**
1g **Protein**

## Ingredients

1½ cup almond flour

¼ cup arrowroot powder

2 tsp cinnamon

1 tsp ground ginger

½ tsp nutmeg

¼ tsp cloves

1 tsp baking powder

½ tsp pink salt

¼ cup coconut oil, melted and cooled

¼ cup dark molasses

⅓ cup coconut sugar

1 tsp vanilla extract

¼ cup crystallized ginger, minced

## Directions

1. Preheat the oven to 350°F. In a bowl, whisk together the dry ingredients, breaking up any clumps. In a separate large bowl, whisk the coconut oil, molasses, coconut sugar, and vanilla until the sugar is completely dissolved.
2. Slowly add in the dry mix, a little at a time. Gently mix until no flour clumps remain. Add in the chopped crystallized ginger and stir to distribute.
3. Line cookie sheets with parchment paper. To form the cookies, roll 1 tablespoon of dough into a ball, place on the cookie sheet, and flatten lightly with your fingers. You can sprinkle the cookie with large sugar crystals if you'd like. You can also roll out the dough and use cookie cutters to create fun and festive shapes.
4. Bake for 12–14 minutes until the edges start to crisp. Be sure to let them cool before removing them from the cookie sheet or they'll fall apart.

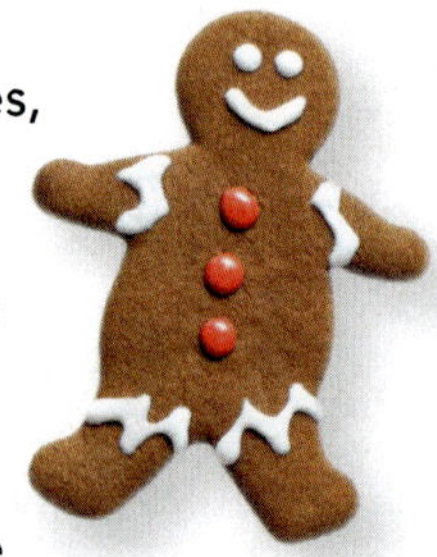

**Pro Tip:** These cookies freeze well, so go ahead and double or triple your batch!

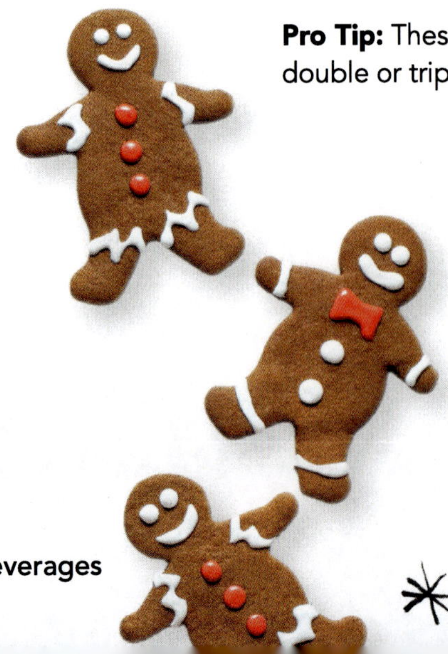

Chef Alexia Hall, RDN

# Hot Spiced Apple Cider

**Makes 8 servings:** each ~1¼ cup, 275 grams

**15** CAL

0g **Fat**
3g **Net Carb**
0g **Protein**

## Ingredients

64 oz (1 gal) filtered water

½ cup Bragg organic apple cider vinegar

1½ tsp Better Stevia liquid sweetener or alternative sweetener

3 tbsp mulling spice mix

1 whole Fuji or Red Delicious apple, cored and sliced thin

**Garnish recommendation:**

6 cinnamon sticks

## Directions

1. Boil water in a kettle. Place mulling spice in the center of a 4"x4" square of cheesecloth. Tie all 4 sides together with a string.
2. Pour the gallon of boiling water into a slow cooker. Add the mulling spices and the apple cider vinegar to the slow cooker, then add the stevia and stir well.
3. Core the apple, then slice thin with the skin on. Float the apple slices on top of the cider mixture. Turn the slow cooker on high for at least 30 minutes before you plan to serve. Remove the mulling spices after an hour or so.
4. To serve, pour into heat-safe mugs and garnish with apple slices and cinnamon sticks.

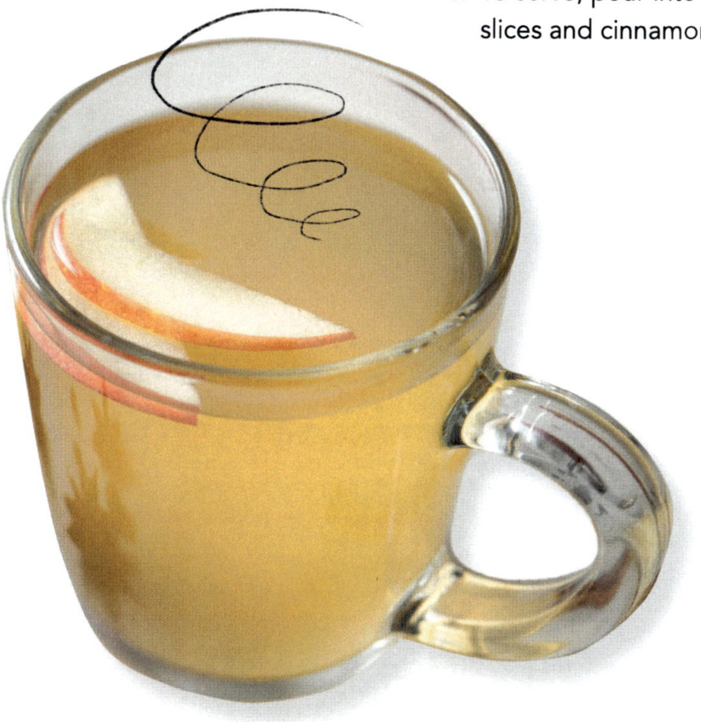

### Fierce Foods Facts

This very low-carb drink provides the tart delicious taste of hot spiced cider with almost no blood sugar impact. For those who must follow a keto diet, simply choose not to eat the apple slices. The apple cider vinegar will provide a nice source of probiotics, especially if raw, unfiltered, and not heated to very high temperatures. Vinegar also contains cancer-fighting polyphenols.

Chef Andrew Johnson

# Lemon Coconut Zucchini Bread

**Makes 12 servings:** each ~1" slice, 82 grams

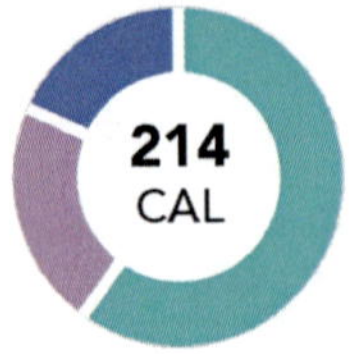


17g **Fat**
6g **Net Carb**
5g **Protein**

## Ingredients

⅓ cup butter or dairy-free alternative (e.g. Miyoko Creamery vegan butter)

½ cup honey or carb-conscious alternative (e.g. Pyure Hunny)

2 eggs

½ cup water or milk of choice (e.g. Tempt unsweetened hemp milk)

2 tbsp lemon juice

1 lemon zest (approx. 2 tsp)

1 tsp baking soda

1 tsp ground cinnamon

¼ tsp nutmeg

2 tsp vanilla extract

½ tsp salt

1 cup zucchini (approx. 2 medium), finely shredded with skin on

1 cup almond flour

¼ cup shredded coconut flour

½ cup unsweetened coconut, shredded

¼ cup ground flaxseed

## Directions

1. Preheat the oven to 325°F. Oil and flour a 9"x5" loaf pan. In a large mixing bowl, combine the butter and honey and beat with a whisk until they are combined, then add the eggs and beat well.
2. Add the milk, baking soda, cinnamon, vanilla, salt, nutmeg, lemon juice, and zest, and whisk to blend. Stir in the zucchini, then add the almond and coconut flours, ground flaxseed, and shredded coconut and stir just until combined.
3. Pour the batter into the prepared loaf pan and sprinkle lightly with additional cinnamon. Bake for 55–60 minutes, or until a toothpick inserted into the center comes out clean. Let the bread cool in the loaf pan for 10 minutes, then transfer it to a wire rack to cool for 20 minutes before slicing it with a sharp, serrated knife.

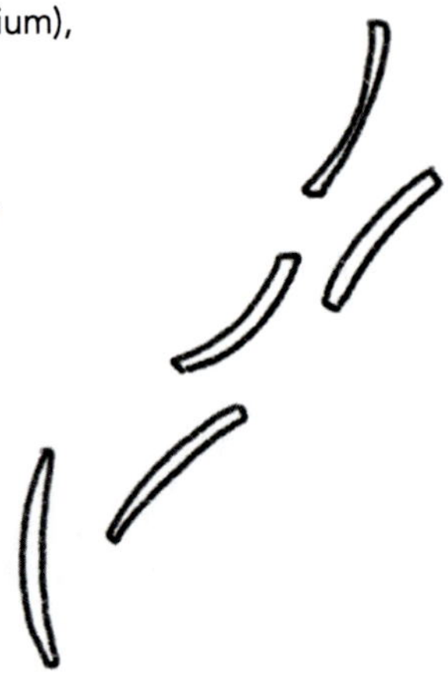

### Fierce Foods Facts

Have your cake and eat it too, especially with zucchini! This flavorful fall bread has almost 10 grams of microbiome-supporting fiber thanks to the zucchini as well as the almond, flax, and coconut flours. And all that for less than 6 net grams of carbohydrates per slice! It also has a nice amount of B vitamins, and almost 17% of your immune-supporting and anti-inflammatory daily requirement of vitamin E.

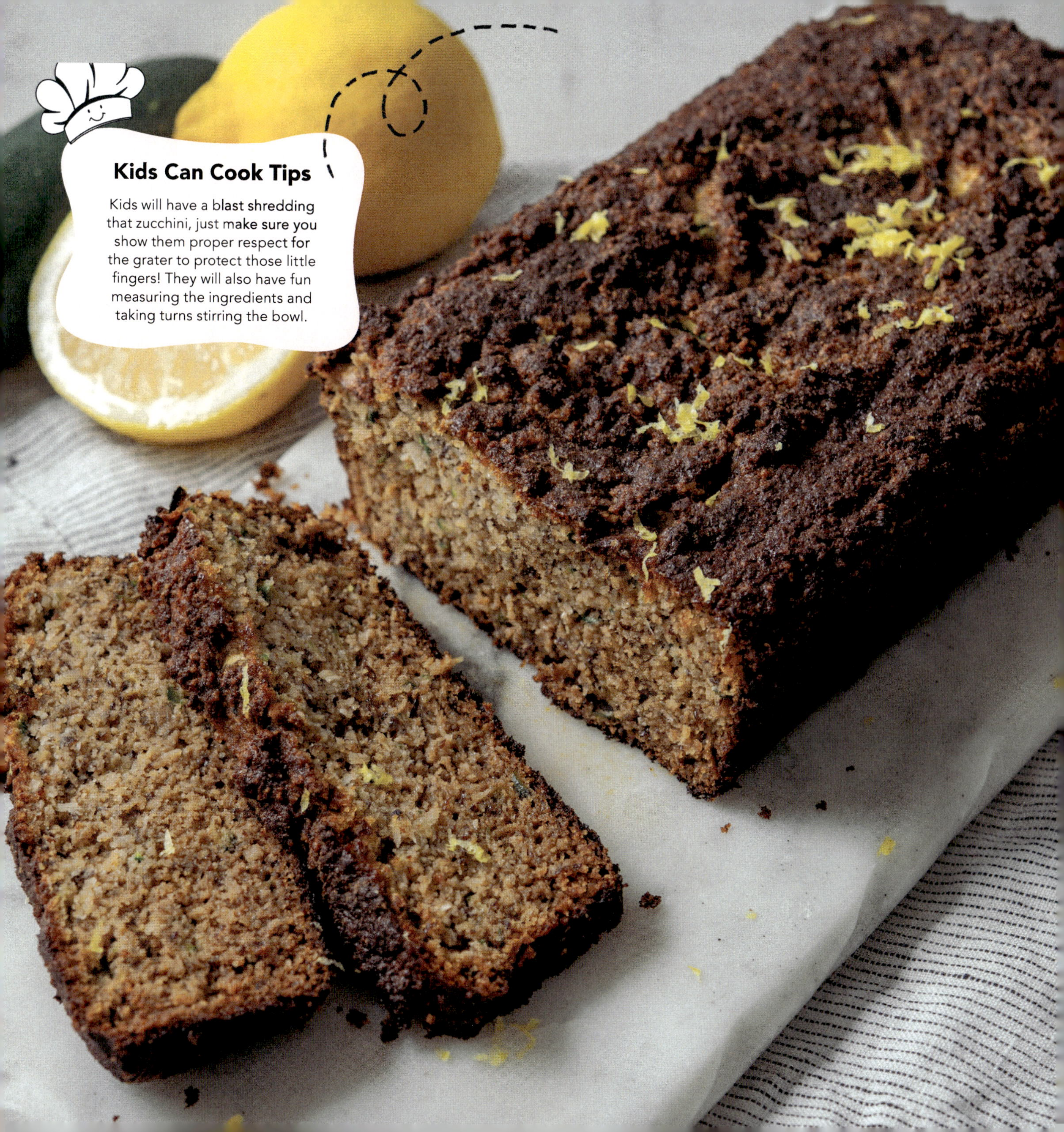

## Kids Can Cook Tips

Kids will have a blast shredding that zucchini, just make sure you show them proper respect for the grater to protect those little fingers! They will also have fun measuring the ingredients and taking turns stirring the bowl.

Chef Andrew Johnson

# Lime Coconut Bars

**Makes 12 servings:** 1 bar each, 79 grams

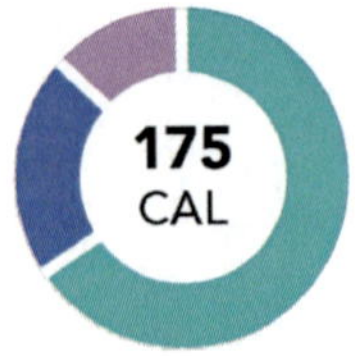


16g **Fat**
3g **Net Carb**
5g **Protein**

## Ingredients

### Crust

¾ cup superfine blanched almond flour

½ cup pecans, finely chopped

¼ cup unsweetened shredded coconut

⅓ cup powdered monk fruit sweetener or powdered coconut sugar

1 lime, zested

⅛ tsp sea salt

¼ cup unsalted grass-fed butter, ghee, or coconut oil, softened

### Filling

1 cup lime juice

½ cup coconut milk

½ cup alternative sweetener (consider Allulose for cake-like texture)

1 tbsp coconut oil

1 tsp lime, zested

1 drop lime essential oil (optional)

5 large eggs, beaten

### Garnish

2 tbsp powdered monk fruit sweetener or alternative powdered sugar

2 tsp lime, zested

1 lime, sliced into 12 quarter-moon shapes

## Directions

1. Preheat oven to 350°F. Use butter or coconut oil to prepare an 8"x8" oven-safe baking dish. Using a large bowl, stir almond flour, pecans, coconut, sweetener, lime zest, and salt in a large bowl. Using a pastry fork, blend the butter with the mixture until well combined.
2. Press the crust mixture firmly and evenly into the bottom of the prepared baking dish, and bake until lightly browned, (10–12 minutes).
3. Using a medium saucepan, whisk the lime juice, coconut milk, sweetener, butter, zest, and essential oil. Whisk over medium heat until the sweetener dissolves, then remove from heat.

4. Using a small bowl, whisk eggs until well combined. Temper eggs by adding a small amount of heated mixture into the bowl with eggs, whisking until well combined. Return the combined egg mixture to the saucepan and whisk well.
5. Pour final filling mixture over the crust, then bake for 10–15 minutes, or until the filling has set. Allow to cool, then refrigerate until ready to serve. Right before serving, garnish with powdered Lakanto sweetener, lime zest, and half-moon sliced lime.

## Fierce Foods Facts

This low-sugar dessert has a nice amount of immune-supporting vitamin C. The nutty crust also offers some balancing protein and fiber as well as nourishing vitamin E thanks to the pecans and almond flour.

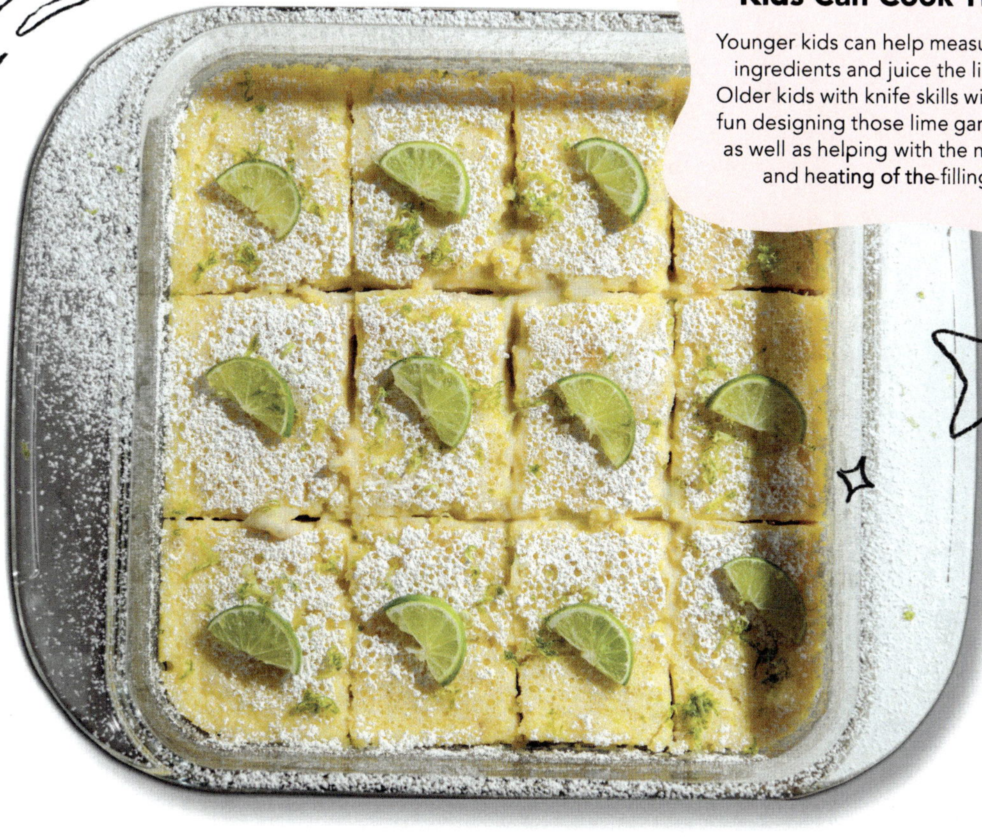

## Kids Can Cook Tips

Younger kids can help measure the ingredients and juice the limes. Older kids with knife skills will have fun designing those lime garnishes as well as helping with the mixing and heating of the filling.

Chef Andrew Johnson

# No-Bake Pumpkin Cheesecake

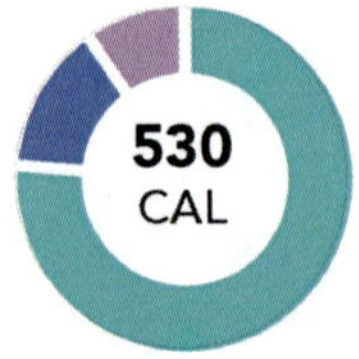


52g **Fat**
6g **Net Carb**
9g **Protein**

**Makes 8 servings:** each ~⅔ cup or 162 grams

## Ingredients

### Crust

1½ cups almond flour, finely ground

½ cup pecans, toasted and chopped

¼ cup butter, melted

½ cup allulose alternative sweetener

½ tsp salt

½ tsp cinnamon

1 tsp vanilla extract

### Filling

1 cup heavy cream, ice-cold

16 oz cream cheese

1 can (15 oz) unsweetened pumpkin purée

1 cup powdered sugar or alternative sweetener (e.g. monk fruit)

1 tsp cinnamon

½ tsp nutmeg

¼ tsp cloves

## Directions

1. Using a large bowl, combine almond flour, toasted chopped pecans, salt, cinnamon, and alternative sweetener. Slowly add melted butter and vanilla and stir to combine well. Firmly press the mixture into a springform pan if you have one (a round pie pan or a bar pan will also work just as well).
2. In a medium bowl with a stand mixer (or handheld mixer), beat cold heavy cream until stiff peaks form. In a separate bowl, beat cream cheese until fluffy, then slowly add pumpkin purée, and beat until well combined. Add powdered sugar slowly, and continue beating until no clumps remain. Mix in the spices until combined.
3. Using just a spatula or large spoon, fold in the whipped cream, then pour the cheesecake mixture over the crust and refrigerate overnight to set. To store, loosely cover in the refrigerator for up to 5 days.
4. For a fun and festive "crustless" cheesecake, add filling to a small hollowed-out pumpkin and refrigerate overnight.

**Dairy-free option:** Consider using coconut whipping cream, Kite Hill almond cream cheese, and Miyoko Creamery faux vegan butter.

## Fierce Foods Facts

This recipe is loaded with some beautiful fat-soluble vitamins providing over 40% of the day's vitamins A and E, which is great for the skin, eyes, and immune system. It also has a nice mix of the minerals selenium and zinc, which are also helpful for the immune system.

### Kids Can Cook Tips

Hollow out a mini pumpkin for kids to decorate with sharpies and paints. Use this to serve the mini cheesecake chilled within its own bowl. Kids will also enjoy adding each ingredient to the mixing bowl, layering it inside the pumpkin, and adding a light sprinkle of spices to finish their decoration.

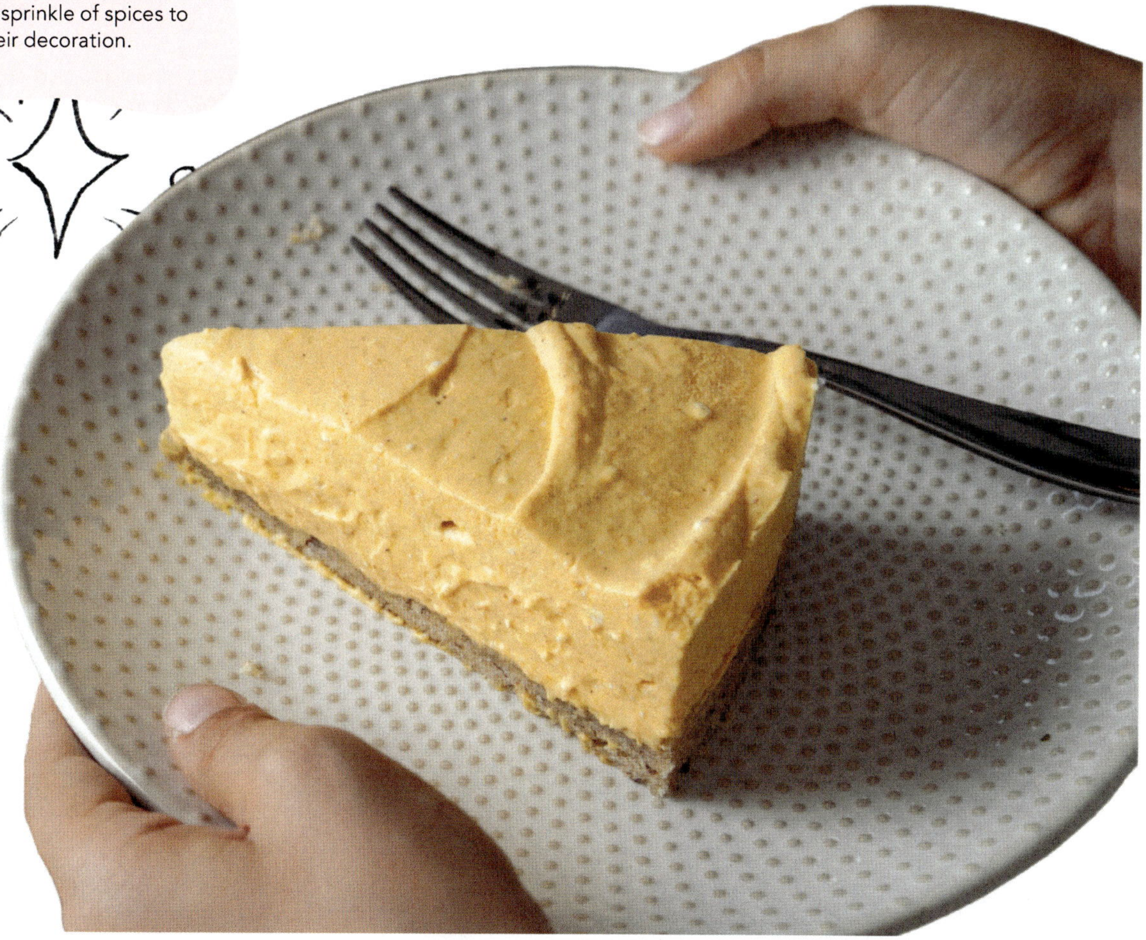

Chef Audra DiPadova Wilford

# No Sugar No Grain (NSNG) Chocolate Bakes

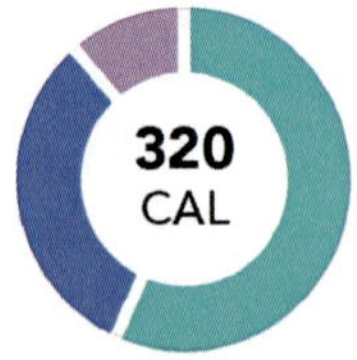


27g **Fat**
5g **Net Carb**
15g **Protein**

**Makes 12 servings:** 2"x2" square each, 110 grams

## Ingredients

16 oz (~2 cups) roasted nut butter

8–11 eggs

2 tbsp apple cider vinegar

2 cups of erythritol (e.g. organic erythritol with stevia or Lakanto brand)

Drop of stevia glycerite to taste

1 cup of cocoa powder

2 tsp baking soda

¼ tsp sea salt

**Note:** You can use this batter to make brownies, cakes, muffins, and waffles.

## Directions

1. Prepare a baking dish or bread pan with coconut oil. Blend together the nut butter and eggs in a food processor until very smooth. Add erythritol, stevia, and salt, then mix until well combined.
2. Mix in the cocoa powder, then add the apple cider vinegar and baking soda and blend well. Taste the batter and be sure it's to your liking.
3. For breads and cakes, pour the batter into the baking dish of your choice. Bake at 350°F for 45 minutes. Cool on a cooling rack for 2 hours.
4. For cupcakes or muffins, pour the batter into prepared muffin tins until ⅔ full. Bake for 18–20 minutes or until firm to touch.
5. For waffles, thin the batter slightly with milk or alternative until pourable. Place in a hot waffle iron, and watch carefully for the end of steam which will indicate that the waffle is done.

### Flavor variations

**Cream Cheese Ripple:** Place a ½ cup of cream cheese in a small bowl and whip until smooth. Using a spoon or butter knife, swirl cream cheese through the batter in the pan prior to baking.

**Strawberry:** Replace the cocoa powder with an even amount of strawberry powder, and bake as usual.

### Fierce Foods Facts

This is a grainless option for those on restricted diets that will enable a chocolatey sweet treat. There are 16 grams of sugar alcohols, which when subtracted can provide a very low net carb option for those that are on a ketogenic diet. This batter will also work for lots of other dessert options!

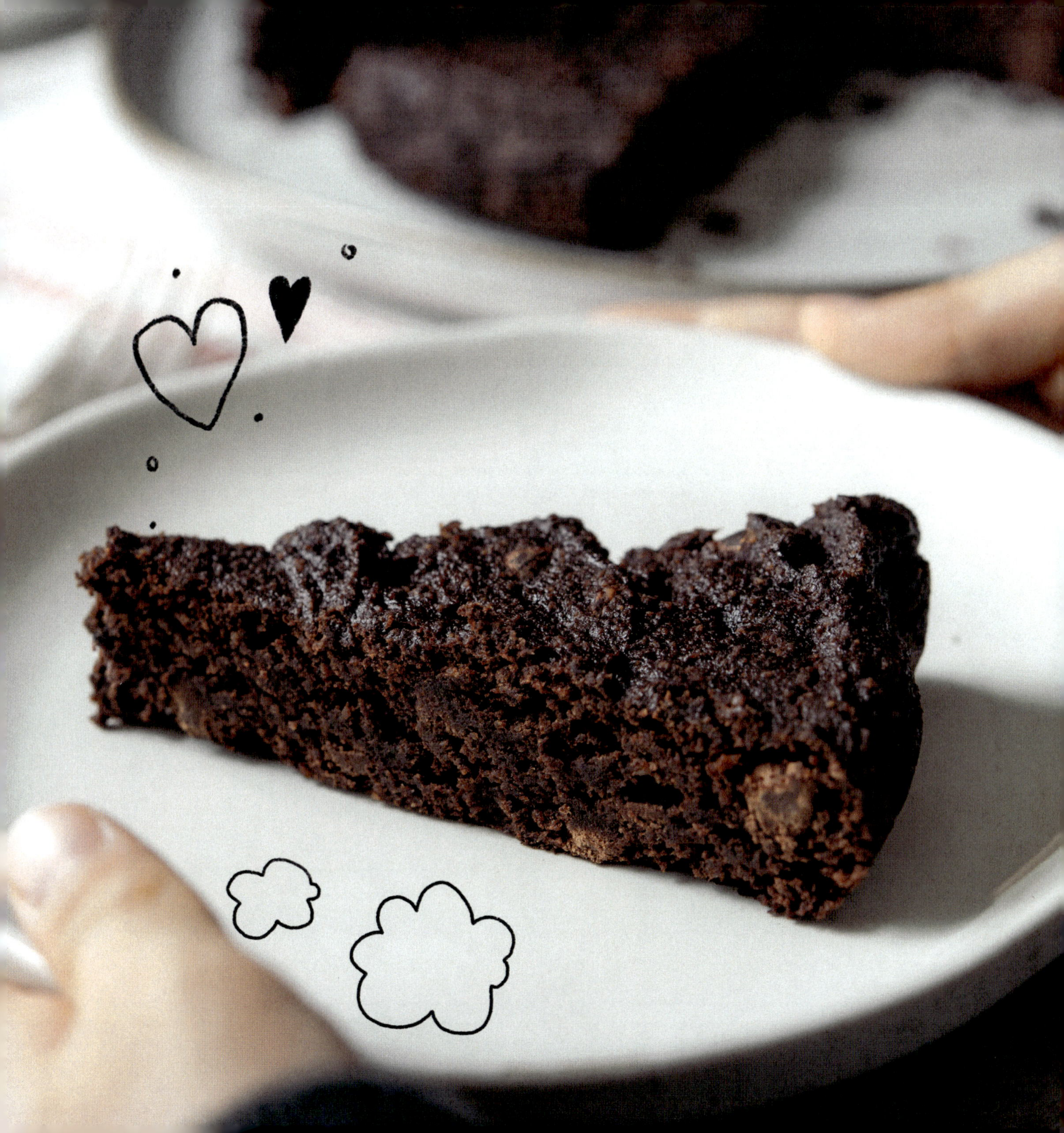

Chef Andrew Johnson

# Apricot Strawberry Coconut Cream Popsicles

103 CAL

7g Fat
7g Net Carb
2g Protein

**Makes 12 servings:** each ~1 popsicle, 115 grams

## Ingredients

3 cups strawberries, sliced

1 can (15 oz) full-fat coconut milk

½ cup Greek yogurt or dairy-free alternative, unsweetened

3–4 tbsp honey or alternative

(e.g. Pyure Hunny)

1 tsp vanilla extract

2 cups apricots, washed and cut into ⅛-¼" slices, skin-on

1 tsp cardamom

### Fierce Foods Facts

This low sugar fruit-filled summer snack is a huge crowd pleaser and the color options are endless. Loaded with vitamins A and C, they are sure to keep those summer sniffles away by bolstering the immune system.

## Directions

1. In a blender, purée the strawberries with 2 tablespoons of honey. Rinse the blender, using it again to combine coconut milk, yogurt, remaining honey to taste, and vanilla extract. Process until smooth.
2. Slice apricots and toss with cardamom. Insert 3–5 whole apricot slices directly into each popsicle mold. Alternately pour coconut milk mixture and strawberry mixture over the apricots in the mold. Using a popsicle stick or small spoon, swirl through colors to create a design.
3. Gently tap the molds on the countertop to remove air bubbles. Insert popsicle sticks, and freeze for several hours (5–6) or overnight. Alternatively, may consider pouring the mixture into a large plastic container and freezing, defrosting slightly, and then scooping to serve.
4. Consider using silicone popsicle molds. May run under warm water for 15 seconds to help loosen the mold.

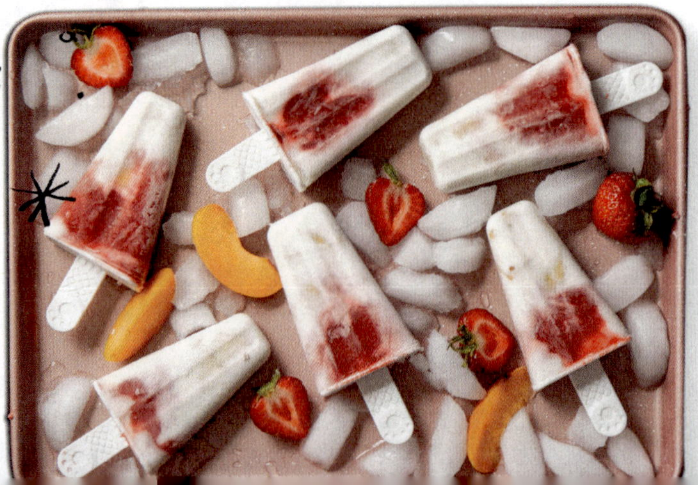

Chef Anne Watson

# Russell and Mom's Favorite Healthy Brownies

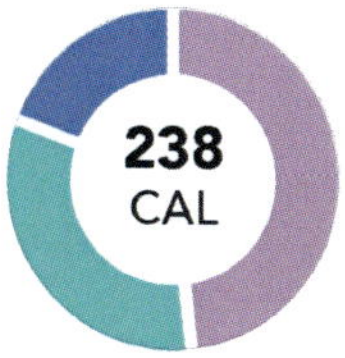


12g Fat
18g Net Carb
7g Protein

**Makes 12 servings:** 1 each, 82 grams

## Ingredients

1½ cup fine-ground almond flour

½ cup cocoa powder or nutrient-dense option (e.g. Navitas Organics cacao powder)

1 tsp baking soda

1½ cup pitted dates

¾ cup water

⅓ cup almond milk

1 tbsp cornstarch

2 tsp vanilla extract

¼ tsp xanthan gum

¾ cup sugar-free dark chocolate chips (e.g. Lily's dark chocolate baking chips)

## Fierce Foods Facts

This delicious healthy brownie packs an impressive 11 grams of fiber per serving thanks to the dates, almond flour, and cocoa. As a bonus, it also has a nice amount of iron, 25% of the daily vitamin E, and plenty of magnesium. Already a low carbohydrate option, carbs can be made even lower with the allulose sugar alternative, a sweetener that will help it retain its wonderful cake-like texture.

## Directions

1. Preheat the oven to 325°F, then grease and line your baking pan. For a more rustic look, use a cast iron pan.
2. Sift together the almond flour, cocoa or cacao powder, and baking soda in a medium bowl and set aside.
3. Place the dates, water, and almond milk in a high-speed blender and blend into a smooth paste, then blend in the corn-starch, vanilla, and xanthan gum for approximately 1 minute to activate the thickeners.
4. Fold the wet mixture from the blender into the dry mixture in the bowl and stir until smooth. Gently fold in the chocolate chips and then spread evenly in your pan.
5. Bake for approximately 25–30 minutes, or until a knife inserted in the center comes out clean. When serving, these brownies go perfectly with fresh berries, especially when the brownies are still warm.

**Carb-conscious options:**
Swap the pitted dates for 1½ cups allulose sweetener. This provides 5 net carbs per serving. For a no-sugar, no-grain option, look at our **NSNG Chocolate Bakes.**

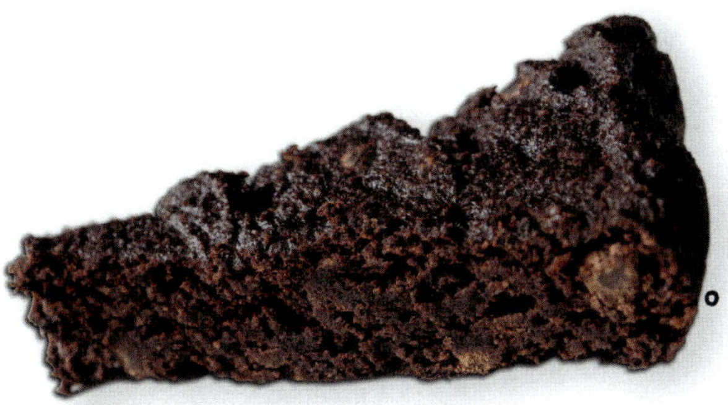

Chef Andrew Johnson

# Sugar-Free Spiced Cocoa

**Makes 4 servings:** each ~1 cup, 271 grams

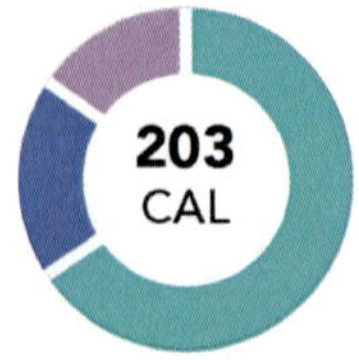


18g **Fat**
4g **Net Carb**
5g **Protein**

## Ingredients

### Cocoa

8 tbsp cocoa powder, unsweetened

6 tbsp monk fruit sweetener or coconut sugar, divided

1 tsp ground cinnamon

1 tsp ground ginger

½–1 tsp dark chili powder

Pinch of salt

4 cups Tempt Hemp Milk or heavy cream, unsweetened

### Whipped Cream

½ cup heavy cream or coconut whipping cream

1 tsp vanilla extract

## Directions

1. Using a small saucepan over medium-low heat, whisk together the cocoa powder, 4 tablespoons of sweetener, salt, cinnamon, ground ginger, and chili powder with about 2 tablespoons milk in a small saucepan until the cocoa and sugar dissolve completely.
2. Whisk in the rest of the milk and heat it over medium heat, whisking occasionally, until it is hot. If you like it frothy, blend it with a hand blender.
3. This can be made in larger batches by doubling dry ingredients. Add 1 cup of milk and 1 tablespoon of dry ingredients per serving.
4. For the whipped cream, combine heavy cream, the remaining 2 tablespoons of sweetener, and vanilla extract in a medium chilled bowl. Use a hand mixer or stand mixer to beat on high for 1–2 minutes until soft peaks form.

### Fierce Foods Facts

Finally, a delicious mug of holiday hot chocolate that contains all the calcium, phosphorus, and magnesium you need without all the sugar you don't!

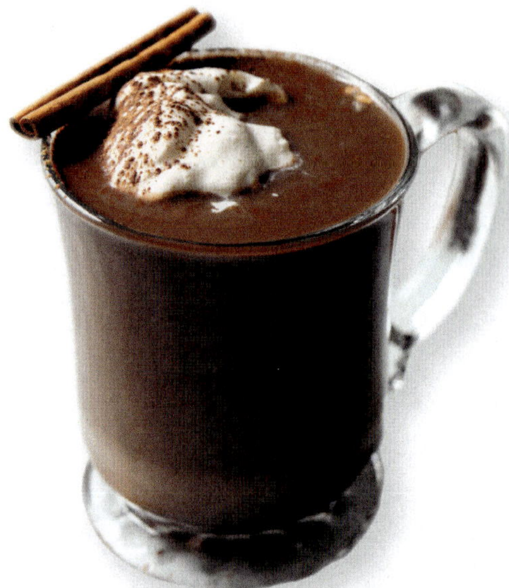

Chef Audra DiPadova Wilford

# Very Cold Cream and Eggs AKA Ice Cream

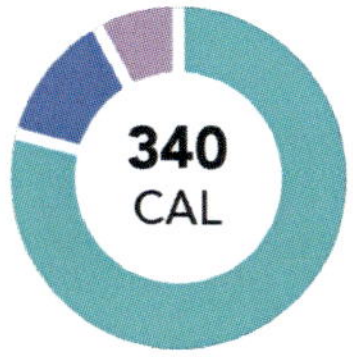


33g Fat
3g Net Carb
5g Protein

**Makes 7 servings:** each ~½ cup, 120 grams

## Ingredients

2½ cups heavy cream

3 eggs

Generous pinch of salt

½ cup of ZSweet

Several drops stevia glycerite to taste

1¼ tbsp vegetable glycerine (totally safe to eat, makes ice cream really creamy)

## Directions

1. Mix eggs vigorously with ZSweet, then add glycerin, stevia, salt, and vanilla. Mix well, add cream, then mix again to get everything blended before pouring it into the ice cream machine.
2. Store in an airtight container in the freezer until ready to enjoy.

### Fierce Foods Facts

There are 14 grams of sugar alcohol in this recipe, and when subtracted from the total carbohydrate count, it provides a very low (and very delicious) carbohydrate option. This recipe is super nutritious and perfect for keto-kids—go ahead and have ice cream for breakfast! This is also a great choice for those who need to gain weight, or just need a little comfort when suffering from a fever.

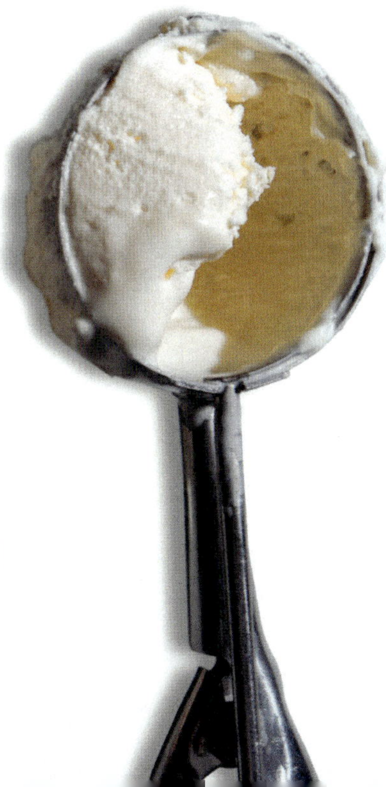

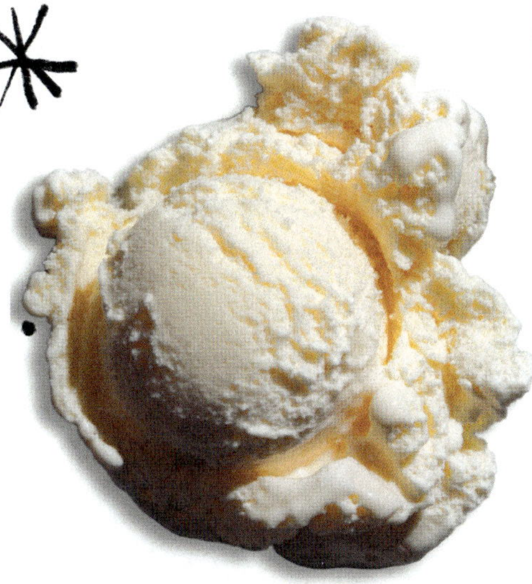

Chef Andrew Johnson

# Thumbprint Cookies

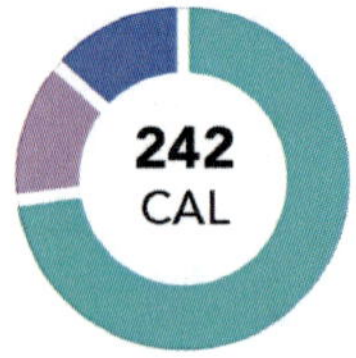


23g Fat
4g Net Carb
4g Protein

Makes 48 cookies, 12 servings: 2 cookies each, 59 grams

## Ingredients

½ cup unsalted grass-fed butter, ghee, or coconut oil, softened

⅔ cups powdered monk fruit sweetener or powdered coconut sugar

1⅔ cups superfine blanched almond flour

1 tsp vanilla extract

Pinch of fine sea salt

1 tsp unsweetened almond milk

1 cup finely chopped pecans (or process into flour if desired)

½ cup jam, flavor of choice, no sugar added (e.g. Nature's Hollow Sugar Free Jam)

### Fierce Foods Facts

These traditional holiday cookies have a nice balance of protein and fat while lowering the overall sugar content thanks to the nuts and nut flours along with a little help from the alternative sweetener. They also come with a very nice amount of Vitamin E, which supports heart and immune function and lowers the risk of cancer.

## Directions

1. Using a stand mixer, hand mixer, food processor, or a fork in a large bowl, cream together the butter/ghee/coconut oil with the powdered sweetener (tasting for desired sweetness) until light and fluffy.
2. Add the vanilla, almond flour, and salt and mix until the dough is well incorporated. Then, stir in chopped (or ground) pecans and mix again until combined.
3. Use your hands to knead the dough until it forms a large dough ball. If your dough is too dry and won't come together, add a small amount of milk. If the dough seems too wet, add small amounts of almond flour until you reach the desired consistency.
4. Preheat the oven to 375°F. Line a baking sheet with parchment paper, then, using a cookie scoop or 2 teaspoons, roll dough into tablespoon-sized dough balls and place on a prepared cookie sheet about 2" apart. Make a small indentation in the middle of each cookie ball with your thumb, then spoon about ½ teaspoon of jam into the center of each cookie.
5. Place cookies in the oven and bake for 10–12 minutes until bottoms are golden, rotating pans halfway through. Be careful not to over-bake.
6. Remove from oven and cool on baking pan for about 3–4 minutes until you can handle them comfortably with your hands.
7. Store cookies in an airtight container for up to 3 days or freeze for up to a month.

**Note:** This dough will also work for Linzer cookies, Mexican wedding cookies, or cookie crusts for treats like pumpkin bars.

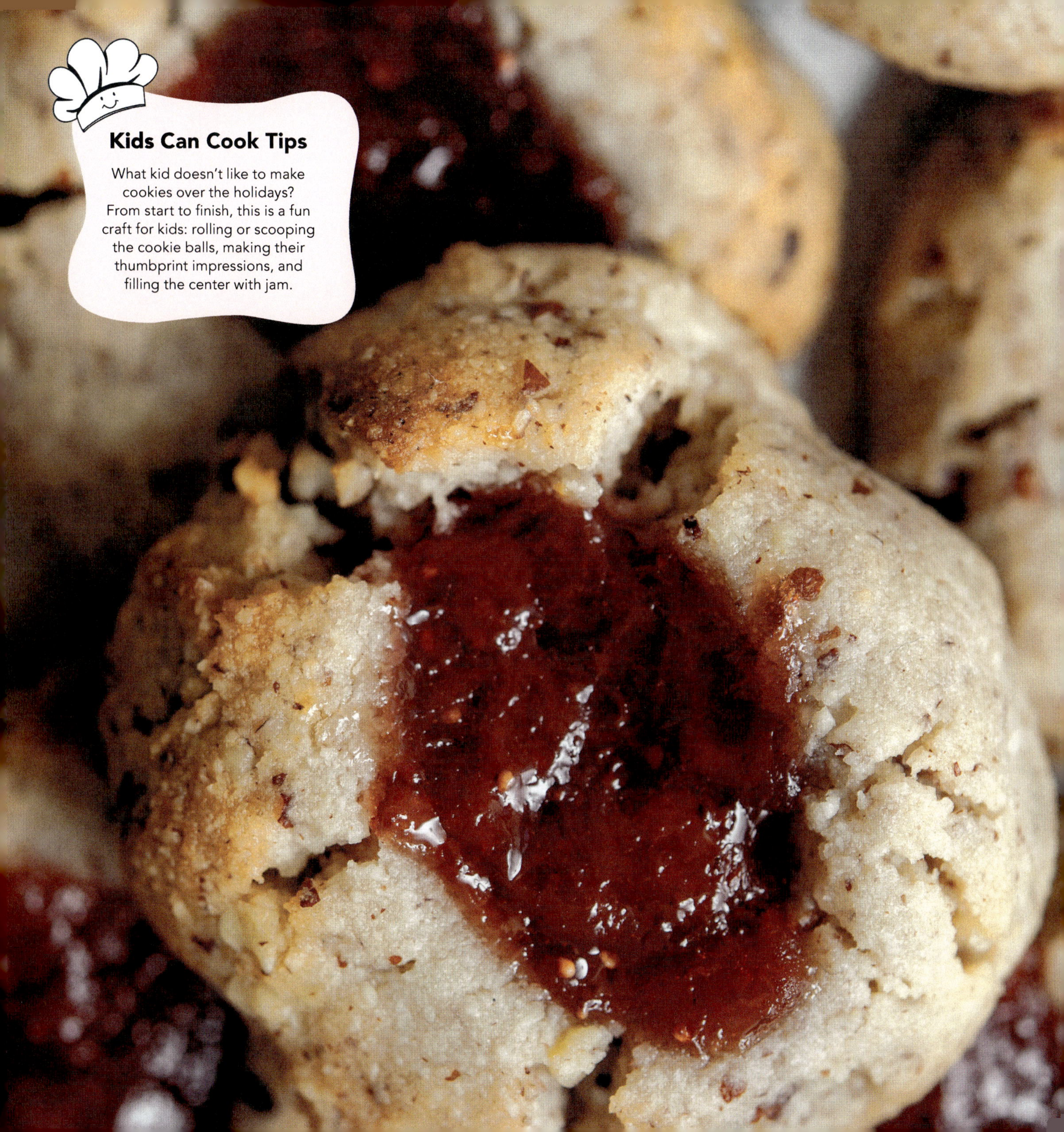

### Kids Can Cook Tips

What kid doesn't like to make cookies over the holidays? From start to finish, this is a fun craft for kids: rolling or scooping the cookie balls, making their thumbprint impressions, and filling the center with jam.

Chef Alexia Hall, RDN

# Avocado Ice Cream in a Bag

**Makes 1 serving:** 222 grams

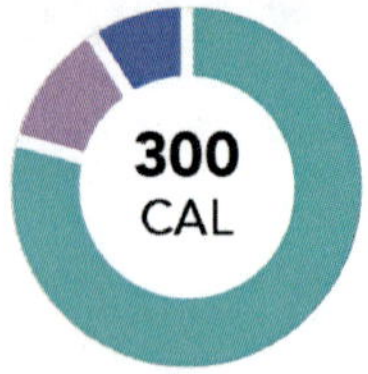


29g **Fat**
4g **Net Carb**
3g **Protein**

## Ingredients

6 tbsp kosher or rock salt

2 tsp coconut sugar or alternative (e.g. Lakanto gold monk fruit sweetener)

½ cup full-fat coconut milk, refrigerated overnight (or consider ½ cup heavy cream)

½ avocado, pitted and peeled

1 tsp lemon juice (use immediately on avocados after cutting to prevent browning)

## You'll also need

1 gal Ziploc bag

1 pint Ziploc bag

Enough ice to fill the gallon-sized bag halfway

### Fierce Foods Facts

This fun, kid-friendly recipe is so easy for all ages and is loaded with healthy fats for brain and heart health. It also has a nice amount of folate and vitamins C and K thanks to the avocado. This recipe is also a good source of potassium, great for staying hydrated during the hot summer months!

## Directions

1. Fill the gallon-sized Ziploc bag halfway with ice. Add the salt, mixing until evenly distributed.
2. In the smaller Ziploc bag, add the sugar, coconut milk, avocado, and lemon juice. Seal the small Ziploc baggie and knead the mixture by hand to combine thoroughly. If a more even texture is preferred, place the contents in a blender and blend on low for 2 minutes, then return to the small bag and ensure it is properly sealed.
3. Place the small bag inside the large bag and make sure it is covered on all sides by the ice and salt mixture. Seal the gallon bag and shake vigorously for 5 minutes. Use a towel to hold the bags to prevent slippery or uncomfortably cold hands.
4. This recipe may be scaled to make larger batches. For the larger batches, blended the mixture on high, then pour the mixture into an aluminum or stainless steel loaf pan that has been in the freezer for at least half an hour. Cover mixture and freeze until firm.

**Flavor variations:**

**Mint Chocolate Chip:** Add 1 teaspoon minced mint leaves and 1 teaspoon chocolate chips

**Chocolate:** Add 1 tablespoon cacao powder, omit the lemon juice and add ½ teaspoon vanilla extract

**Nuts:** Add 1 tablespoon finely chopped toasted pistachios or almonds

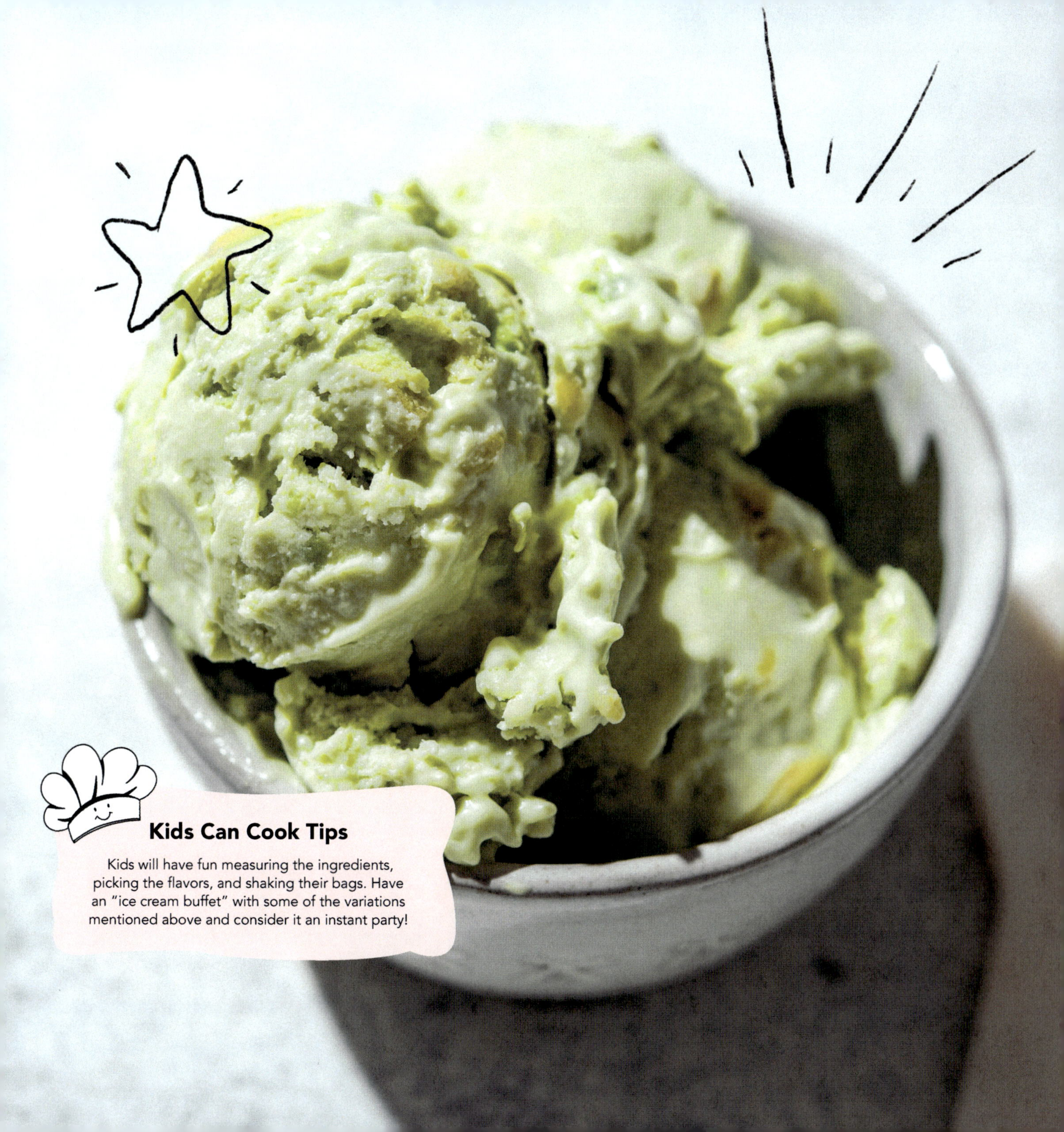

### Kids Can Cook Tips

Kids will have fun measuring the ingredients, picking the flavors, and shaking their bags. Have an "ice cream buffet" with some of the variations mentioned above and consider it an instant party!

# Contributors

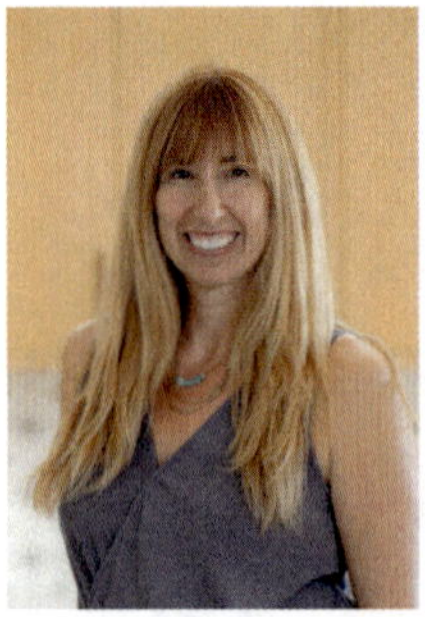

### Anne Watson

It's hard to say which came first, Anne's love of food or her love of photography. Anne has always had a passion for the culinary world and her style comes out of a deep love and understanding of the food culture of Southern California and the places she has lived and traveled, from Europe to Asia, Africa, Australia, and all over North America.

With a background working in professional kitchens, she now combines her unique skillset into a one-stop-shop for recipe development and testing, cooking, food styling, and food photography that she runs out of her custom built home studio kitchen on The Watson Ranch in North San Diego County, California.

Anne's award-winning work has been featured in internationally celebrated magazines, newspapers, online outlets, and cookbooks. When not behind the camera lens, Anne also owns and operates Watson Ranch Vineyards, LLC where she is the Head Winegrower and Wine Seller for her family's three-acre Cabernet Sauvignon estate vineyard. She also runs Watson Wellness, LLC, a holistic healing business where she is a Reiki Master Practitioner, Yogic Lifestyle Coach, and Mindfulness Meditation Teacher. Anne is a mother to her nine-year-old son, and an "animal mom" to over 50 rescue animals including pigs, chickens, dogs, and tortoises, whom she lovingly raises on her farm.

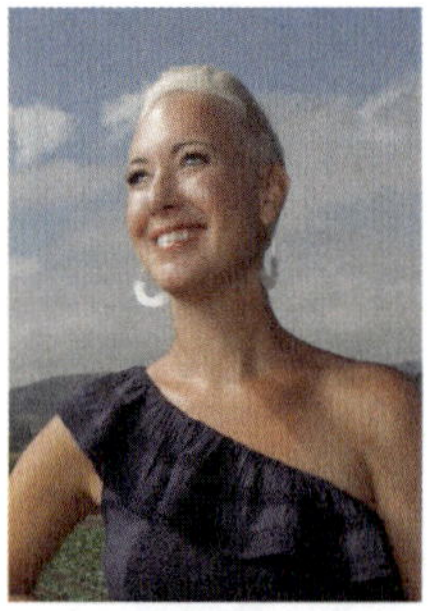

### Audra DiPadova Wilford

Audra DiPadova Wilford is the Chief Hope Officer of Max-Love Project. Classically trained in the culinary arts in Scottsdale, Arizona, Audra became a skilled cook at four-star restaurants before she was 20 years old. In both Arizona and Maine, she worked several positions from grill to sauté to saucier, and discovered that her passion for food went beyond the kitchen. She jumped to the "front of the house" and became both a server and bartender while finishing her college degree with a focus on political science, public policy, and health disparities.

After finishing college, she went to graduate school, earning a degree in philosophy and education from Columbia University with the goal of becoming an educator. Audra moved into leadership training in higher education, but her passion for food never waned. Instead of cooking for hundreds of people a night, her focus turned to cooking alongside her husband for their two children.

Then, just over ten years ago, Audra's son Max was diagnosed with brain cancer. She reflexively fell back on her culinary training and turned to food as medicine. Alongside, intensive brain surgeries, a year-and-a-half of chemotherapy, 30 rounds of radiation, Gamma Knife radiation treatment, and a targeted checkpoint inhibitor, Audra used the kitchen as her tool to help Max thrive in the face of cancer.

As Audra met other moms with children in cancer treatment, she heard the consistent need for culinary education, nutrition science education, and integrative medicine resources. Listening to these needs, and right in the middle of Max's chemotherapy treatment, Audra started the MaxLove Project (MLP), a nonprofit designed to help parents use nutrition and integrative medicine to help their children thrive in treatment and beyond.

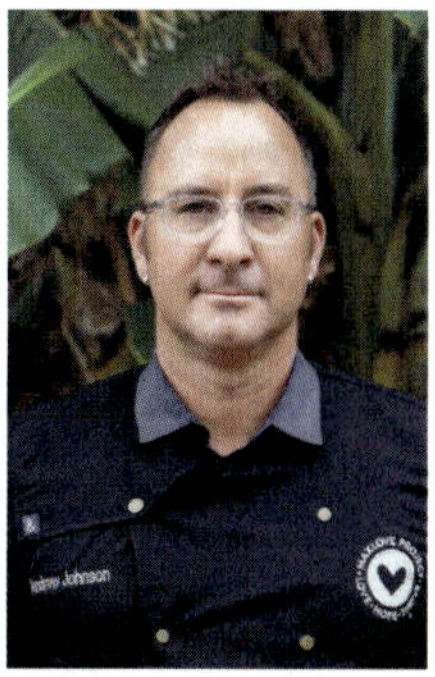

**Andrew Johnson**

Chef Andrew Johnson has over three decades of knowledge working in and around professional kitchens, education, healthcare, and local farms. He is the Nourishment Program Director for the Anneliese Schools in Laguna Beach and operates a personal chef and dietitian business, Kitchen Curative, specializing in meal services, catering, and cooking classes.

Andrew is the Culinary Medicine Chef for MaxLove Project, teaching cooking classes for cancer survivor families and developing recipes and other culinary content for several platforms. He was also recently employed as a chef in residence for The Ecology Center, where he cooks farm-to-table for the 28-acre certified organic farm.

Andrew was the Executive Chef and Co-Founder of The Meal Prep, which offered healthy meal delivery services to Orange County and Los Angeles, and manages and teaches urban agriculture with the City of Irvine's Great Park @ the Farm + Food Lab.

Other previous roles include Director & Culinary Instructor at the International Culinary School, Executive Sous Chef of a multi-unit hospital/health system, Food & Beverage Director of an assisted living community, and Regional Food & Beverage Director for a golf club.

Andrew is a certified Master Food Preserver from the University of California Agriculture and Natural Resources, and teaches food preservation techniques to the communities of Orange County. He has a master's degree in business administration with a focus in sustainability, a bachelor's degree in hospitality manage-ment, and an associate's degree in culinary arts. He also carries certificates as a Servsafe manager/instructor/proctor, a member of the American Culinary Federation, and a HACCP manager and aquaponics.

Diagnosed at an early age, Andrew is a compliant type 1 diabetic but has successfully managed his disease through healthy food choices and an active lifestyle. As a champion for his own personal wellness needs, he has organically gravitated to professional roles where he can thrive at the intersection of food, education, and wellness. He believes in growing our own food, choosing local food producers, and the holistic concept of foods as medicine.

### Alexia Hall

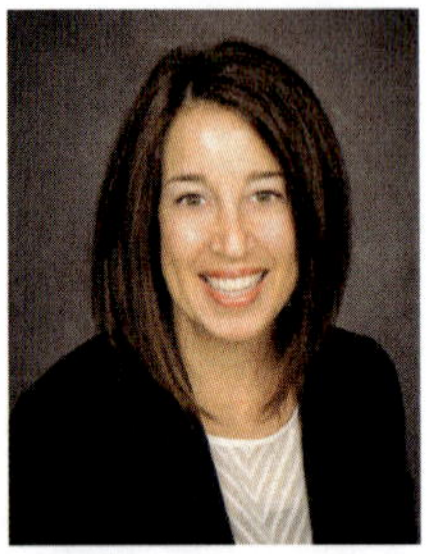

Alexia Hall is a Registered Dietitian who is a fervent supporter of the concept of "Food as Medicine." She witnessed how nutrition therapy improved the lives of those in her own family and works hard to bring her training, knowledge, and passion to those in her practice.

She received her BS in Dietetics from Sacramento State University, with a minor in Biology, and completed her Dietetic Internship at UC Davis Medical Center. She holds certifications in Food Allergy Management and Integrative and Functional Nutrition and is pursuing an additional credential for Nutrigenetics Counseling.

Alexia owns a private practice and is the Co-Founder of Kitchen Curative, a personal dietitian and chef service. She is also grateful to co-lead the Fierce Foods Academy; the nutrition-based instructional classroom founded by the MaxLove Project.

Alexia is dedicated to sharing evidence-based nutrition information and hopes to always offer inspiration that will empower others to thrive.

### Cathy McKnight

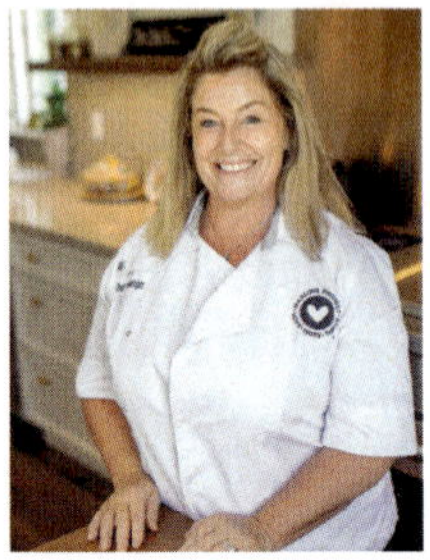

Chef Cathy McKnight is committed to cultivating a regenerative food culture and encouraging people to cook with abundant love and respect for the earth. She connects chefs, butchers, ranchers, and farmers in an effort to reach the larger community of home cooks. Cathy was raised in Northern California and her connection to the Slow Food Movement began as a small child. She grew up with a large garden and was surrounded by local orchards and ranches that her family sourced from. She was obsessed with Alice Waters, and once she stepped into the Chez Panisse kitchen, her future was determined.

Cathy graduated from UC Davis intent on pursuing a criminal law career—but her passion for cooking led her to the kitchen, and What A Dish catering was born. Her boutique catering company and cafe never strayed from local sourcing, which led to her relationship with The Ecology Center, where she is honored to be a Community Accord Chef.

Cathy, along with other like-minded chefs from Orange County, made a commitment to source local, whole foods within a 250-mile radius of the San Juan Capistrano organic farm. This departure from standard restaurant sourcing practices has led to a network of ranchers, farmers, and other food artisans who are committed to regenerative agriculture and sustaining our earth.

She has appeared on the Food Network's program "Chopped," continues to collaborate with The Ecology Center as a community table chef, and is on the Board of Directors for the MaxLove Project, contributing recipes and ideas that contribute to the philosophy that food is medicine. Cathy was the founding executive chef for Model Meals, a food delivery company embracing the Whole 30 lifestyle. She was the consulting executive chef for Eilo's Kitchen, working with founder Aileen Kruidenier to bring whole foods to guests with autoimmune issues. Eilo's concept crystallized Cathy's vision that it is possible to eat delicious and highly nutritious foods without the added sugar and grains commercial food companies push on the consumer.

She uses her vast network of high-level athletes and celebrities in her quest to dismantle the SAD (Standard American Diet) and bring quality nourishment to her table and the tables of her clients. Her latest projects include Kitchen 415, which aims to use food and education to disrupt current restaurant and home food practices, and is also a menu and sourcing consultant for new restaurant concepts.

Cathy says, "My life is an open cookbook, and I am inspired everyday by the abundance that Mother Earth supplies for us. Eat with love and respect for her and know that every dollar you spend on food can enrich our earth."

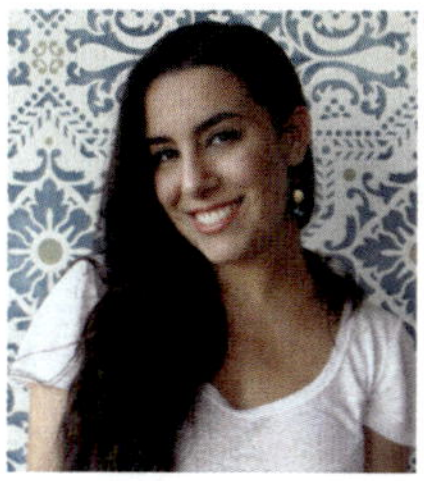

**Jordan Nishkian**

Jordan Nishkian is a writer and editor based in Southern California who has worked for a number of publications, including *LOCALE Magazine, Sauté Magazine, Nobleman Magazine,* and *Yes Collective.*

After earning her bachelor's degrees in Creative Writing and Anthropology from CSU Long Beach, it didn't take long for Jordan to discover her passion for crafting editorial stories, especially those centered around food and the exploration of culinary culture.

Jordan has had the pleasure of writing about restaurants and chefs for most of her career, and some of her favorite interviews have included celebrity chef Aarti Sequeira and rapper, activist, and chef Hugh Augustine.

Jordan is the Editor-in-Chief of *Mythos* literary magazine and Co-Founder of Ink and Quill Publications. When she's not working on copy for websites, brands, and magazines, she can be found crafting poetry and short stories, which have been featured in national and international publications.

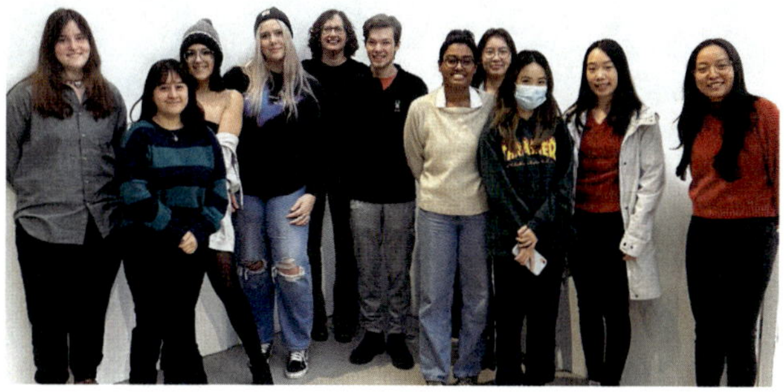

**Massachusetts College of Art and Design**

The Community Partnership Design class has been offered since 2001, when it was started by Professor Lisa Rosowsky. Students in this class partner with one organization each year, most often in the healthcare or public health space, learning about printing and print production in the process. MassArt, located in Boston, is the nation's oldest freestanding public four-year college of art and design; in 2023 it celebrates its 150th anniversary.

***Left to right:***
*Emmy Kelley*
*Domenica Alcivar*
*Hannah Kourbage*
*Serene Desisto*
*Lisa Rosowsky*
*Tyler Roads*
*Shreya Kodi*
*Anny Nguyen*
*Yingxin Li*
*Yici Ma*
*An Nguyen*

# MaxLove Cookbook Index

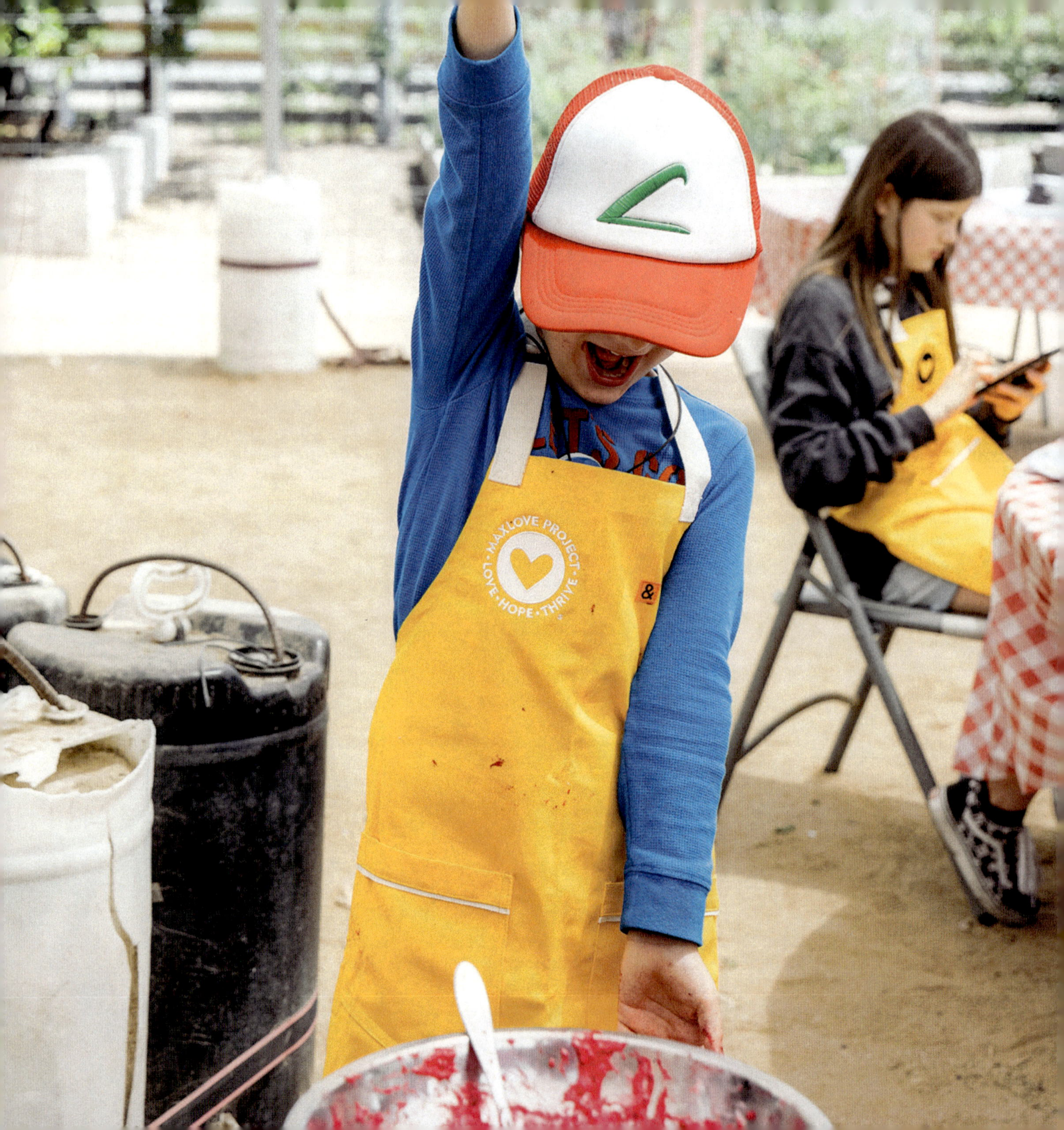
MAXLOVE PROJECT
LOVE • HOPE • THRIVE

Made in the USA
Middletown, DE
28 August 2024

59882598R00135